Clinical Pediatrics

Clinical Pediatrics

Edited by **Alice Kunek**

hayle
medical

New York

Published by Hayle Medical,
30 West, 37th Street, Suite 612,
New York, NY 10018, USA
www.haylemedical.com

Clinical Pediatrics
Edited by Alice Kunek

International Standard Book Number: 978-1-63241-411-3 (Hardback)

The publisher's policy is to use permanent paper from mills that operate a sustainable forestry policy. Furthermore, the publisher ensures that the text paper and cover boards used have met acceptable environmental accreditation standards.

Trademark Notice: Registered trademark of products or corporate names are used only for explanation and identification without intent to infringe.

Printed in the United States of America.

Contents

Preface   IX

Chapter 1   **Sickle Cell Anaemia: Errors in Haemoglobin Genotyping: Impact on Parents of Children Attending Two Hospitals in South East Nigeria**   1
J. M. Chinawa, P. C. Manyike, A. E. Aronu, H. A. Obu and A. T. Chinawa

Chapter 2   **A Case Report of Pediatric Epstein Barr Virus (EBV) Related Cholestasis from Al-Adan Hospital, Kuwait**   6
Fawaz Al-Refaee, Sarah Al-Enezi, Enamul Hoque and Assad Albadrawi

Chapter 3   **Double Aortic Arch in Adolescence: A Case Report**   10
Sri Endah Rahayuningsih, Rahmat Budi Kuswiyanto, Mira Haryanti and Evelyn Phangkawira

Chapter 4   **Anesthetic Technique for Transesophageal Electrophysiology Studies in Pediatric Patients with Wolff-Parkinson-White Syndrome**   15
George M. Gilly, Walter J. Hoyt, Donald E. Harmon, Eric H. Busch, Bobby D. Nossaman, David M. Broussard and Christopher S. Snyder

Chapter 5   **Breastfeeding Status and Effective Factors in 21 - 27 Months Iranian Infants**   21
Fatemeh Nayeri, Mamak Shariat, Hosein Dalili, Farima Raji and Akram Karimi

Chapter 6   **One Stage Reconstruction of Esophageal Atresia and Distal Tracheoesophageal Fistula in a 3250-gm Neonate: A Case Report**   29
Bijay Upadhyay, Xuedong Wu, Jun Li, Ning Wang, Shanshan Zhang and Na Li

Chapter 7   **Epidemiology, Clinical Aspects and Management of Cleft Lip and/or Palate in Burkina Faso: A Humanitarian Pediatric Surgery-Based Study**   33
Kisito Nagalo, Isso Ouédraogo, Jean-Martin Laberge, Louise Caouette-Laberge and Jean Turgeon

Chapter 8   **Calcium Intake in Relation to Body Mass Index and Fatness in Thai School-Aged Children**   41
Uruwan Yamborisut, Wanphen Wimonpeerapattana, Nipa Rojroongwasinkul, Atitada Boonpraderm, Sayamon Senaprom, Wiyada Thasanasuwan, Ilse Khouw and Paul Deurenberg

Chapter 9   **Verbal Autopsy of Stillbirths and Neonatal Deaths in a Rural Area of Burkina Faso**   50
Fla Koueta, Kisito Nagalo, Leatitia Ouedraogo, François Housseini Tall and Diarra Ye

Chapter 10   **Correlation between Vitamin C Deficiency and Hydroxyproline Amino Acid in Young Children of Northern Part in Palestine**   57
Maen Mahfouz, Ismail Masri, Haneen Mahfouz and Yara Mahfouz

Chapter 11   **Education of Parents when a Child Born with an Imperforate Anus; Does it Improve the Health of the Child?**   62
Thi Hoa Chu and Thi Hoa Duong

Chapter 12   **Allergies in Children: What's New? — A Cross-Sectional Descriptive Study**   71
Daniela Simoncini, Anna Peirolo, Alberto Macchi, Stefania Porcu, Daniela Graziani and Luigi Nespoli

Chapter 13   **Prevalence of Neural Tube Defects: Moroccan Study 2008-2011**   79
Mohammed Amine Radouani, Naima Chahid, Loubna Benmiloud, Leila El Ammari, Aicha Kharbach, Larbi Rjimati, Laila Acharrai, Khalid Lahlou, Hassan Aguenaou and Amina Barkat

Chapter 14   **On Relationship Between Pediatric Shi Ji and Fever**   87
Xiangyu Hu and Lina Hu

Chapter 15   **Establishment of Growth Curves to Full Term Newborns: A Moroccan Study**   91
Mohamed Amine Radouani, Salem Ananou, Mustapha Mrabet, Aicha Kharbach, Hassan Aguenaou and Amina Barkat

Chapter 16   **Resolution of Late Steroid-Responsive Nephrotic Syndrome in a Patient with Alport Syndrome Treated with Atorvastatin**   102
Jia-Feng Chang, Wei-Ning Lin and Chien-Chen Tsai

Chapter 17   **NPHS2 Gene Mutation and Polymorphisms in Indonesian Children with Steroid-Resistant Nephrotic Syndrome**   107
Dedi Rachmadi, Ani Melani and Leo Monnens

Chapter 18   **Management of Specific Complications after Congenital Heart Surgery (I)**   114
A. Sánchez Andrés, C. González Miño, E. Valdés Diéguez, L. Boni and J. I. Carrasco Moreno

Chapter 19   **Seroprevalence of Dengue Virus IgG among Children 1 - 15 Years, Selected from an Urban Population in Karachi, Pakistan: Population Based Study**   125
Shakeel Ahmed, Syed Rehan Ali and Farhana Tabassum

Chapter 20   **Herpes Zoster in Childhood**   131
Alexander K. C. Leung and Benjamin Barankin

Chapter 21   **The Differences of Urinary Neutrophil Gelatinase-Associated Lipocalin (NGAL) Levels Between Asphyxiated and Non-Asphyxiated Neonates**   137
Nur Dian Firmani, Tetty Yuniati and Dedi Rachmadi

Chapter 22   **Hepatitis B, Hepatitis C and HIV among Children 6 to 59 Months in the Community in the Democratic Republic of Congo**   142
Jeff Maotela Kabinda,Tony Shindano Akilimali, Ahuka Serge Miyanga, Philippe Donnen, Dramaix-Wilmet Michèle

Chapter 23   **Association of Body Mass Index and Lipid Profiles in Children**   **150**
Gülsen Meral, Ayşegül Uslu, Ali Ünsal Yozgatli and Faruk Akçay

Chapter 24   **The Correlation of Urine Retinol Binding Protein-4 and Serum HbA$_{1c}$ with**
Glomerular Filtration Rate in Type 1 (Insulin-Dependent) Diabetic
Children: A Perspective on the Duration of Diabetes   **156**
Edy Novery, Susi Susanah and Dedi Rachmadi

Chapter 25   **Neonatal Nutrition and Later Outcomes of Very Low Birth Weight and**
Preterm Infants <32 Gestational Age at a Tertiary Care Hospital of Portugal   **163**
Conceição Costa, Teresa Torres and Andreia Teles

Chapter 26   **Neonatal Graves' Disease and Cholestatic Jaundice: Case Series and Review of**
the Literature   **172**
Osama Almadhoun, Teresa Rivera-Penera and Lauren Lipeski

Chapter 27   **Preventative Strategies in the Management of ROP: A Review of Literature**   **178**
Irina Livshitz

Chapter 28   **Effectiveness of Music Therapy on Social Skill Growth in Educable Intellectual**
Disability Boys   **185**
Peyman Hashemian and Mansoureh Mohammadi

Chapter 29   **Outcomes of Severely Malnourished Children Aged 6 - 59 Months on Outpatient**
Management Program in Kitui County Hospital, Kenya   **189**
Dorothy Mbaya, Lucy Kivuti Bitok, Anna K. Karani, Boniface Osano and
Michael Habtu

Chapter 30   **Hereditary Vesicoureteral Reflux: A Study of 66 Families**   **197**
Zsuzsa I. Bartik, Agneta Nordenskjöld, Sofia Sjöström, Rune Sixt and Ulla Sillén

Chapter 31   **Performance of Children and Adolescents from a School of the City of Sogamoso**
on a Decision-Making Test   **207**
Patricia Bernal, Johanna Montaña, Rocio Acosta and Yonathan Rojas

Chapter 32   **Syrup versus Drops of Iron III Hydroxide Polymaltose in the Treatment of Iron**
Deficiency Anemia of Infancy   **216**
Ayala Yahav, Chaim Kaplinsky, Miguel M. Glatstein, Yaakov Shachter,
Aryeh Simmonds, Yakov Shiff, Dennis Scolnik and Nechama Sharon

Chapter 33   **Specific Injuries Management in the Postoperative of Congenital Heart Diseases**
(II): Univentricular Hearts   **221**
A. Sánchez Andrés, C. González Miño, E. Valdés Diéguez, L. Boni and
J. I. Carrasco Moreno

Chapter 34   **Changes in Congenital Anomaly Incidence in West Coast and Pacific States**
(USA) after Arrival of Fukushima Fallout   **230**
Joseph Mangano and Janette D. Sherman

Permissions

List of Contributors

Preface

This book has been a concerted effort by a group of academicians, researchers and scientists, who have contributed their research works for the realization of the book. This book has materialized in the wake of emerging advancements and innovations in this field. Therefore, the need of the hour was to compile all the required researches and disseminate the knowledge to a broad spectrum of people comprising of students, researchers and specialists of the field.

This book traces the progress of the field of pediatrics and highlights some of its key concepts and applications. It discusses the fundamentals as well as modern approaches of this field. Pediatrics refers to a branch of medical science which deals with the diagnosis and treatment of disorders and diseases in infants, children, pre-teens and teens. The aim of this field is to prevent infections, control death rates, reduce chronic diseases and promote general hygiene in adolescents, infants, and children till the age of 18. This book includes detailed explanations of the various theories and techniques that pediatricians use to treat diseases. It consists of contributions made by international experts. Students, doctors, pediatricians, researchers and all those interested in this subject will find this text beneficial.

At the end of the preface, I would like to thank the authors for their brilliant chapters and the publisher for guiding us all-through the making of the book till its final stage. Also, I would like to thank my family for providing the support and encouragement throughout my academic career and research projects.

Editor

Sickle Cell Anaemia: Errors in Haemoglobin Genotyping: Impact on Parents of Children Attending Two Hospitals in South East Nigeria

J. M. Chinawa[1,2], P. C. Manyike[3,4], A. E. Aronu[1,2], H. A. Obu[1,2], A. T. Chinawa[5]

[1]College of Medicine, Department of Pediatrics, University of Nigeria, Nsukka, Nigeria
[2]University of Nigeria Teaching Hospital (UNTH), Ituku, Nigeria
[3]College of Medicine, Ebonyi State University, Abakalki, Nigeria
[4]Department of Pediatrics, Federal Teaching Hospital, Abakiliki (FETHA), Abakiliki, Nigeria
[5]College of Medicine, Department of Community Medicine, Enugu State University of Science and Technology, Enugu, Nigeria
Email: maduabuchichinawa@yahoo.com

Academic Editor: Carl Friedrich Classen, University Children's Hospital Rostock, Germany

Abstract

Objectives: The study is aimed at determining that errors in assigning genotypes to intending couples do exist; and the impact of these errors on parents. Methods: The study was conducted at the children clinics in Enugu and Abakiliki, south east Nigeria. It is a cross-sectional retrospective study in which a review of the records of all the children attending 2 private clinics in Enugu and Abakiliki of Enugu and Ebonyi states respectively, over a 3-year period was done. Results: A total of 6006 children attended the children clinics over the study period. Twenty three (23) of them had sickle cell anaemia. Out of the 23 cases 10 (43.5%) were males and 13 (56.5%) were females. Male to female ratio was 1:1.3. The commonest features were abdominal and leg pains, involving 20 (87%) and 21 (91.3 %) respectively. Among the 23 parents that had their genotypes repeated, 9 males had different genotypes from what they had during courtship or before marriage. The genotypes of all the females that could recall their genotypes before marriage or during courtship were the same after a repeat test. Conclusions: There exist errors in assigning genotypes to parents which at the end made them have children with sickle cell anemia, unwittingly, with serious consequences bordering on strained relationship between the parents with the children bearing the brunt.

Keywords

Sickle Cell Anaemia, Children, Errors

1. Introduction

Sickle cell anaemia (SCA) is a genetic haematological disorder characterized by red blood cells that assume an abnormal, rigid, sickle shape [1]. This hereditary disorder contributes the equivalent of 3.4% mortality among under 5 children worldwide [2].

Sickle cell disorders were originally found in the tropics and subtropics but are now common worldwide due to migration of people from tropical to temperate zones [2]. The prevalence of sickle cell anaemia in Nigeria ranges from 0.4% - 3% affecting about 20 per thousand newborns [3].

Episodic attacks of pain are the most common features of sickle cell anaemic crises and are the most frequent reason for hospitalization [4]. Vaso occlusive crises among children with sickle cell anemia present in different forms with different prevalence rates. For instance, hand foot swelling (dactylitis) occurs in about 30% of children in the first 3 years of life; avascular necrosis of the femoral head affects children over 13 years of age probably due to the hypoxic ischaemic necrosis and occlusion of the vessels that supply neck of femur [5]. The central nervous system infarction could present as cerebrovascular accidents (CVA) in about 4.01% of sickle cell anaemia patients [6].

Genotyping is the process of determining differences in the genetic make-up of an individual by examining the individual's DNA sequence using biological assays and comparing it to another individual's sequence or a reference sequence [6]. Genotyping error is defined as the proportion of mistyping of called genotypes [7]-[10]. This may occur due to non-specificity of experimental assay, inappropriate allele calling, or random assay instability [7]-[10].

Unfortunately, majority of the work on Sickle cell anaemia were carried out in teaching hospitals. Much has not been documented on the topic in a private hospital setting. This study is also aimed at establishing the fact that errors in assigning genotype to intending couples do exist as these parents who thought they had no problems with their genotypes before marriage end up having children with SCA after marriage. However when a repeat genotype was done for the parents, it was different from what was obtained hitherto.

2. Methods

2.1. Study Area and Period

The study was conducted in two children clinics in Enugu and Abakaliki, south east Nigeria. The clinics which are located in highly dense areas provide only outpatient and inpatient care.

The clinics provide care for children and also handle all cases in general pediatrics. Enugu and Ebonyi States of Nigeria have populations of about 3.3 million and 2.2 million people respectively, according to the national census of 2006 [11].

2.2. Study Design and Study Procedure

This is a cross-sectional retrospective study where a review of the records of all children attending the clinics over a 3-year period was undertaken. The folders of these children were retrieved from the clinics' records and examined individually by the investigators. Haemoglobin genotypes of the children were determined by haemoglobin electrophoresis using cellulose acetate at a PH of 8.6 as has been recommended [12]. Cellulose strips measuring 140×120 mm were soaked in buffer and gently bloated. The strips were placed in an electrophoretic tank and secured at each side by a double layer of whitman filter paper [12].

Haemoglobin solution was applied in a 2 cm-line midway between the centre of the strip and at the cathode. Another haemoglobin solution with a known electrophoretic pattern was similarly applied to another cellulose strip to serve as control. Electrophoresis was carried out for 2 hours at 5 MA and a potential of 220 V across the strip. Thereafter, the membrane was removed with a pair of forceps and dried for 10 - 30 minutes. The electrophoretic band was then inspected [12].

The parents provided their genotype results before marriage or at the time of courtship. Their genotypes were repeated when we found that their children are HBSS genotype after presenting with crisis.

The families were assigned socioeconomic classes using the recommended method (modified) by Oyedeji [13].

2.3. Data Analysis

Rates and proportions were calculated with 95% confidence intervals (CI). Level of significance was set at $P < 0.05$.

3. Results

A total of 6006 children attended the children clinics over the study period. Twenty three (23) of them had sickle cell anaemia. Out of the 23 cases 10 (43.5%) were males and 13 (56.5%) were females. Male to female ratio was 1:1.3. The commonest features were abdominal and leg pains, involving 20 (87%) and 21 (91.3 %) of the 23 cases respectively with one case of acute osteomyelitis confirmed by clinical findings and X-rays (**Table 1**).

Age group ranged from (one) 1 year to 17 years (**Table 2**).

Among the 23 parents that had their genotypes repeated, 9 males had a different genotype from what they had during courtship or before marriage. The genotypes of all the females that could recall their genotypes before marriage or during courtship were the same after a repeat test.

About 2 males and 1 female did not know their genotypes before marriage (**Table 3**). One of the parents had a twin and the twins are of HBSS genotype.

Table 1. Common features of presentation of cases.

Symptoms	Number of cases	Percentage (%)
Abdominal pains	20	87
Lower limb pains	21	91.3
Complications		
Acute Osteomylities	1	4.3

Table 2. Percentages distribution of the children by sex and parents' social class.

Sex of children	Frequency n = 23
Female	13
Male	10
Total	**23**
Social class of parents	
Upper	2
Middle	19
Lower	2

Table 3. Errors on genotyping.

Gender of Parent	Genotype before wedding (n)	Repeated genotype of parents after child was ill
Male	AA 23	**AS 9, AA 14**
	AS 0	AS 0
	SS 0	SS 0
Female	AS 21	AS 21
	Don't Know 2	

4. Discussion

Sickle cell disorder affects millions of people worldwide and is particularly common among people of African descent [14]. The commonest presentation among children with sickle cell anemia is vaso-occlusive crisis. This is also in keeping with that of Chinawa *et al.* [15]. Other studies also corroborated these findings [16] [17].

We noted with interest from this study that majority of children with sickle cell anemia are from middle and low socio economic classes. The reason for this finding could be that children whose parents are from high socio-economic class are well taken care of, well fed and followed up regularly, so hospital visits are reduced to the barest minimum [18].

It is pertinent to note from this study that some parents presented with different genotypes from what they had before marriage. Genotype error has caused a lot of havoc among married couples especially when parents are assigned genotypes of AA and AS with some of their children having recurrent illnesses in their early childhood. These recurrent illnesses are usually mistaken for malaria or enteric fever since no one will ever think of sickle cell crises. In all our cases, the children had been treated either for drug resistant malaria or gastritis for abdominal pains. However, when this fever and leg pains occurred repeatedly, a genotype was ordered, not minding that the known genotypes of the parents can't suggest sickle cell in their children. Surprisingly, the children were all SS. Their parents had their genotypes redone and were all found to be both AS. The reason for these errors in genotyping may not be known, but reasons ranging from suboptimal laboratory conditions at the time of the first analysis, file confusion, lab methodology and mis-reporting of the men have been adduced. However, further analysis of these reasons may be an area for further study.

We noted with interest that the genotypes of the female parents were the same before and after marriage while that of the male parents at courtship were not the same after marriage. Errors in relaying the information on genotype status from the laboratory scientist to the females or possibly denial and/or shame on the females in accepting results could account for the male/female differences.

Errors in assigning genotypes to parents affect both the parents and children in so many ways. This is shown as anger and frustration and at times less love for the wife and even the children by the father. This is exacerbated by the extra money paid on hospital bills of the children with sickle cell anemia. The mother also shows anger and frustration, and gripped by fear of divorce. This could lead to serious family strife with the children bearing the brunt.

Although genotyping errors affect most parents and can cause family schism, it is too often neglected. Errors have various causes other than that mentioned above, but their occurrence and effect can be limited by considering these causes during haemoglobin electrophoresis. Procedures that have been developed for dealing with errors such as linkage studies, forensic analyses and non-invasive genotyping should be applied more broadly to any genetic study [19].

For instance, the recently released Gene Chip Mapping 10K array offers the ability to genotype over 10,000 SNPs on a single array [20] [21]. This technology uses an innovative assay that eliminates the need for locus-specific PCR and requires only 250 of ng DNA for each sample [20] [21]. This result suggested a fairly high degree of accuracy. In all the laboratories where the genotypes of the parents were done both before and after marriage, Hb electrophoresis was used; a more refined high performance liquid chromatography may have reduced these errors. For instance, it is noted that high-performance liquid chromatographic methods which was developed for either screening or confirmation of hemoglobinopathies has relatively high sensitivity or specificity when compared with Hb electrophoresis [21].

We recommend a protocol for estimating error rates and propose that these measures be systemically reported to attest its reliability. We also recommend incorporation of genotyping in school health program. This will at least clarify the genotypes of the students way before marriage.

5. Conclusion

There exist errors assigning genotype to parents which at the end make them have children with sickle cell anemia, unwittingly, with serious consequences bordering on strained relationship between the parents, with the children bearing the brunt.

Limitation

A study of errors in genotyping in a wider population or in a community would be worthwhile.

References

[1]   Quirolo, K. and Vichinsky, E. (2004) Haemoglobin Disorders. In: Behrmen, R.E., Kliegman, E.M., Jenson, H.B., Eds., *Nelson Text Book of Paediatrics*, 17th Edition, Saunders Company, Philadephia, 1623-1634.

[2]   Livingstone, F.B. (1975) Abnormal Haemoglobins in Human Populations. Vol. 25, Aldine, Chicago, 1-12.

[3]   Araba, A.B. (1976) A Survey of Haematological Variable in 600 Healthy Nigerians. *Nigerian Medical Journal*, **6**, 49-53.

[4]   Kambel, M. and Chatravedep, P. (2000) Epidemiology of Sickle Cell Disease in a Rural Hospital of Central India. *India J Paediatr*, **37**, 391-396.

[5]   Ebong, WW. (1977) Avascular Necrosis of the femoral Head Associated with Haemoglobinopathy. *Trop Geogr Med*, **29**, 19-23.

[6]   Ohene-Frempong, K., Weiner, S.J., Sleeper, L.A., Miller, S.T., Embury, S., Moohr, J.W., kinney, S.T. and Platt, O.S. (1998) Cerebrovascular Accidents in Sickle Cell Disease: Rates and Risk Factors. *Blood*, **9**, 288-294.

[7]   Genotyping—Wikipedia, the Free Encyclopedia. http://en.wikipedia.org/wiki/Genotyping

[8]   Abecasis, G.R., Cherny, S.S. and Cardon, L.R. (2001) The Impact of Genotyping Error on Family-Based Analysis of Quantitative Traits. *European Journal of Human Genetics*, **9**, 130-134. http://dx.doi.org/10.1038/sj.ejhg.5200594

[9]   Abecasis, G.R., Cherny, S.S., Cookson, W.O. and Cardon, L.R. (2002) Merlin— Rapid Analysis of Dense Genetic Maps Using Sparse Gene Flow Trees. *Nature Genetics*, **30**, 97-101. http://dx.doi.org/10.1038/ng786

[10]   Akey, J.M., Zhang, K., Xiong, M., Doris, P. and Jin, L. (2001) The Effect That Genpyping Errors Have on the Robiustness of Common Linkage Disequilibrium Measures. *The American Journal of Human Genetics*, **68**, 1447-1456. http://dx.doi.org/10.1086/320607

[11]   National Population Commission (2006) Provisional Census Figures. *Census News*, 31, 14.

[12]   Roberts, S., Kenneth, A. and Henry, M. (2005) Measurement of Coagulation Factors. In: Marc, S., Robert, P. and Patrick, C., Eds., *Haematology in Clinical Practice*, 4th Edition, McGraw-Hill Medical Publishers, London, 329-330.

[13]   Oyedeji, G.A. (1985) Socio-Economic and Cultural Background of Hospitalized Children in Ilesha. *Nigerian Journal of Paediatrics*, **12**, 111-117.

[14]   Organização Mundial de Saúde (2006) Sickle-Cell Anaemia. *59th World Health Assembly*, 11, 26-27.

[15]   Chinawa, J.M., Chukwu, B.F., Ikefuna, A.N. and Emodi, I.J. (2013) Musculoskeletal Complications among Children with Sickle Cell Admitted in University of Nigeria Teaching Hospital Ituku-Ozalla Enugu: A 58 Month Review. *Annals of Medical & Health Science Research*, **3**, 564-567. http://dx.doi.org/10.4103/2141-9248.122110

[16]   What Gender Does Sickle Cell Affect? http://www.answers.com/Q/What_gender_does_Sickle_cell_affect

[17]   Ikefuna, A.N. and Emodi, I.J. (2007) Hospital Admission of Patients with Sickle Cell Anaemia Pattern and Outcome in Enugu Area of Nigeria. *Nigerian Journal of Clinical Practice*, **10**, 24-29.

[18]   Okany, C.C. and Akinyanju, O.O. (1993) The Influence of Socio-Economic Status on the Severity of Sickle Cell Disease. *African Journal of Medicine and Medical Sciences*, **22**, 57-60.

[19]   Pompanon, F., Bonin, A., Bellemain, E. and Taberlet, P. (2005) Genotyping Errors: Causes, Consequences and Solutions. *Nature Reviews Genetics*, **6**, 847-846. http://dx.doi.org/10.1038/nrg1707

[20]   Kennedy, G.C., Matsuzaki, H., Dong, S.L., Liu, W.-M., Huang, J., *et al* (2003) Large-Scale Genotyping of Complex DNA. *Nature Biotechnology*, **21**, 1233-1237. http://dx.doi.org/10.1038/nbt869

[21]   Matsuzaki, H., Loi, H., Dong, S.L., Tsai, Y.-Y., Fang, J., Law, J., *et al.* (2005) Parallel Genotyping of over 10,000 SNPs Using a One-Primer Assay on a High-Density Oligonucleotide Array. *Genome Research*, **14**, 414-425. http://dx.doi.org/10.1101/gr.2014904

2

A Case Report of Pediatric Epstein Barr Virus (EBV) Related Cholestasis from Al-Adan Hospital, Kuwait

Fawaz Al-Refaee*, Sarah Al-Enezi, Enamul Hoque, Assad Albadrawi

Department of Pediatrics, Al-Adan Hospital, Ministry of Health, Kuwait, Kuwait
Email: *dralrefaee@gmail.com

Abstract

Infectious mononucleosis is an acute illness due to Epstein Barr virus infection, which occurs commonly in young adults. Liver involvement in acute EBV infection occurs in up to 95% of patients between the 6th and 15th day of illness and is usually mild [1]. Here we report on a 7-year-old girl treated by Gastroenterology, Hepatology, and Nutrition Unit of Al-Adan Hospital pediatric Department, presented with prolonged fever, lymphadenopathy, generalized edema, hyperbilurubinemia and elevated liver enzymes secondary to EBV infection. This case represents a rare presentation of common viral infection in pediatric population.

Keywords

Epstein Barr Virus (EBV)

1. Introduction

Epstein-Barr virus (EBV) infection typically causes the clinical syndrome of infectious mononucleosis. Liver involvement is usually mild, and resolves spontaneously [2]. Hepatitis with mild transient elevations in serum aminotransferases is often reported in Epstein-Barr virus (EBV) infectious mononucleosis. Mild jaundice develops in approximately 5% of cases and may result from cholestasis or virus-induced hemolysis [3]. However, the majority of patients recover without apparent sequelae and most patients will need only supportive treatment.

2. Case Report

A 7-year-old girl previously well was admitted to our hospital with a history of fever for 10 days, decreased ap-

---
*Corresponding author.

petite, malaise and abdominal pain. No history of vomiting or diarrhea, no skin rash, and no headache. In the first 5 days of her illness prior of admission, she was evaluated by a family physician and found to have pharyngitis and she was treated with oral Amoxicillin Clavulanate 45 mg/kg/day every 12 hours for 7 days.

On admission she was looking well but irritable, hydrated, febrile T: 40c, HR: 140/min RR: 30/min, BP: 101/65 mmgh, Capillary refilling time was 2 seconds. She had bilateral palpable cervical lymph nodes 5 mm size each. Abdominal examination revealed tenderness all over the abdomen with no signs of peritonitis, liver was enlarged 3 cm below costal margin and spleen was not palpable. The rest of the clinical examination was unremarkable.

Initial blood investigation showed, CBC white count of 9×10^9/L, Hb: 109 g/L, platelet 126. Liver function test (LFT) showed: LDH 587 U/L, ALT 126 U/L, ALP 315 U/L, AST 124 U/L, total bilirubin 18.10 micromol/L, direct bilirubin 12.5 micromol/L. Renal function and serum electrolyte were normal, CRP: 60, ESR: 11 mm/hr, paracetamol level was within normal range. Coagulation profile showed INR: 1.3 seconds.

Widal test normal and Brucella antibody was negative. Urine and blood culture were negative. Blood virology (EBV, CMV, Hepatitis A, B and C) were taken. Ultrasound of the abdomen done at Emergency Room with no evidence of gallstones or ascites or other abnormal findings.

Patient was treated as a case of pyrexia from unknown origin (PUO) and covered with Intravenous broad spectrum antibiotics, but with no improvement in her symptoms. Few days later, she had ever abdominal pain with fever, so U/S abdomen was repeated and revealed hepatosplenomegaly, contracted gallbladder with thick edematous wall, mild free fluid in the abdomen and the right iliac fossa. Computed Tomography (CT) abdomen with contrast was done which showed minimal fluid in the pelvis with no other abnormalities, so surgical causes needed to be rolled out at this point.

Furthermore, a diagnostic laparoscopy was normal, with unremarkable peritoneal fluid analysis and culture. She became clinically jaundiced and developed generalized edema. Her clinical examination at that time revealed irritable, febrile, pale and icteric young girl, but no signs of chronic liver disease were elicited. She had remarkable edema of face, abdomen and extremities. Her vital signs showed, RR: 30/min, P: 125/min, oxygen saturation was: 98% in room air and BP 100/60 mmhg. Abdomen was distended with generalized tenderness, moderate enlargement of the liver and spleen noted and evidence of shifting dullness were present. Other systemic examination was unremarkable.

Blood investigation was repeated, complete blood count revealed elevated white count with lymphocyte predominance and borderline platelet count at 154×10^9. Peripheral blood film showed reactive lymphocytosis. A repeat of her liver profile showed total: Bilirubin: 103 micromol/L with predominant direct fraction of 89.3 micomol/l. Her liver enzymes showed mainly a cholestatic pattern with significant elevation of GGT and ALP 427 U/L and 867 U/L respectively.

Albumin was low at 24 g/l. Her serum glucose, renal function test and electrolytes were normal. A repeat of coagulation profile: showed significant coagulopathy consistent with acute liver failure of INR 2.2.

Blood virology previously done confirmed acute EBV infection (PCR + IgM).

She was treated conservatively with Albumin infusions, Ursodeoxycholic acid, fresh frozen plasma and intravenous Vitamin K.

The patient continued to have high grade fevers along with the presence of generalized lymphadenopathy, bone marrow examination was done showed marginally increased relative proportion of lymphocytes with presence of 8 - 10 atypical (reactive) lymphocytes, no evidence of blast cells and no evidence of hematological malignancy was present.

Finally, after two weeks of admission, she had gradual clinical improvement. Liver enzymes and total bililrubin were dropping and she was discharged in stable condition. The patient underwent a repeat of liver function tests and ultrasound abdomen two weeks after discharge both of which were normal (**Table 1**).

3. Discussion

EBV is a ubiquitous human herpesvirus that is usually transmitted through close personal contact among young children and via intimate oral contact among adolescent and young adults [4]. Contact of Epstein-Barr virus (EBV) with oropharyngeal epithelial cells allows replication of the virus, release of EBV into the oropharyngeal secretions, and infection of B cells in the lymphoid-rich areas of the oropharynx [5].

The incubation period prior to the development of symptoms averages four to eight weeks [6]. The cardinal

Table 1. The patient's laboratory parameters overtime.

Parameters	At admission	At day 8	On discharge	References range
Hemoglobin	109	90	90	100 - 140 g/L
Total white count	10.67	22.6	18.6	$5 - 19.5 \times 10^9$
Neutrophil	23	9.4	8.8	30% - 50%
Lymphocyte	61	86.2	87	38% - 58%
Total bilirubin	18	132.6	50.5	0 - 17 Micmol/L
Direct bilirubin	12.8	111.9	39.7	0 - 7 Micmol/L
ALT	126	40	46	7 - 55 U/L
AST	124	87	120	8 - 48 U/L
ALP	315	799	759	45 - 115 U/L
GGT	-	400	601	9 - 48 U/L
PT	14.8	24.5	13.3	9.5 - 13.8 seconds
INR	1.3	2.2	1.2	0.8 - 1.2
Albumin	31	24	38	35 - 55 g/dL

Abbreviations: ALT: alanine transaminase; AST: aspartate aminotransferase; ALP: alkalinephosphatase; GGT: γ glutamyltransferase; PT: prothrombin time; INR: international normalized ratio; U/L: units per liter.

symptoms of infectious mononucleosis are the well-known triad of fever, pharyngitis, and peripheral lymphadenopathy, especially involving the posterior cervical chains. A minority of patients have splenomegaly, gastrointestinal symptoms, rash, and headache [7].

Our patient had initially the clinical presentation of infectious mononucleosis but the prolonged fever and cholestatis made us think about other differential diagnosis like autoimmune hepatitis, alpha-1 antitrypsin deficiency and other. Recently EBV-induced hepatitis has been recognized as an important cause of cholestasis [8]. Sever cholestasis is rare and the mechanism is unknown. High concentrations of enzyme-inhibiting autoantibodies against the antioxidative enzyme, manganese-superoxide dismutase (MSD), have been postulated to play a role [9], but support for this concept is limited. In adults, Hepatitis caused by EBV is common, mild, and self limiting, although fulminant hepatic failure has been reported in 17 patients worldwide, with an overall mortality of 85% [10].

During the acute stage of her illness, our patient had serial abdominal sonography which was done because of the persistant abdominal pain throughout hospital admission. However, all of them had shown edematous gallbladder with thickened wall. Gallbladder wall thickening is rare in infectious mononucleosis syndromes and has been proposed as a sign of severity of the infectious mononucleosis and as an indicator for the need to carefully monitor the clinical course [11].

EBV has been associated with a variety of malignancies, particularly lymphoma. Many of these infections are subclinical, but Hodgkin lymphoma has been associated with a history of infectious mononucleosis [6], based on that, this girl had bone marrow examination to rule out possible hidden malignancies. Although of all of these complications and liver involvement, this girl responded well to the supportive treatment.

4. Conclusion

Atypical presentations of Epstein-Barr virus (EBV) infection are more common with increasing age but can also be seen in young children. All pediatricians should be aware of various presentations of common viral childhood infection in order to provide a comprehensive cascade of investigation and supportive management for those children. The good news is that most of the viral infections are self limited and rarely can lead to significant morbidity and mortality in immunocompotent patients.

References

[1]   Rapp Jr., C.E. and Hewetson, J.F. (1978) Infectious Mononucleosis and the Epstein-Barr Virus. *American Journal of Diseases of Children*, **132**, 78-86.

[2]   Barlow, G., Kilding, R. and Green, S. (2000) Epstein-Barr Virus Mimicking Extra-Hepatic Biliary Obstruction. *Journal of the Royal Society of Medicine*, **93**, 316-318.

[3]   Jenson, H.B. (2000) Acute Complications of Epstein-Barr Virus Infectious Mononucleosis. *Current Opinion in Pediatrics*, **12**, 263-268. http://dx.doi.org/10.1097/00008480-200006000-00016

[4]   Hoagland, R.J. (1955) The Transmission of Infectious Mononucleosis. *The American Journal of the Medical Sciences*, **3**, 229-262.

[5]   Anagnostopoulos, I., Hummel, M., Kreschel, C. and Stein, H. (1995) Morphology, Immunophenotype, and Distribution of Latently and/or Productively Epstein-Barr Virus-Infected Cells in Acute Infectious Mononucleosis: Implications for the Interindividual Infection Route of Epstein-Barr Virus. *Blood*, **85**, 744-750.

[6]   Aronson, M.D. and Auwaerter, P.G., Hirsch, M.S., Kaplan, S.L. and Mitty, J., Eds. Infectious Mononucleosis in Adults and Adolescents. UpToDate.

[7]   (1972) General Features of Infectious Mononucleosis (Roundtable Discussion). In: Glade, P.R., Ed., *Infectious Mononucleosis*: *Proceedings of Symposium*, New York, 7 April 1972, Philadelphia, JB Lippincott, 1-18.

[8]   Shaukat, A., Tsai, H.T., Rutherford, R. and Anania, F.A. (2005) Epstein-Barr Virus Induced Hepatitis: An Important Cause of Cholestasis. *Hepatology Research*, **33**, 24-26. http://dx.doi.org/10.1016/j.hepres.2005.06.005

[9]   Juttner, H.U., Ralls, P.W., Quinn, M.F., *et al.* (1982) Thickening of the Gall-Bladder Wall in Acute Hepatitis: Ultrasound Demonstration. *Radiology*, **142**, 465-466. http://dx.doi.org/10.1148/radiology.142.2.7054838

[10] Patel, S., Zuckerman, M. and Smith, M. (2003) Real-Time Quantitative PCR of Epstein-Barr Virus *BZLF1* DNA Using the LightCycler. *Journal of Virological Methods*, **109**, 227-233. http://dx.doi.org/10.1016/S0166-0934(03)00076-4

[11] Yamada, K. and Yamada, H. (2001) Gallbladder Wall Thickening in Mononucleosis Syndromes. *Journal of Clinical Ultrasound*, **29**, 322-325. http://dx.doi.org/10.1002/jcu.1042

3

Double Aortic Arch in Adolescence: A Case Report

Sri Endah Rahayuningsih, Rahmat Budi Kuswiyanto, Mira Haryanti, Evelyn Phangkawira

Department of Child Health, Faculty of Medicine, Padjadjaran University/Hasan Sadikin General Hospital, Bandung, Indonesia
Email: endah.perkani@gmail.com

Abstract

Introduction: Double aortic arch (DAA) is the most frequently encountered vascular ring malformation characterized by a complete encirclement of the trachea and esophagus by the aortic arch with a wide clinical spectrum. Objective: The aim of this study is to describe a case of DAA in adolescents. Case Presentation: An 11-year-old boy was admitted for chronic productive cough which initially was diagnosed with pulmonary arterial hypertension. The final diagnosis was DAA which was established after chest computed tomography (CT) scan. Conclusion: Establishing a diagnosis of DAA in adolescents requires thorough understanding and clinical skills in performing diagnostic steps. The management of heart failure symptoms and other comorbidities is essential while preparing for its definite therapy.

Keywords

Adolescent, Double Aortic Arch

1. Introduction

Vascular ring is a congenital anomaly in which the trachea and esophagus (or its atretic remnant) are completely surrounded by vessels. Vascular rings, which constitute less than 1% of congenital heart diseases, were first identified by Gross in 1945 [1]. Double aortic arch (DAA) is the most frequently encountered vascular ring malformation characterized by a complete encirclement of trachea and esophagus by the aortic arch. Classically, DAA has three types; right dominant aortic arch, left dominant aortic arch, and balanced-type aortic arch. In 75% of the cases, the right arch is dominant, whereas the left arch is dominant in approximately 20% of the cases, and the remaining 5% of cases, both arches are equally dominant [2] [3].

Double aortic arch may be sufficiently tight to cause clinical symptoms or loose enough to be asymptomatic.

For children aged less than 2 years, symptoms are typically respiratory in nature, while older children and adults frequently present with dysphagia and rarely show respiratory symptoms [4].

Diagnosing DAA is challenging because it has a wide clinical spectrum. Double aortic arch is usually diagnosed in infants with life-threatening respiratory symptoms due to severe trachea compression. However, when it is minimal, DAA may remain undiagnosed until adulthood.

We report a case of a teenager with DAA which is diagnosed incidentally during a CT evaluation for chronic productive cough and pulmonary arterial hypertension.

2. Case Presentation

An 11-year-old Sundanese boy was admitted to the emergency Room of the Child Health Department, Hasan Sadikin Hospital, Bandung for breathing difficulty. Additionally, he also experienced swelling in all over his body that was initially prominent on both legs accompanied with bluish discoloration of the lips and nails. The boy had been suffering from frequent episodes of productive cough, exertional dyspnea, and fatigue for 1 year.

Physical examination showed that the patient was alert, had tachypnea, tachycardia. He looked weak and cyanotic, without noticeable dysmorphic appearance. He was overweight (45 kg and 142 cm high) and microcephaly. On heart auscultation, there was no audible murmur. Laboratory findings were unremarkable. Chest radiograph showed slightly increased pulmonary vascular marking with cardiomegaly (**Figure 1**), while electrocardiography revealed right axis deviation and right ventricular hypertrophy without strain. Echocardiography demonstrated mild tricuspid regurgitation, severe pulmonary hypertension, good left and right ventricular contractility; no intracardiac defect was found. The patient was initially diagnosed with heart failure due to idiopathic pulmonary arterial hypertension (PAH). To exclude abnormalities in the lungs and heart, the patient underwent chest CT, spirometry, sputum analysis, and right cardiac catheterization. He was treated with sildenafil and furosemide as we explored the etiology of PAH.

The chest CT and right cardiac catheterization revealed DAA surrounding the trachea and esophagus with right arch dominance and compression to trachea. No intracardiac defect was seen on both the CT and angiogram (**Figure 2** and **Figure 3**). Besides DAA, chest CT results also revealed bronchiectasis. No compression of esophagus was seen in barium esophagogram. Spirometry test showed severe restrictive lung abnormalities, whereas sputum culture and antibiotic resistance test revealed *Streptococcus viridans*, which was sensitive to cefotaxime, cefazolin, erythromycin, and meropenem.

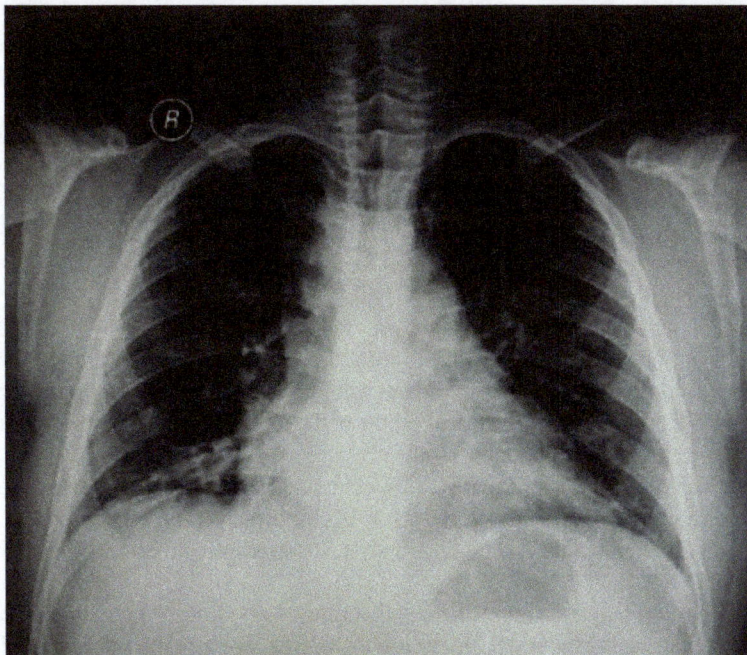

Figure 1. Chest radiograph showed increased pulmonary vascular marking, cardiomegaly, no pulmonary edema, and cuffing sign (white arrows).

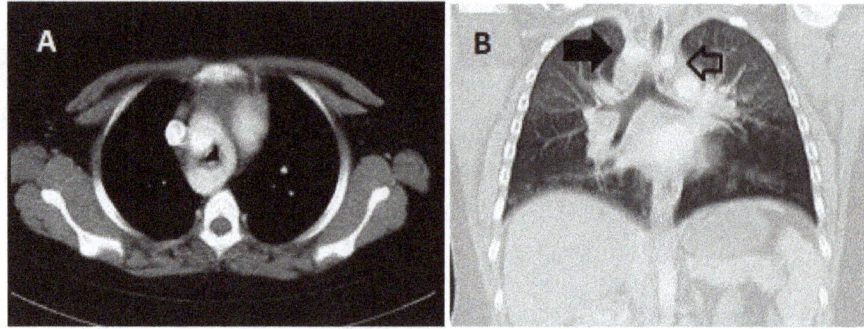

Figure 2. Chest computed tomography showed double aortic arch. Coronal view (A); Sagital view, right aortic arch (black arrow), left aotic arch (unfilled arrow) (B).

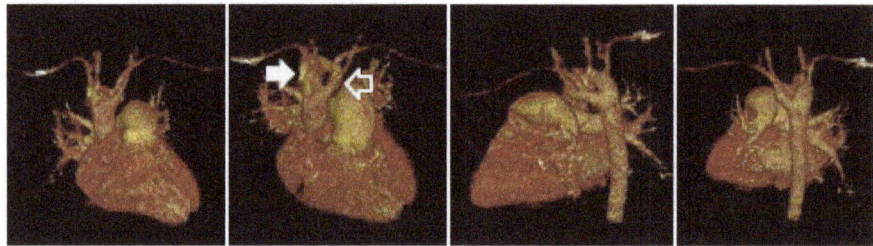

Figure 3. Reconstruction of patient's chest computed tomography, right aortic arch (white arrow), left aortic arch (unfilled arrow).

In addition, the patient was also mentally retarded because there was a delay in language development and self-reliance. The patient was then consulted to paediatric nutrition and metabolic disease divisions for obesity management and to a psychologist for intellegence testing. We arranged a regular chest physiotherapy to manage the bronchietasis and referred him to a cardiac surgeon. Up till we report this case he was still waiting for surgical repair.

3. Discussion

Double aortic arch (DAA) is reported to account for less than 1% of congenital heart diseases [3]. In DAA, both of the aortic arches form a complete vascular ring encircling the trachea and oesophagus due to failure of regression of the right aortic arch. Each aortic arch passes the ipsilateral mainstem bronchus superiorly and enters the descending aorta, which is more commonly located on the left side than on the right side of the spine. Both aortic arches are often different in size and position. The right aortic arch is usually larger and located higher than the left. The left aortic arch may be degenerated and atretic or remains as a fibrous band. In our case, both aortic arches reunite to form the descending aorta located in front of the spine, with the right aorta being larger than left [1] [3] [5].

A report analyzed a series of DAAs over a period of 16 years, between 1987 and 2003. The main symptoms were stridor, dysphagia, choking episodes, and life-threatening apneic spells. Diagnosis was established by barium studies, bronchoscopy, echocardiogram, angiogram, computed tomography (CT), and magnetic resonance imaging (MRI). From this report, early surgical repair of DAA is associated with low mortality, and resulted in marked symptomatic relief in most patients.

Embryologically, the ventral and dorsal aortas are connected by aortic arches which persist or involute to give rise to the normal aortic arch. The fourth right aortic arch normally involutes at about 36 - 38 days when the embryo size is 16 mm, while the left aortic arch persists. Persistence of the fourth right and left aortic arches led to DAA [2] [5].

Classically, DAA is divided into three forms depending on both size and dominance of either of the arch. Sometimes, there is a partial atresia in one of the arch. Dominance cannot be determined if the size difference is not more than 5%, and it is referred as balance DAA. Intracardiac defects can be present in 20% of DAA patients [6]. In our case, the right aortic arch is dominant and the patient did not have any intracardiac defects.

Patients with DAA may experience respiratory and gastrointestinal symptoms due to the formation of a vascular ring around the trachea and esophagus [4]. If the vascular ring compresses the trachea, respiratory symptoms may include snoring, shortness of breath, cough, recurrent respiratory infections, apnea, and cyanosis, which mainly occur in the newborn period. Gastrointestinal symptoms may consist of feeding problems, vomiting, and failure to thrive due to the compression of the esophagus. These symptoms may appear later in life due to an enlargement of the aortic structure caused by atherosclerotic changes [4] [6]. Our patient experienced persistent cough due to trachea compression.

Bronchiectasis is suspected if there are symptoms of chronic productive cough (>12 weeks) and chest x-ray abnormality that persist despite prompt treatment. The diagnosis requires a confirmation of chest CT-scan. Children who have symptoms of bronchiectasis but have not undergone evaluation are referred to as having chronic suppurative lung disease (CSLD) [7] [8]. The pathogenesis of bronchiectasis begins with the presence of acute ulceration in the bronchial wall that occurs after infection of the bronchi, such as bronchopneumonia. Destruction of the mucous membrane is soon followed by ulcerations, which then involves muscular structure, elastic tissue and cartilage, eventually leading to abnormal bronchial wall, being partially covered by healthy tissue, and alveolar wall collapse.

Within 4 - 6 weeks, granulation tissue will be present in the damaged areas of bronchial wall. Further growth will occur in the epithelium of non-ulcerated area. This can be both normal ciliated epithelium, more often non-ciliated cuboidal, squamous, or transitional cells. Cartilage, muscular and elastic tissue do not regenerate, hence the granulation tissue will be replaced by fibrous tissue. If the infection becomes chronic, fibrosis extends so that most of the lung tissue is replaced by fibrous tissue and dilated bronchi [9] [10]. In our patient, bronchiectasis may occur because of chronic tracheal constriction that disrupts lung defense and ultimately the mucociliary clearance. The evidence of infection is supported by the discovery of *Streptococcus viridans* in respiratory secret, probably due to chronic marginal gingivitis as the consequence of bad oral hygiene.

Our patient experienced PAH due to alveolar hypoxia caused by bronchiectasis. Chronic reduction in the oxygen tension in the alveolar capillary region (alveolar hypoxia) elicits a strong pulmonary vasoconstrictor response, which is stronger than vasoconstriction due to a low oxygen tension in the PA. In normal conditions, the balance between the release of nitric oxide (NO), vasodilator, and endothelin, a vasoconstrictor released by endothelial cells, regulates the pulmonary circulation. Reduced production of NO that occurs in chronic hypoxia causes pulmonary vasoconstriction and vascular remodeling. Conversely, plasma levels of endothelin is increased in association with hypoxia.

To manage pulmonary hypertension, in addition to bosentan which is an endothelin receptor antagonist, sildenafil is also commonly used. It works by blocking the phosphodiesterase enzyme, and therefore has a strong selective vasodilator effect on the pulmonary vasculature with comparable efficacy to the inhaled NO in adults [11]. A previous study showed that 12 month administration of sildenafil for the pediatric population resulted in significant improvements in both idiopathic and secondary PAH [12]-[15]. In our patient, we gave only sildenafil because bosentan was unavailable in our setting.

In our patient, obesity risk factors might include exercise limitation due to his medical condition, psychosocial problems, and adolescence period. Adolescence is a transitional period that begins with puberty and is marked by dynamic physiological and psychological changes that makes it a critical period for weight gain. Obesity hypoventilation syndrome is suggested to be associated with pulmonary hypertension. An obese child may have respiratory insufficiency due to multiple factors, such as decreased lung compliance and development, reduced inspiratory muscle strength, abnormal thoracic cage, and lung vital capacity. The resulted alveolar hypoventilation may lead to pulmonary hypertension, which in turn may cause right ventricular dysfunction.

Besides planning a corrective surgery, bronchiectasis management is also important for our patient. To manage bronchiectasis, the following measures are recommended: airway clearance maneuvers and chest physiotherapy, avoidance of biomass smoke exposure, including second-hand smoking exposure, identification and management of complications and comorbidities, and annual influenza immunization. Up till the publishing date of this report, the patient is still on hold for surgery. This is due to the long waiting list, and the availability of such operation is limited only at pediatric heart centre in Jakarta.

4. Conclusion

Establishing DAA diagnosis in adolescents is challenging, because of its diverse clinical spectrum and low prevalence. It requires a thorough understanding and clinical skills in performing diagnostic steps. The management of heart failure symptoms and other comorbidities are essential apart from investigating and performing definite therapy for DAA.

References

[1] Gross, R.E. (1955) Arterial Malformations Which Cause Compression of the Trachea or Esophagus. *Circulation*, **11**, 124-134. http://dx.doi.org/10.1161/01.CIR.11.1.124

[2] Kau, T., Lesnik, G., Eicher, W., Sinzig, M., Gasser, J., Rabitsch, E., *et al.* (2007) Aortic Development and Anomalies. *Seminars in Interventional Radiology*, **24**, 141-152. http://dx.doi.org/10.1055/s-2007-980040

[3] Baraldi, R., Address, S.S., Bighi, S. and Mannella, P. (2004) Vascular Ring Due to Double Aortic Arch: A Rare Cause of Dysphagia. *European Journal of Radiology*, **52**, 21-24. http://dx.doi.org/10.1016/j.ejrex.2004.06.001

[4] Umegaki, T., Sumi, C., Nishi, K., Ikeda, S. and Shingu, K. (2010) Airway Management in an Infant with Double Aortic Arch. *Journal of Anesthesia*, **24**, 117-120. http://dx.doi.org/10.1007/s00540-009-0850-4

[5] Weinberg, P.M. (2006) Aortic Arch Anomalies. *Journal of Cardiovascular Magnetic Resonance*, **8**, 633-643.

[6] Lowe, G.M., Donaldson, J.S. and Backer, C.L. (1991) Vascular Rings: 10-Year Review of Imaging. *Radographics*, **11**, 637-646. http://dx.doi.org/10.1148/radiographics.11.4.1887119

[7] Chang, A.B., Redding, G.J. and Everard, M.L. (2008) Chronic Wet Cough: Protracted Bronchitis, Chronic Suppurative Lung Disease and Bronchiectasis. *Pediatric Pulmonology*, **43**, 519-531. http://dx.doi.org/10.1002/ppul.20821

[8] Chang, A.B., Grimwood, K., Maguire, G., King, P.T., Morris, P.S. and Torzillo, P.J. (2008) Management of Bronchiectasis and Chronic Suppurative Lung Disease in Indigenous Children and Adults from Rural and Remote Australian Communities. *Medical Journal of Australia*, **189**, 386-393.

[9] McNeil, C., MacGregor, A.R. and Alexander, W.A. (1929) Studies of Pneumonia in Childhood: I. Statistical Analysis of Pneumonia and Bronchitis. *Archives of Disease in Childhood*, **4**, 12-32.

[10] King, P.T. (2009) The Pathophysiology of Bronchiectasis. *International Journal of Chronic Obstructive Pulmonary Disease*, **4**, 411-419. http://dx.doi.org/10.2147/COPD.S6133

[11] McLaughlin, V.V., Archer, S.L., Badesch, D.B., Barst, R.J., Farber, H.W., Lindner, J.R., *et al.* (2009) ACCF/AHA 2009 Expert Consensus Document on Pulmonary Hypertension: A Report of the American College of Cardiology Foundation Task Force on Expert Consensus Documents and the American Heart Association: Developed in Collaboration with the American College of Chest Physicians, American Thoracic Society, Inc., and the Pulmonary Hypertension Association. *Circulation*, **119**, 2250-2294.

[12] Widlitz, A. and Barst, R.J. (2003) Pulmonary Arterial Hypertension in Children. *European Respiratory Journal*, **21**, 155-176. http://dx.doi.org/10.1183/09031936.03.00088302

[13] Barst, R., Maislin, G. and Fishman, A. (1999) Vasodilator Therapy for Primary Pulmonary Hypertension in Children. *Circulation*, **99**, 1197-1208. http://dx.doi.org/10.1161/01.CIR.99.9.1197

[14] Zeng, W.J., Sun, Y.J., Gu, Q., Xiong, C.M., Li, J.J. and He, J.G. (2012) Impact of Sildenafil on Survival of Patients with Idiopathic Pulmonary Arterial Hypertension. *Journal of Clinical Pharmacology*, **52**, 1357-1364.

[15] Daniels, S.R., Arnett, D.K., Eckel, R.H., Gidding, S.S., Hayman, L.L., Kumanyika, S., *et al.* (2005) Overweight in Children and Adolescents Pathophysiology, Consequences, Prevention, and Treatment. *Circulation*, **111**, 1999-2012. http://dx.doi.org/10.1161/01.CIR.0000161369.71722.10

Anesthetic Technique for Transesophageal Electrophysiology Studies in Pediatric Patients with Wolff-Parkinson-White Syndrome

George M. Gilly[1], Walter J. Hoyt[2], Donald E. Harmon[1], Eric H. Busch[1], Bobby D. Nossaman[1], David M. Broussard[1], Christopher S. Snyder[3*]

[1]Department of Anesthesiology, Ochsner Clinic Foundation, New Orleans, LA, USA
[2]Division of Pediatric Cardiology, University of Virginia, Charlottesville, VA, USA
[3]Department of Pediatrics, Division of Pediatric Cardiology, Rainbow Babies and Children's Hospital, Case Western Reserve School of Medicine, Cleveland, OH, USA
Email: *Christopher.Snyder@UHhospitals.org

Academic Editor: Carl E. Hunt, George Washington University School of Medicine and Health Sciences, USA

Abstract

Objective: Patients with Wolff-Parkinson-White (WPW) Syndrome require risk assessment to determine their potential for sudden cardiac death. Transesophageal electrophysiology studies (TEEPS) are an effective risk stratification tool. The purpose of this study is to describe a minimially invasive, effective anesthetic technique to employ during transesophageal electrophysiology studies. Methods: A retrospective review of anesthetic technique utilized during TEEPS. Inclusion criteria; WPW on ECG; age <18 years; and no history of tachycardia, palpitations, or syncope and patient had TEEPS under monitored anesthesia care (MAC). Midazolam, Fentanyl, and Propofol were used in various combinations. Sevoflurane was used during induction period in all GA cases and discontinued 10 minutes prior to initiation of TEEPS. Results: Inclusion criteria were met by 20 patients with an average age of 11.9 years, average weight of 48.9 kg and average height of 149.2 cm. IV sedation was performed on 15%, MAC on 10% and GA in remainder. Airway management techniques included 13.3% LMA, 20% endotracheal tube (ETT) and 66% mask. IV sedation, the initial anesthetic, was found to be cumbersome and uncomfortable. Next was ETT and LMA but trouble pacing was encountered due to positional change of the esophagus relative to the left atrium during ventilation. Mask induction was then performed in remaining 10 patients with TEEPS probe inserted through a nare while anesthesiologist continued mask ventilation. All mask

*Corresponding author.

procedures were successful without complications. Conclusions: Induction of anesthesia to perform TEEPS procedures on pediatric patients with Wolff-Parkinson-White syndrome underwent numerous attempts to make the procedure easy, reliable and reproducible for anesthesia and electrophysiologist. The eventual technique that proved to meet these criteria during a transesopheagel electrophysiology procedure was utilization of mask induction with continuous IV sedation.

Keywords

Wolff Parkinson White, Transesophagel Electrophysiology Study

1. Introduction

Wolff-Parkinson-White syndrome (WPW) is an electrocardiographic abnormality that manifests on the electrocardiogram with a short PR interval, presence of a delta wave, and episodes of supraventricular tachycardia [1]. These findings are due to the presence of an accessory pathway (AP) that bridges the electrical activity of the atrium to the ventricles and bypassing the normal conduction delay of the atrio-ventricular node. Many patients with WPW are asymptomatic without complaints of syncope, near-syncope, palpitations, supraventricular tachycardia, atrial fibrillation, or sudden cardiac death (SCD) and are identified only by "routine" electrocardiogram. Regardless, all patients with WPW have risk of SCD due to rapid conduction down their accessory pathway during atrial fibrillation. Due to this risk, current recommendations state that patients with WPW on their ECG undergo formal assessment to determine their risk of SCD. The methods of risk stratification include exercise stress testing, transesophageal electrophysiology studies (TEEPS), and transvenous electrophysiology studies (TVEPS). TVEPS is currently accepted as the most effective way to assess the risk of these patients; however, this procedure is associated with increase cost, time, invasiveness, and risk. In contrast, a TEEPS is easy to perform, less costly, with less risk and excellent success rates [2].

When performing invasive risk assessment on a patient with WPW, the anesthetic plan must be carefully designed to avoid interference with the conduction properties of the accessory pathway (AP) as well as assure a painless and safe procedure for the patient. Traditional anesthetic agents such as Propofol, Fentanyl, and Midazolam have been shown to have negligible effects on the AP conduction [3]-[8]. In contrast to these agents, the volatile anesthetics Sevoflurane and Isoflurane have been shown to increase AP-effective refractory period (AP-ERP), make them conduct better, and therefore it increases the shortest preexcited R-R interval during Afib, potentially taking a patient from no-risk of sudden death into a group that has risk [3] [6] [8] [9]. To date, no safe and effective anesthetic technique has been described for use during the minimally invasive TEEPS procedures. The purpose of this study is to describe our evolution of anesthetic technique to arrive at a safe and effective method of anesthetizing patients for the minimally invasive transesophageal electrophysiology studies during risk assessment of asymptomatic Wolff-Parkinson-White syndrome patients.

2. Methods

A retrospective chart review was performed on all patients with asymptomatic WPW that underwent TEEPS procedure at our institution. Inclusion criteria included evidence of preexcitation on ECG (WPW); age < 18 years; and no history of tachycardia, palpitations, or syncope. Data collected included patient age, weight, height, TEEPs results, anesthetic medications and technique(s) utilized. TEEPS studies were performed as part of the risk assessment protocol on asymptomatic WPW patients with the goal of inducing Afib.

Anesthesia was utilized during the study for patient comfort and ease of performing the study. The anesthetic technique evolved during the study as shortfalls were encountered. Initially, the technique was simple IV sedation administered by the performing electrophysiologist. This evolved into the monitored anesthesia care (MAC), or general anesthesia (GA). Each patient had a single anesthesiologist during their case. Anesthetic technique (MAC vs. GA) as well airway management decisions were left to the clinical judgment of the performing anesthesiologist. The anesthetic agents used during the procedure were, Midazolam, Fentanyl, and Propofol alone or in combination. Sevoflurane was also used during the immediate induction period in all GA cases. Airway management included mask ventilation, laryngeal mask airway (LMA), or endotracheal intubation [10] [11].

3. Results

Inclusion criteria were met by 20 patients with average age of 11.9 years (2 - 17), average weight of 48.9 kg (13.5 - 104) and average height of 149.2 cm (89 - 178). The methods of anesthesia included; IV sedation in 3 (15%), MAC in 2 (10%), and GA on remaining 15 (75%). In addition, multiple methods of airway management were employed including Laryngeal Mask Airway (LMA) in 2 (13%), ETT in 3 (20%), and pure mask technique in 10 (67%). The method of anesthesia and airway management had no effect on the final results of the procedure since Afib was induced in 18 of 20 patients. The cases were afib could not be induced were: 1 sedation and 1 GA with LMA.

In the first three cases, IV sedation was utilized but was found to be cumbersome to perform the procedure and uncomfortable for the patient. The issues encountered during its use were difficulty making the patient comfortable and positioning the TEEPS probe without anesthesia. In addition, once the probe was positioned, it required higher thresholds for capture (18 vs. 15 millivolts) with in turn resulted in patient discomfort. Afib was not inducible in one of these patients due to the inability to position the probe in a place where capture of the heart could be reliably obtained. Due to the difficulty of probe placement and sedation, anesthesia was involved in the subsequent patients (17) to anesthetize the patient and allow the electrophysiologist performed the TEEPS.

General anesthesia was performed on next 15 patients. Depending on the age and overall disposition of the patient, IV access was obtained in either the pre-operative suite or after mask induction. In addition, pre-operative Midazolam (IV or PO) was administered to 13 of 15 patients prior to their receiving general anesthesia. Sevoflurane was used to induce general anesthesia on all patients with the highest end tidal recorded of 6. After induction of general anesthesia and brief maintenance, Sevoflurane was discontinued to avoid any issues with AP conduction. Maintenance of anesthesia was then continued with a combination of IV Propofol and Fentanyl (**Table 1**). No anesthetic complications were noted.

General anesthetic with endotracheal intubation (GETA) was performed on the first 3 patients that underwent general anesthesia. No anesthetic complications were noted but the electrophysiologist noted difficulty properly positioning the TEEPS probe. The issue positioning the TEEPS probe was felt to be due to a small positional change of the esophagus relative to the left atrium after intubation with a cuffed endotracheal tube and the use of positive pressure ventilation.

For this reason, the anesthesiologist attempted general anesthesia with an LMA for the next 2 patients. Due to the age of the patients (13 and 16 years old), both patients underwent IV induction. Sevoflurane was initially used for maintenance of anesthesia before switching to Propofol, Fentanyl, and Midazolam. No anesthetic complications were noted with this method. As with the previous GETA cases, the TEEPS probe was inserted through the nare; and the LMA was placed and inflated. During both cases, the inflation of the LMA moved the TEEPS probe out of position. Afib was not induced in one patient, so the study was converted to TVEPs with successful induction of Afib.

Due to TEEPS probe positioning problems with the endotracheal tube and the LMA, the subsequent procedures were performed with general mask anesthesia on 10 of 20 patients. Mask induction was performed on 5 of 10 patients with IV placement after induction; the remainder of the patients had IV access placed in the pre-operative area. Pre-operative Midazolam and intraoperative Fentanyl were administered to 8 of 10 patients. Two patients received no anxiolytics or narcotics in the pre-operative or intra-operative period. All 10 patients, regardless of IV status, underwent mask induction. The TEEPS probe was inserted through a nare and properly positioned by the electrophysiologist. The anesthesiologist secured the probe in the proper position while continuing to mask ventilate the patient. The procedure was performed and the probe was removed. There were no anesthetic complications in any of these patients.

The remaining 2 patients underwent the TEEPS study under MAC anesthesia which was performed by the pediatric anesthesia team. The patients were 16 and 17 years old and easily tolerated the procedure. Overall, 18 of 20 (90%) patients underwent successful TEEPS studies as defined by induction of A-fib.

4. Discussion

WPW can manifest as syncope, near-syncope, palpitations, supraventricular tachycardia, atrial fibrillation, or

Table 1. Demographics and anesthetic techniques in twenty patients undergoing TEEPs.

Age	Weight (kg)	Height (cm)	Anesthesia	Airway	Sevoflurane Max (%)	Narcotics	Pre-Op Midazolam	Intra-Op Midazolam	Propofol (mg)	Neuromuscular Blocker
5	25.9	94	General	Mask	1.4	0	5 mg PO	0	0	0
9	32.5	135	IV Sedation	NC	0	Fentanyl 70 mcg	15 mg PO	2 mg IV	60	0
16	48	163	IV Sedation	NC	0	0	0	0	170	0
17	63	170	IV Sedation	NC	0	0	0	6 mg IV	190	0
17	72	178	General	ETT	3.9	Fentanyl 125 mcg	2 mg IV	0	200	Succinylcholine 100 mg
13	47	161	General	Mask	3.5	Fentanyl 100 mcg	0	0	0	0
13	62	160	General	Mask	2	Fentanyl 100 mcg	2 mg IV	0	0	0
15	72.3	179	General	ETT	2	Fentanyl 100 mcg	2 mg IV	0	0	Rocuronium 30 mg
13	58	169	General	LMA	6	Fentanyl 100 mcg	0	2 mg IV	200	0
16	53.8	172	General	LMA	2	Fentanyl 50 mcg	0	2 mg IV	150	0
11	45.1	147	General	Mask	2	Fentanyl 50 mcg	20 mg PO	0	200	0
17	104	173	General	Mask		Fentanyl 200 mcg	2 mg IV	0	0	0
9	34.6	146	General	Mask	3	0	0	0	0	0
16	64.1	156	MAC	MAC	0	Fentanyl 100 mcg	2 mg IV	0	140	0
2	13.5	89	General	Mask	6	0	7 mg PO	0	0	0
17	62.3	180	MAC	MAC	0	Fentanyl 50 mcg	2 mg IV	1 mg IV	200	0
9	28	132	General	ETT	4	Fentanyl 50 mcg	15 mg PO	0	80	Rocuronium 25 mg
5	24	115.5	General	Mask	4	0	12 mg PO	0	0	0
11	50	149	General	Mask	6	0	2 mg IV	0	90	0
6	18.6	115	General	Mask	1.8	0	10 mg PO	0	0	0

MAC: Monitored Anesthesia Care; ETT: Endotracheal Tube; NC: Nasal Canula.

even sudden cardiac death which necessitates risk stratification of asymptomatic patients. Current procedures of risk stratification include exercise stress testing, transesophageal electrophysiology studies (TEEPS), and transvenous electrophysiology studies (TVEPS). Exercise stress testing is a non-invasive test used to rule out asymptomatic ventricular preexcitation (aVPE) but is limited by its sensitivity in patients with WPW. TVEPS is an effective way to risk stratify patients; however, it is hampered by its invasiveness, cost, and potential complications. TEEPS procedures have been shown to be an effective screening tool with potentially less complications; however no consensus anesthetic technique has been proven superior [2]. This study series describes our attempt to find the easiest, most effective anesthetic technique for the TEEPS procedure.

Depending on the age and co-existing diseases of the patient, this procedure can successfully be performed under MAC or GA. In the older pediatric population, MAC is likely the preferred anesthetic technique due to minimal airway manipulation, the ability to bypass phase I recovery, decreased risk of post-operative nausea and vomiting (PONV). If a patient is unable to tolerate MAC, conversion to GA only requires deepening of IV sedation and airway management by mask ventilation. As shown by our case series, pediatric patients who undergo mask induction for the purpose of obtaining IV access tolerate general anesthesia with mask ventilation for maintenance. The advantages of this technique are that the patient's oropharynx is unobstructed for TEEPS probe placement and when necessary the probe can be easily manipulated by the anesthesiologist during the procedure. In our study, TEEPS probe adjustment was more difficult with an ETT or LMA in place.

Techniques such as MAC or mask general that minimize airway manipulation likely decrease the risk of laryngospasm during TEEPS procedure. Laryngospasm did not occur in any patient in this series, regardless of the technique employed. Probe placement should be performed only after IV access is obtained, and the patient is adequately anesthetized to minimize this risk. The results of this case series suggest that MAC or mask general anesthesia is the preferred anesthetic technique for the TEEPS procedure.

5. Conclusion

Induction of anesthesia to perform TEEPS procedures on pediatric patients with Wolff-Parkinson-White syndrome underwent numerous attempts to make the procedure easy, reliable and reproducible for anesthesia and electrophysiologist. The eventual technique that proved to meet these criteria during a transesopheagel electrophysiology procedure was utilization of mask induction with continuous IV sedation.

References

[1]   Wolff, L., Parkinson, J. and White, P.D. (1930) Bundle Branch Block with Short PR Interval in Healthy Young People Prone to Paroxysmal Tachycardia. *American Heart Journal*, **5**, 686-692.
http://dx.doi.org/10.1016/S0002-8703(30)90086-5

[2]   Hoyt, W.J., Thomas, P.E., DeSena, H.C., Steinberg, J.S., Harmon, D.E. and Snyder, C.S. (2012) Atrial Fibrillation Induction by Transesophageal Electrophysiology Studies in Patients with Asymptomatic Ventricular Preexcitation. *Congenital Heart Disease*, **8**, 57-61.

[3]   Lavoie, J., Walsh, E.P., Burrows, F.A., Laussen, P., Lulu, J.A. and Hansen, D.D. (1995) Effects of Propofol or Isoflurane Anesthesia on Cardiac Conduction in Children Undergoing Radiofrequency Catheter Ablation for Tachydysrhythmias. *Anesthesiology*, **82**, 884-887. http://dx.doi.org/10.1097/00000542-199504000-00010

[4]   Sharpe, M.D., Dobkowski, W.B., Murkin, J.M., Klein, G. and Yee, R. (1995) Propofol Has No Direct Effect on Sinoatrial Node Function or on Normal Atrioventricular and Accessory Pathway Conduction in Wolff-Parkinson-White Syndrome during Alfentanil/Midazolam Anesthesia. *Anesthesiology*, **82**, 888-895.
http://dx.doi.org/10.1097/00000542-199504000-00011

[5]   Sharpe, M.D., Dobkowski, W.B., Murkin, J.M., Klein, G., Guiraudon, G. and Yee, R. (1992) Alfentanil-Midazolam Anaesthesia Has No Electrophysiological Effects upon the Normal Conduction System or Accessory Pathways in Patients with Wolff-Parkinson-White Syndrome. *Canadian Journal of Anaesthesia*, **39**, 816-821.
http://dx.doi.org/10.1007/BF03008294

[6]   Sharpe, M.D., Dobkowski, W.B., Murkin, J.M., Klein, G., Guiraudon, G. and Yee, R. (1994) The Electrophysiologic Effects of Volatile Anesthetics and Sufentanil on the Normal Atrioventricular Conduction System and Accessory Pathways in Wolff-Parkinson-White Syndrome. *Anesthesiology*, **80**, 63-70.
http://dx.doi.org/10.1097/00000542-199401000-00013

[7]   Pecht, B., Maginot, K.R., Boramanand, N.K. and Perry, J.C. (2002) Techniques to Avoid Atrioventricular Block during Radiofrequency Catheter Ablation of Septal Tachycardia Substrates in Young Patients. *Journal of Interventional Cardiac Electrophysiology*, **7**, 83-88. http://dx.doi.org/10.1023/A:1020828401929

[8]   Pérez, E.R., Bartolomé, F.B., Carretero, P.S., Fernández, C.S., Mateos, E.J. and Tarlovsky, L.G. (2008) Electrophysiological Effects of Sevoflurane in Comparison with Propofol in Children with Wolff-Parkinson-White Syndrome. *Rev Esp Anestesiol Reanim*, **55**, 26-31.

[9]   Caldwell, J.C., Fong, C. and Muhyaldeen, S.A. (2010) Should Sevoflurane Be Used in the Electrophysiology Assess-

ment of Accessory Pathways? *Europace*, **12**, 1332-1335. http://dx.doi.org/10.1093/europace/euq076

[10] Klein, G.J., Bashore, T.M., Sellers, T.D., Pritchett, E.L., Smith, W.M. and Gallagher, J.J. (1979) Ventricular Fibrillation in the Wolff-Parkinson-White Syndrome. *The New England Journal of Medicine*, **301**, 1080-1085. http://dx.doi.org/10.1056/NEJM197911153012003

[11] Bromberg, B.I., Lindsay, B.D., Cain, M.E. and Cox, J.L. (1996) Impact of Clinical History and Electrophysiologic Characterization of Accessory Pathways on Management Strategies to Reduce Sudden Death among Children with Wolff-Parkinson-White Syndrome. *Journal of the American College of Cardiology*, **27**, 690-695. http://dx.doi.org/10.1016/0735-1097(95)00519-6

Breastfeeding Status and Effective Factors in 21 - 27 Months Iranian Infants

Fatemeh Nayeri[1], Mamak Shariat[1], Hosein Dalili[2]*, Farima Raji[2], Akram Karimi[2]

[1]Maternal, Fetal and Neonatal Research Center, Tehran University of Medical Sciences, Tehran, Iran
[2]Breast Feeding Research Center, Tehran University of Medical Sciences, Tehran, Iran
Email: fsnayeri@sina.ac.ir, mshariat@tums.ac.ir, *hoseindalili@yahoo.com, mfnhrc@yahoo.com, mfnhrc@tums.ac.ir

Abstract

The aim of this study was to assess the Breastfeeding status among children aged 21 - 27 moths. A cross sectional study was carried out in South Health Center (Tehran-Iran) in 2010. Four hundred 21 - 27 month breastfed infants entered the study. This study compared some variables in 2 groups; weaning before and after 22 months. The level of significance was considered $P < 0.05$. Mean breastfeeding duration and median (either exclusive or combined) were 19.66 ± 6.40 and 22 months. Among all reasons were cited by mothers, some reasons like insufficient breast milk supply (77.9%), infant restless (77.1%), and Mother's reluctance (75.6%) were the most common causes of exclusive breastfeeding cessation. A significant relation was seen between breastfeeding duration and gestational age or birth trauma (P Value = 0.031, P Value = 0.04). Breastfeeding training and First mother-infant skin to skin contact had significant roles on breastfeeding duration (P Value < 0.05, P Value = 0.001, respectively). It seems lots of public health efforts and policy are needed to improve breastfeeding rate in our country.

Keywords

Infant, Breastfeeding Rate, Iran

1. Introduction

There is no doubt that breastfeeding is ideal infant's nutrition. It is a source of protein, lipid, oligosaccharide, vitamins, elements, hormones, enzymes, growth and immune factors that can adjust over time based on infant's need [1]. Breastfeeding protects children against respiratory tract infections, atopic dermatitis, asthma, type II

---

*Corresponding author.

diabetes, obesity, and sudden infant death syndrome [2]. Suboptimal breastfeeding is responsible for children death (under 5 years old) due to infections (45%), diarrhea (30%) and acute respiratory disease (18%) [3]. Moreover, breastfeeding is beneficial to the mother's health by returning pelvic organs to prior pregnancy condition, delaying next pregnancy and protection against ovarian and breast cancer [4].

In the USA breast feeding rate is 70% at hospital discharge, but this rate declines to 50% in 6 months and 25% in 24 months [5]. Some elements like personal, cultural, social, environmental, and psychological characteristics, acceptance of female role, breastfeeding experience, infant health status and belief of insufficient milk supply affect on breastfeeding tendency [2]. Pre and post natal breastfeeding training are also considered influential [6]. In addition intra partum mothers' training such as rooming-in and skin to skin contact influence on breastfeeding success [7]. American Academy of Family Physicians (AAFP) suggest intra partum training, physicians' support and improving educational breastfeeding methods can promote breastfeeding initiation and duration [8].

Mothers face lots of advertisement about formula and complementary feeding but information about breast pump and milk storage are not enough that can affect on breast feeding trend [9]. Different statistics of breastfeeding rates were published from different Iranian provinces [10]-[12]. This study was to assess breastfeeding frequency in 21 - 27 month infants born in Baby Friendly Hospitals (Tehran-Iran) by characteristics of the child and mother. Evaluation of effective factors can suggest some interventions to promote breastfeeding success.

2. Materials and Methods

A descriptive-cross sectional study was carried out in South Health Center (Tehran-Iran) in 2010. Four hundred 21 - 27 month single (not twin or more) breastfed infants entered the study. Exclusion criteria were mothers' dissatisfaction, separation of mother and baby due to hospitalization, mother's illness or drug consumption with absolute contra indication in breastfeeding period. Exclusive breastfeeding and breastfeeding duration were clarified based on WHO definition [13]. A questionnaire compatible with other studies and confirmed by experts was applied. Veteran and trained midwives completed questionnaires in a pilot study then its validity and reliability were assessed (Cronbach's alpha = 75%).

The aim of the study and its process were described for all participants, and then all demographic data (infants' birth weight, height, and mothers' age, educational level, occupation, past medical and Ob history, drug consumption except from routine prenatal and breastfeeding period medications) were gathered and recorded in the questionnaires.

In next step investigators asked mothers to answer questions about breastfeeding initiation time, exclusive breast feeding, duration of breastfeeding, initiation of formula and their reasons, time of weaning and it's causes, any medical complications like allergies, baby satisfaction, nipple sore, any breastfeeding training in pre, intra and postpartum periods, attendance and non-person training, skin to skin contact, and role of father's support in their breastfeeding.

Patients' data were considered secret and as no interventions were performed in our study, no patient's consent was asked. Ethics approval for the study was obtained from the institutional review board of Tehran University of medical sciences (ID: 12043).

Finally the software package SPSS version 16 was used to perform the statistical analysis. The t-test, Chi square and Pearson Correlation Coefficient were applied where applicable. The power of study was 80% and level of significance was considered $P < 0.05$.

3. Results

Among four hundred, 21 - 27 month infants' mothers with mean gestational age 38.16 weeks, 340 (85%) mothers were under High School diploma and 388 (97%) were unemployed and housekeeper. forty five percent mothers had 1 - 3 abortions. Thirty two mothers (8%) had underlying disease of which 7% used psychological drugs, 1% cardiovascular, 26% antibiotic and 21% took other drugs. Three hundred and eleven mothers were trained by physicians, midwives, family, relatives, press, media and breastfeeding classes in hospitals.

Of 400 breastfed infants born in Baby Friendly Hospitals with mean birth weight 3228 + 438 gram, 216 (54%) were female.

Based on our results unfortunately 25% of mothers have not had any breastfeeding. Of 300 others, 52 mothers (17%) had Exclusive 6 month's breastfeeding, 87% breastfed their infants until 12 while 36% had breastfeeding until 24 months. Participants' breastfeeding trend was shown in **Figure 1**.

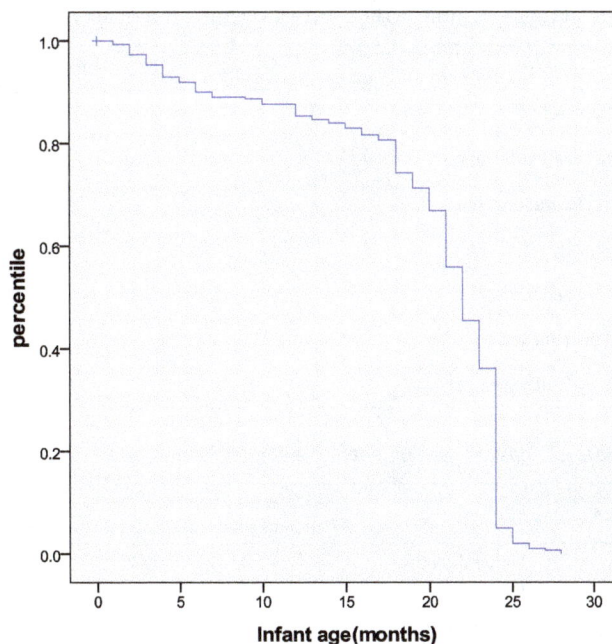

Figure 1. Trend of breastfeeding duration in 22 - 27 months infants' mothers.

Mean breastfeeding duration and median (either exclusive or combined) were 19.66 ± 6.40 and 22 months. Two hundred and forty eight mothers had added formula before 6 months. **Table 1** shows mothers' reasons for formula initiation.

Among all reasons which cited by mothers, Some reasons like insufficient breast milk supply (77.9%), mothers' occupation (73.3%), physician and family's recommendation (74.8%, 76%), infant crying and restless (77.1%), Mother's reluctance (75.6%) and infant refuse (74%) were the most common causes of stopping exclusively breastfeeding until 6 months while vaccination (8.2%), breast congestion (3.2%), oral thrush (1.6%), earache (1.6%), teething (1.7%), and use of cosmetics (1.7%) were the least common causes. In addition no cases reported stop breast feeding due to fast flow milk, breast shaking or blistering and skin inflammation.

As breastfeeding median was 22 months, investigators compared some variables in 2 groups; Group A: weaning before 22 months and Group B: weaning after 22 months. Breastfeeding was stopped in 133 infants in group A and 165 infants in group B. **Table 2** shows comparison of two groups' demographic data.

A significant relation was seen between breastfeeding duration and gestational age (P Value = 0.031). Stopping breast feeding was more frequent in mothers with lower gestational age (in Group A gestational age was 37.73 ± 3.48 while in Group B was 38.49 ± 2.52 weeks). First mother-infant skin to skin contact was seen in 99(60%) cases in group B and 63 (47%) cases in group A, which this difference was significant (P Value = 0.001). A significant correlation was seen between breastfeeding duration and birth trauma (P Value = 0.04). Pre, intra and postpartum breastfeeding training especially private and face to face training by physicians had a significant role on breastfeeding duration (**Table 3**). Besides that father's support was important factor on breastfeeding trend (P Value < 0.05).

In two groups, no significant correlations were observed between weaning or adding formula and some factors mentioned by mothers like mothers' occupation (P Value = 0.804), physicians' encouragement (P Value = 0.299), insufficient breast milk supply (P Value = 0.465), family advice (P Value = 0.423), baby crying (P Value = 0.465), infant refuse (P Value = 0.811), Mothers reluctance (P Value = 0.351).

No relation was seen with infant's birth weight (Group A; 3219 ± 467, Group B 3235 ± 415, P Value = 0.753). More over this study could not find any relation between stop breastfeeding and mother's parity (Group A; 1.59 ± 0.7, Group B; 1.79 ± 1, P Value = 0.059). Maternal age and infant's sex also were not significant factors on mean breastfeeding duration and even breastfeeding initiation time. No relation was found with drug consumption, too (P Value = 0.140).

Table 1. Effective factors on initiation of formula (both Breastfeeding and formula).

Variables	Both breastfeeding and formula total = 248 [n%]
Baby refuse	188 (76)
Insufficient breast milk supply	198 (80)
Mother's return to work	186 (75)
Encourage by physician	191 (77)
Baby cry and restless	198 (80)
Mothers reluctance	191 (77)
Encourage by family members	188 (76)

Table 2. Demographic factors in 2 groups; weaning before and after 22 months.

Demographic characteristics		Weaning before 22 months total = 133 [n%]	Weaning after 22 months total = 165 [n%]	P value
Education	Under diploma Upper diploma	45 (34) 88 (66)	56 (33.9) 109 (66.1)	0.987
Job	Housekeeper Employed	128 (96) 5 (4)	162 (98) 3 (2)	0.758
Underlying disease	Yes No	17 (13) 116 (87)	13 (7.8) 152 (92.2)	0.145
Drug consumption	Yes No	19 (14) 114 (86)	15 (9) 150 (91)	0.140
Breastfeeding experience	Yes No	56 (42) 77 (58)	78 (47) 89 (53)	0.583

Table 3. Effects of training on breastfeeding duration.

Variables	Group A Total = 133	Group B Total = 165	P value
Breastfeeding training	74 (56.2)	118 (72)	0.0001
Training by physicians at office	12 (9.0)	26 (15.6)	0.045
Prenatal training	4 (3.0)	12 (7.2)	0.050
Intra partum training	21 (15.5)	39 (23.4)	0.046
Postpartum training	55 (42.1)	85 (52)	0.047

4. Discussion

The benefits of breast feeding for mother and her infant are well-documented, however, these effects depends on its duration and exclusivity [14]. Our analysis provided further explores the rates of breastfeeding in Teheran-Iran by characteristics of the infant and mother. The main strengths of this study were the large sample size and evaluating the status of breastfeeding in 21 - 27 months infants which had not been done previously in other studies from Iran.

The project found that 17% of our participants were exclusively breastfed by 6 months. Although this prevalence rate was lesser than Saudi Arabia and China, Compared to WHO report (1.7% - 24.4%) it was appropriate. In Saudi Arabia and China exclusive breastfeeding rate were reported 32% - 38% and 70% which seems differences in cultures, believes, training and breastfeeding social supports are responsible for such discrepancies [15] [16]. Maybe in our country exclusive breastfeeding was being replaced by a combination of breast milk and formula.

This study found that the mean breastfeeding duration was 19.66 ± 6.40 which was near to another report from Iran by 20.6 months [12]. Fortunately about 90% of our participants had breastfeeding until 12 months. It shows breast feeding is preferred nutrition for Iranian infants in one and two-years of age. Our religion (Islam) and governmental strategies highly emphasized on breastfeeding, too. Africa and Asia have the highest rate of breast-feeding duration while the USA has the lowest [11].

This study like previous reports indicated that in spite of large number breast feeding initiation rate, this rate declined at 27 months postpartum. Our results consistent to another local study (2014) which showed 65.8% of Iranian mothers had breastfeeding in 4 first months but this rate decreased to 24 months [2]. Spears and Garbarino in their studies also revealed that the prevalence rate of the breastfeeding initiation rate was much more than breast feeding sustaining after 6 months or latter [17] [18].

Our finding indicated that some formula was added for 82.7% of infants in 24 months. Based on mothers' reports initiation of formula was due to family advice, breast refusal by infant, insufficient milk supply, return to work, physicians' recommendation, baby crying and mother's unwillingness. Tararnt et al. (2010) in their study also pointed to husband preference, milk insufficiency and mother's occupation as important factors for adding formula [19]. Another study indicated that initiation of formula may be due to mother's reluctance, baby restless, return to work and milk insufficiency. Although 50% of mothers mentioned inadequacy of their milk, no evidences such as infant weight loss were seen [20] [21]. Providing work places more friendly towards breastfeeding for employed mothers, finding the related factors to perception of insufficient milk, solving problems, use of medications to increase milk supply, and confirmation of milk insufficiency by physicians before initiation of formula can encourage mothers to continue their breastfeeding [22] [23].

A significant relation was seen between mother's gestational age and breastfeeding duration. Breastfeeding duration in mothers with a term infant is longer than a preterm. Nagulesapillai et al. explained that mothers with preterm infants need more attention for breastfeeding continuity [24]. Haschke et al. also reported that in developed and developing countries term in compare to preterm infants benefit more from mother's milk [25]. In addition because preterm infants receive little milk, breastfeeding success need more attempt and support. Mothers preterm infants after hospital discharge did not have enough experience and knowledge due to bottle milk or formula feeding which started in the hospital [26].

This study of mothers in Tehran has identified the important role of face to face training by physicians at private office. Physicians' supportive and educational program, guidance on breast-feeding techniques and ways to resolve problems bedside increasing the rate of exclusive breastfeeding, decrease cessation of breastfeeding at birth time, first month and 1 to 5 months of life [27]. Honda et al. showed in their investigation that physicians have a key role in mothers' inspiration and training [28]. Moreover based on Albernaz's report face to face consultation increases exclusive breastfeeding rate because of continuous support, breastfeeding technical training and mothers' problem solving [29]. This finding shows more deliberate need for policy makers. Every day tens of public classes are held in private and public prenatal clinics and hospitals to improve breastfeeding knowledge, attitude and practice. This help received by women was not always useful. Moreover, in Baby Friendly Hospitals different methods like brochures, films, and health staff consultation are usually applied simultaneously to increase efficacy of training program, which should be revised. It is considered that mothers trust their doctors and one of the most effective factors on breastfeeding duration may be physicians' face to face training during different time periods.

Father's supports also were independently associated with breastfeeding continuity. A number of previous studies have confirmed our finding; Meedya et al. in 2010 and Sherriff et al. in 2014 demonstrated that beside mothers' intention and decision, social factors particularly fathers' supports in breastfeeding initiation and continuance are crucial [30] [31]. Breastfeeding seems a team work efforts which fathers' physical, practical, emotional, psychological attendance and supports are undeniable [32]. Kenosi found that children with short breastfeeding period had fathers with very restricted knowledge about breastfeeding and its advantages [33].

Immediately after birth, skin to skin contact was found as another efficient factor in this study. Based on UNICEF report (2006) infant and mother skin to skin contact in first hour of life is one of ten steps in breastfeeding success [34]. It has been reported that skin to skin contact is an effective intervention to promote babies' sucking ability, weight gain, body temperature stability and mother's satisfaction [35].

Our results on the influence of mother's birth trauma on breastfeeding duration are generally in line with those reported in other studies. It is considered that birth trauma causes some troubles and discomfort on mother's position. Brown et al. in their study confirmed that complications during labor and delivery may increase risk of specific physical difficulties with more breastfeeding failure. Both pain due to birth trauma and associated medications decrease breastfeeding duration [36] [37].

Despite the fact that our study highlights the status of breastfed infants born in Baby Friendly Hospitals (which are significant and well established in Iran), not evaluate all the related factors such as delivery status, economic factor and ethnicity in this study. Participants in our study were from urban areas and therefore are not representative of all Tehran population.

5. Conclusion

To determine the causes of short breastfeeding duration, this study was performed. Based on results, some reasons like insufficient breast milk supply, mothers' occupation, physician and family's recommendation, infant crying and restless, Mother's reluctance and infant refuse were the most common causes of stopping exclusively breastfeeding. On the other hand, training course particularly physician's face to face education and father's support can influence on exclusive breastfeeding and breastfeeding duration significantly. It seems lots of public health efforts and policy are needed to improve breastfeeding rate in our country.

Acknowledgements

The authors would like to thank Fetal, Maternal and Neonatal Research Center for financial support.

Authors' Contribution

Dr Nayeri and Dr Dalili were responsible for concepts, design, editing Manuscript and Experimental studies, Dr Shariat and Dr Raji did Literature search, Data acquisition, Data analysis, and Statistical analysis and Dr Karimi prepared and reviewed manuscript.

References

[1] Şencan, I., Tekin, O. and Mansur, T.M. (2013) Factors Influencing Breastfeeding Duration: A Survey in a Turkish Population. *European Journal of Pediatrics*, **172**, 1459-1466. http://dx.doi.org/10.1007/s00431-013-2066-8

[2] Assarian, F., Moravveji, A., Ghaffarian, H., Eslamian, R. and Atoof, F. (2014) The Association of Postpartum Maternal Mental Health with Breastfeeding Status of Mothers: A Case-Control Study. *Iranian Red Crescent Medical Journal*, **16**, e14839. http://dx.doi.org/10.5812/ircmj.14839

[3] http://www.who.int/maternal_child_adolescent/news_events/news/2012/30_07_2012

[4] Froehlich, J., Boivin, M., Walter, K.C., Bloch, M.K., Rice, D., McGraw, K. and Munson, E. (2013) Influencing University Students' Knowledge and Attitudes toward Breast Feeding. *Journal of Nutrition Education and Behavior*, 1-3.

[5] Li, R., Zhao, Z., Mokdad, A., Barker, L. and Grummer-Strawn, L. (2003) Prevalence of Breastfeeding in the United States: The 2001 National Immunization Survey. *Pediatrics*, **111**, 1198-1201.

[6] Perez-Escarnilla, R., Lutter, C., Segall, A.M., *et al.* (1995) Exclusive Breast-Feeding Duration Is Associated with Attitudinal, Socioeconomic and Biocultural Determinants in Three Latin American Countries. *Nutrition Journal*, **12**, 2972.

[7] Rosenberg, K.D., Eastham, C.A. and Kasehagen, L.J. (2008) Marketing Infant Formula through Hospitals: The Impact of Commercial Hospital Discharge Packs on Breast Feeding. *American Journal of Public Health*, **98**, 290-295. http://dx.doi.org/10.2105/AJPH.2006.103218

[8] http://www.aafp.org/online/en/home

[9] Dalili, H., Farsar, A., Barakati, H., Raij, F., Shariat, M., Pourmalek, F., *et al.* (2014) Frequency of Exclusive Breastfeeding and Its Affecting Factors in Tehran, 2011. *Acta Medica Iranica*, **52**, 552-556.

[10] The Ministry of Health IR of Iran, Breastfeeding Office. http://www.bfps.ir/(i5emlr45w1kdeg45tov0ysem)/Persian/Home.aspx

[11] Marandi, A., Afzali, H.M. and Hossaini, A.F. (1993) The Reasons for Early Weaning among Mothers in Teheran. *Bulletin of the World Health Organization*, **71**, 561-569.

[12] Veghari, G.H., Mansourian, A. and Abdollahi, A. (2011) Breastfeeding Status and Some Related Factors in Northern Iran. *Oman Medical Journal*, **26**, 342-348. http://dx.doi.org/10.5001/omj.2011.84

[13] World Health Organization (1991) Indicators for Assessing Breast-Feeding Practices. World Health Organization, Geneva.

[14] Wenru, W., Ying, L., Aloysius, C. and Kin, S.C. (2014) Breast-Feeding Intention, Initiation and Duration among Hong Kong Chinese Women: A Prospective Longitudinal Study. *Midwifery*, **30**, 678-687.

http://dx.doi.org/10.1016/j.midw.2013.07.015

[15] Al Juaid, D.A., Binns, C.W. and Giglia, R.C. (2014) Breastfeeding in Saudi Arabia: A Review. *International Breast-feeding Journal*, **9**, 1-9. http://dx.doi.org/10.1186/1746-4358-9-1

[16] Liu, P., Qiao, L., Xu, F., Zhang, M., Wang, Y. and Binns, C.W. (2013) Factors Associated with Breastfeeding Duration: A 30-Month Cohort Study in Northwest China. *Journal of Human Lactation*, **29**, 253-259. http://dx.doi.org/10.1177/0890334413477240

[17] Spear, H.J. (2004) Nurses' Attitudes, Knowledge, and Beliefs Related to the Promotion of Breastfeeding among Women Who Bear Children during Adolescence. *Journal of Pediatric Nursing*, **19**, 176-183. http://dx.doi.org/10.1016/j.pedn.2004.01.006

[18] Garbarino, F., Morniroli, D., Ghirardi, B., Garavaglia, E., Bracco, B., Gianní, M.L., Roggero, P. and Mosca, F. (2013) Prevalence and Duration of Breastfeeding during the First Six Months of Life: Factors Affecting an Early Cessation. *La Pediatria Medica e Chirurgica*, **35**, 217-222. http://dx.doi.org/10.4081/pmc.2013.30

[19] Tarrant, M., Fong, D.Y., Wu, K.M., Lee, I.L., Wong, M.E., *et al.* (2010) Breast Feeding & Weaning Practices among Hong Kong Mothers, a Prospective Study. *BMC Pregnancy & Childbirth*, **10**, 1-12.

[20] Li, R., Fein, S.B., Chen, J. and Grummer, S. (2008) Why Mothers Stop Breast Feeding: Self Reported Reason for Stopping during First Year. *Pediatrics*, **122**, S69-S76. http://dx.doi.org/10.1542/peds.2008-1315i

[21] Amir, L.H. and Cwikel, J. (2005) Why Do Women Stop Breastfeeding? A Closer Look at "Not Enough Milk" among Israeli Women in the Negev Region. *Breastfeed Re*, **13**, 7-13.

[22] Amir, L.H. (2006) Breastfeeding, Managing Supply Difficulties. *Australian Family Physicians*, **35**, 686-689.

[23] Ong, G., Yap, M., Li, F.L. and Choo, T.B. (2005) Impact of Working Status Ion Breastfeeding in Singapore. *European Journal of Public Health*, **15**, 424-430. http://dx.doi.org/10.1093/eurpub/cki030

[24] Nagulesapillai, T., McDonald, S.W., Fenton, T.R., Mercader, H.F. and Tough, S. (2013) Breastfeeding Difficulties and Exclusivity among Late Preterm and Term Infants: Results from the All Our Babies Study. *Canadian Journal of Public Health*, **104**, 351-356.

[25] Haschke, F., Haiden, N., Detzel. P., Yarnoff, B., Allaire, B. and Haschke-Becher, E. (2013) Feeding Patterns during the First 2 Years and Health Outcome. *Annals of Nutrition and Metabolism*, **62**, 16-25. http://dx.doi.org/10.1159/000351575

[26] Niela-Vilén, H., Axelin, A., Melender, H.L. and Salanterä, S. (2014) Aiming to Be a Breastfeeding Mother in a Neonatal Intensive Care Unit and at Home: A Thematic Analysis of Peer-Support Group Discussion in Social Media. *Maternal & Child Nutrition*. http://dx.doi.org/10.1111/mcn.12108

[27] Haroon, S., Das, J.K., Salam, R.A., Imdad, A. and Bhutta, Z.A. (2013) Breastfeeding Promotion Interventions and Breastfeeding Practices: A Systematic Review. *BMC Public Health*, **13**, 20. http://dx.doi.org/10.1186/1471-2458-13-S3-S20

[28] Handa, D. and Schanler, R.J. (2013) Role of the Pediatrician in Breastfeeding Management. *Pediatric Clinics of North America*, **60**, 1-10. http://dx.doi.org/10.1016/j.pcl.2012.10.004

[29] Albernaz, E. and Victora C.G. (2003) Impact of Face-to-Face Counseling on Duration of Exclusive Breast-Feeding: A Review. *Revista Panamericana de Salud Pública*, **14**, 17-24. http://dx.doi.org/10.1590/S1020-49892003000600004

[30] Meedya, S., Fahy, K. and Kable, A. (2010) Factors That Positively Influence Breastfeeding Duration to 6 Months: A Literature Review. *Women and Birth*, **23**, 135-145. http://dx.doi.org/10.1016/j.wombi.2010.02.002

[31] Sherriff, N., Panton, C. and Hall, V. (2014) A New Model of Father Support to Promote Breastfeeding. *The Journal of Community Practice*, **87**, 20-24.

[32] Tohotoa. J., Maycock, B., Hauck, Y.L., Howat, P., Burns, S. and Binns, C.W. (2009) Dads Make a Difference: An Exploratory Study of Paternal Support for Breastfeeding in Perth, Western Australia. *International Breastfeeding Journal*, **4**, 15. http://dx.doi.org/10.1186/1746-4358-4-15

[33] Kenosi, M., Hawkes, C.P., Dempsey, E.M. and Ryan, C.A. (2011) Are Fathers Underused Advocates for Breastfeeding? *Irish Medical Journal*, **104**, 313-315.

[34] Grizzard, T.A., Bartick, M., Nikolov, M., Griffin, B.A. and Lee, K.G. (2006) Policies and Practices Related to Breastfeeding in Massachusetts: Hospital Implementation of the Ten Steps to Successful Breastfeeding. *Maternal and Child Health Journal*, **10**, 247-263.

[35] Srivastava, S., Gupta, A., Bhatnagar, A. and Dutta, S. (2014) Effect of Very Early Skin to Skin Contact on Success at Breastfeeding and Preventing Early Hypothermia in Neonates. *Indian Journal Public Health*, **58**, 22-26. http://dx.doi.org/10.4103/0019-557X.128160

[36] Brown, A. and Jordan, S. (2013) Impact of Birth Complications on Breastfeeding Duration: An Internet Survey. *Journal of Advanced Nursing*, **69**, 828-839. http://dx.doi.org/10.1111/j.1365-2648.2012.06067.x

[37] Khabbal, Y., Zaoui, S. and Cherrah, Y. (2013) Medicines and Breastfeeding: Assessing the Risk of Medicines to Infants. *Eastern Mediterranean Health Journal*, **19**, 186-191.

One Stage Reconstruction of Esophageal Atresia and Distal Tracheoesophageal Fistula in a 3250-gm Neonate: A Case Report

Bijay Upadhyay, Xuedong Wu*, Jun Li, Ning Wang, Shanshan Zhang, Na Li

Department of Pediatric Surgery, Affiliated Hospital of Dali University, Dali, China
Email: *xuedong3288@sina.com

Abstract

Esophageal atresia (EA) occurs when the upper part of the esophagus does not connect with the lower part of esophagus and stomach. Tracheoesophageal fistula (TEF) is an abnormal connection between the upper part of the esophagus and the trachea. Treatment for esophageal atresia has advanced over several decades due to improvements in surgical techniques and neonatal intensive care. The aim is to share our experience regarding the treatment of esophageal atresia with tracheoesophageal fistula. A 4-day-old neonate suffering from esophageal atresia with type IIIB tracheoesophageal fistula underwent one stage esophageal reconstruction and obtained good outcome without any complications. In this paper, a simple intra-operative technique for tracheal fistula repair and end to end esophageal anastomosis is discussed. We used a simple technique that we have found useful for ligation of tracheal fistula. Anastomosis of lower and upper esophagus without any complication like anastomotic leakage or stricture/stenosis of the neonate with EA/TEF (type IIIB), was proved to be safe and effective.

Keywords

Esophageal Atresia, Tracheoesophageal Fistula, Esophageal Reconstruction, End to End Anastamosis

1. Introduction

Esophageal atresia (EA) with or without tracheoesophageal fistula (TEF) is a fairly common congenital disorder that doctor should consider in the differential diagnosis of a neonate who develops feeding difficulties and res-

---

*Corresponding author.

piratory distress in the first few days of life. It is often associated with other congenital anomalies, most commonly congenital cardiac defects. EA/TEF is a life threatening condition as well as esophagus reconstruction for the patients, prompt recognition, appropriate clinical management to prevent aspiration, and swift referral to an appropriate tertiary care center have resulted in a significant improvement in the rates of morbidity and mortality in these infants over the past 50 years. But the leakage of anastomosis and esophageal stenosis are still the main complications after operation. A neonate with EA and TEF underwent one stage reconstruction and who got good outcome was reported in this paper and the complications prevention management was discussed.

2. Case Report

The patient was 4-day-old, 3250 gm, female, born after 39 weeks and 6 days gestational age by uncomplicated primary lower segmental cesarean section. Because vomiting and respiratory distress after birth, progressive abdominal distention was noticed, a nasogastric tube could not be passed into the stomach and esophagogram was made through injected iodine oil via nasogastric tube given, contrast not visible under the level of 4th thoracic vertebra, forming an enlarged blind end and gas intra-alimentary tract can be found, the diagnosis of EA/TEF with gross type III was established (**Figure 1(a)** and **Figure 1(b)**) smooth round pouch like structure and coiling of Ryle's tube seen (**Figure 1**). No other anomalies exist through total physical examination and investigations; surgical Correction was scheduled for the baby treatment.

General anesthesia was given without muscle relaxant and then an endotrecheal tube was inserted and gradually pushed until breath sounds can be heard both left and right lungs means the tube was in its right position. Then the patient was placed into the left lateral position. Horizontal S-shaped incision was given at the 6th intercostal space, thoracic cavity was opened and posterior mediastinum was exposed, the azygos vein was divided and cut down to reveal the underlying EA/TEF. The blind end of esophagus and the fistula were found and made label respectively (**Figure 2**).

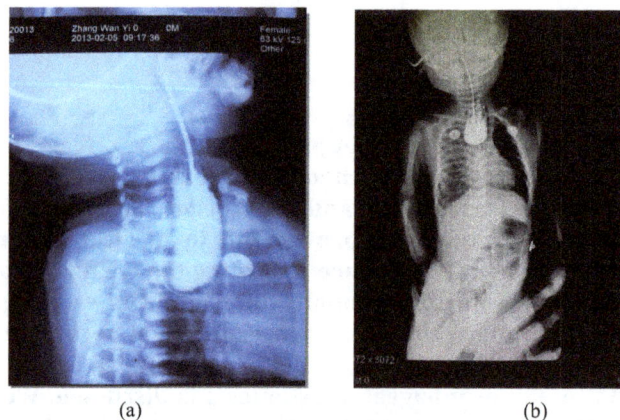

(a) (b)

Figure 1. (a) Lateral view; (b) A/P view. Both X-ray esophagogram shows contrast not visible beyond the level of T4 vertebrae.

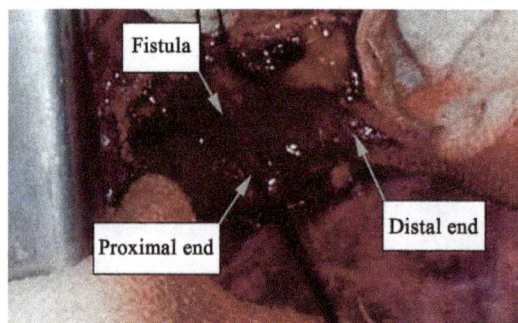

Figure 2. Operative photography showing the blind end of esophagus and fistula and labeled them respectively.

The TEF was dissected circumferentially and its attachment to the membranous portion of trachea is taken down. The tracheal fistula opening and definition with diameter 0.5 cm was ligated and the end to tracheal was closed with nonabsorbable suture but the connective tissue between two pouches was not cut down completely. The gap between two ends was 1.5 cm, the proximal esophagus pouch was mobilized as high as possible to afford a tension free esophageal anastomosis, The blood supply to the upper esophageal pouch is generally robust and is based on arteries derived from the thyrocervical trunk. However, the blood supply to lower esophagus is more tenuous and segmental, originating from intercostal vessels. As such, significant mobilization of the lower esophagus is avoided to prevent ischemia at the esophageal anastamosis.

After opened the proximal end the anastomosis was performed by interrupted suturing the posterior mucosal layer first with 6 - 0 absorbable vircryl and then Ryle's tube was inserted into stomach and anterior mucosal layer was sutured and then outer layer was sutured to give strength to the anastomosis with 6 sutures, connective tissue around the esophagus was not separated apart so that it can give strength and release the tension of anastamosis. No active bleeding in operative field and a chest tube was inserted at the seventh intercostal space to the right posterior axillary line. Incision was sutured layer by layer.

Surgical process went well with less bleeding and effective anesthesia. Patient was sent back to ward when awake and endotrecheal tube was put out. Antibiotics coverage and fluids management was done post operation and recovery was smoothly and uneventfully. Nasogastric tube was removed 2 weeks after operation and feed milk normal, contrast chest x-ray with iodine oil feed shows normal chest and esophagus through with no leakage (**Figure 3(a)**). Patient was discharged after 16 days of operation. Contrast (iodine oil) chest x-ray followed up at 3 months after operation with no abnormal constriction and stenosis noted (**Figure 3(b)**) and the patient weight was 5000 gm. Up to now, the patient was followed-up for 2 years regularly without any swallowing difficulty and any other complains.

3. Discussion

Esophageal artesia with tracheoesophageal fistula is a life threatening condition occurs in one of 3000 to 5000 births with a complicated prognosis. Although survival in patients of EA with/without TEF has markedly improved due to advances in surgical techniques and neonatal intensive care, complications often occur and morbidities after treatment are still regarded as an important issue. The reasons for high morbidity associated with esophageal atresia are well known [1]-[3]. Associated anomalies, low birth weight or prematurity, and likelihood of pneumonia are common findings with esophageal artesia and affect treatment outcome. In addition, variations in the type of Artesia, anatomical differences, anastomotic tension induced by long gap of esophageal atresia and lack of surgical experience are also considered as potential risk.

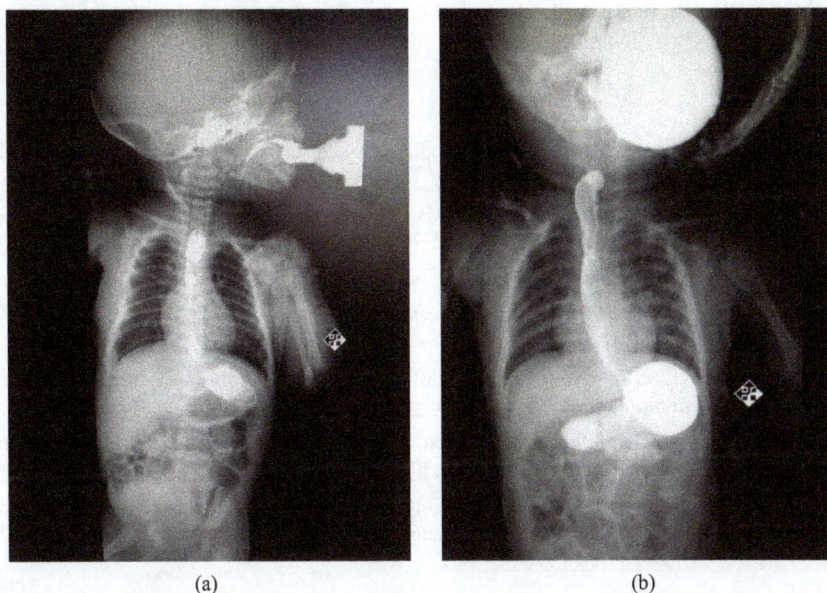

(a)   (b)

Figure 3. Both esophagogram shows no leakage and stenosis, contrast freely flowed to the stomach.

Doctors who care for neonates should be aware of both the clinical presentation and management of neonates with these conditions. It may be suspected prenatally if ultrasound examination reveals polyhydramnios, absence of a fluid-filled stomach, a small abdomen. Lower than expected fetal weight and distended esophageal pouch. Fetal MRI may be used to confirm the presence of EA/TEF. EA may be detected postnataly by failure to pass nasogastric tube and radiographs that demonstrate coiling of the NG tube in the pouch, tracheal compression and deviation on plain chest radiographs, absence of a gastric bubble on plain radiographs, which may suggest EA without a TEF or EA with a proximal TEF. Three dimensional CT scanning, administration of contrast into the esophagus followed by chest radiographs can confirm the diagnosis.

As soon as the diagnosis is made patient need to be prepared for prompt surgical treatment for optimal outcome in which it's out-comes are mainly depends on the surgery. Treatments of EA have gradually evolved due to not only better pre-operative and postoperative neonatal intensive care but also the application of meticulous and precise surgical technique. Recently, the mortality rate associated with EA was reported to be less than 10% and high risk neonates now have better prognosis [4].

Many procedures can be selected for esophageal repair with one or two stages according to different type of the malformation, but anastomotic stricture or leak are still both of the most common complications after operation. The suture material, type of anastomosis, anastomotic tension, ischemia, anastomotic leak and the presence of GER are the main factors affecting the development of anastomotic strictures [4]-[7]. The technique intra-operation and the way of anastomosis are very important for post-operative complications preventing.

As in this case, EA/TEF, type III, one stage reconstruction was performed immediately after clinical diagnosis was established. The distal esophageal segment was less mobilized due to the risk of damage to the connective tissue and occult arterial supply. This was imperative to prevent additional damage to the arterial supply, so as to prevent ischemia that may lead to anastomosis leakage. The ansatomosis was performed using single layer of mucosa to mucosa anastomosis technique with interrupted absorbable sutures. The Ryle's tube was inserted into the stomach after the posterior mucosal layer was sutured. Then only anterior mucosal layer was sutured. The outer adventitia layer was strengthened with few non absorbable sutures. The Ryle's tube was kept in situ for 2 weeks. This technique was found to be effective for anastomotic strictures and leakage prevention. As a result, no anastomotic leakage and uneventful recovery was achieved in the post-operative period. Regular 2 years follow up showed no complain with deglutition.

4. Conclusion

In this case, we used a simple technique by sparing the connective tissue around the esophagus and single layer mucosa to mucosa anastomosis technique. We have found this useful for end to end esophageal anastomosis. Ligation of tracheal fistula with nonabsorbable sutures was also very effective. Anastomosis of lower and upper esophagus without any complication of anastomotic leakage or stricture/stenosis of the neonate with EA/TEF (type IIIB), was proved to be safe and effective.

References

[1] Lopez, P.J., Keys, C., Pierro, A., et al. (2006) Oesophageal Atresia: Improved Outcome in High-Risk Groups? Journal of Pediatric Surgery, 41, 331-334. http://dx.doi.org/10.1016/j.jpedsurg.2005.11.009

[2] Castilloux, J., Noble, A.J. and Faure, C. (2010) Risk Factors for Short- and Long-Term Morbidity in Children with Esophageal Atresia. Journal of Pediatrics, 156, 755-760. http://dx.doi.org/10.1016/j.jpeds.2009.11.038

[3] Townsend, B., et al. (2012) The Biological Basis of Modern Surgical Practice. 2, 1837-1839.

[4] Spitz, L. (2007) Oesophageal Atresia. Orphanet Journal of Rare Diseases, 2, 24. http://dx.doi.org/10.1186/1750-1172-2-24

[5] Singh, S.J. and Shun, A. (2001) A New Technique of Anastomosis to Avoid Stricture Formation in Oesophageal Atresia. Pediatric Surgery International, 17, 575-577. http://dx.doi.org/10.1007/s003830100579

[6] Chang, A.C. and Orringer, M.B. (2007) Management of the Cervical Esophagogastric Anastomotic Stricture. Seminars in Thoracicand Cardiovascular Surgery, 19, 66-71. http://dx.doi.org/10.1053/j.semtcvs.2006.11.001

[7] Upadhyaya, V.D., Gangopadhyaya, A.N., Gupta, D.K., et al. (2007) Prognosis of Congenital Tracheoesophageal Fistula with Esophageal Atresia on the Basis of Gap Length. Pediatric Surgery International, 23, 767-771. http://dx.doi.org/10.1007/s00383-007-1964-0

Epidemiology, Clinical Aspects and Management of Cleft Lip and/or Palate in Burkina Faso: A Humanitarian Pediatric Surgery-Based Study

Kisito Nagalo[1,2*], Isso Ouédraogo[2,3], Jean-Martin Laberge[4,5], Louise Caouette-Laberge[4,6], Jean Turgeon[4,7]

[1]Service of Pediatrics, Clinique El Fateh-Suka, Ouagadougou, Burkina Faso
[2]Training and Research Unit of Health Sciences, University of Ouagadougou, Ouagadougou, Burkina Faso
[3]Department of Pediatric Surgery, Charles De Gaulle Pediatric University Teaching Hospital, Ouagadougou, Burkina Faso
[4]Mission Sourires d'Afrique, Montreal, Canada
[5]Department of Pediatric Surgery, McGill University, Montreal, Canada
[6]Department of Surgery, University of Montreal, Montreal, Canada
[7]Department of Pediatrics, University of Montreal, Montreal, Canada
Email: *kiki_nagalo@yahoo.fr

Abstract

Background: Cleft lip and/or palate are the most common orofacial malformations. Many studies, especially in developed countries have been conducted on this malformation, but in Burkina Faso, data are scarce and they are not specific to children. The aim of this study was to report the epidemiological, clinical and therapeutic aspects of cleft lip and/or palate in children in a low-income country. Materials and Method: The authors conducted a retrospective descriptive study based on data of three humanitarian missions of pediatric reconstructive facial surgery which took place in 2007, 2010 and 2014 at Clinique El Fateh-Suka in Ouagadougou, Burkina Faso. All children of 0 - 14 years of age, presenting with cleft lip and/or palate, were included in the study. Results: A total of 185 cases of cleft lip and/or palate were seen during these three humanitarian surgery missions. There were 100 boys and 85 girls. The average age of the children was 2.4 ± 3.2 years [0 - 12 years]; there were 8.7% newborns. The commonest type of cleft was cleft lip and palate (49.7%) followed by isolated cleft lip (48.7%) and isolated cleft palate (1.6%). The left side was the most affected (49.2%). In 21.1% of cases, clefts were associated with other congenital malformations. In total, 150 of 185 (81.1%) children underwent surgery and there were no postoperative complications reported. Conclusions: Epidemiological and clinical characteristics of cleft lip and/or palate

---

*Corresponding author.

observed in this study are not very different from those described elsewhere in Africa. However, in our conditions, there are circumstances and structural factors which hinder the diagnosis and constitute challenges that must be addressed for adequate management of this congenital, highly disfiguring malformation.

Keywords

Orofacial Clefts, Cleft Lip and/or Palate, Congenital Malformations, Humanitarian Surgery, International Cooperation

1. Introduction

Cleft lip and/or palate (CL/P) are an embryonic syndrome which consists of cleft lip, cleft lip and palate, and cleft palate, and which accounts for 65% of all the congenital malformations of the head and the neck [1]. Ethnic and geographical variations show a high prevalence between 0.55 and 2.50/1000 births in Mongolian populations, between 0.69 and 2.35/1000 in Caucasians; a lower prevalence of between 0.18 and 0.82/1000 in Afro-Americans is reported [2]. In Africa, the prevalence is also lower, estimated at 0.5/1000 in Nigeria [3]. The etiology of this malformation is complex and includes both genetic and environmental factors. Data on orofacial clefts actually are sparsely available in respect of Africa, and this is even truer in Burkina Faso where there are no published studies on CL/P dedicated to the pediatric subpopulation. It is a recent study which revealed that CL/P constituted 70.6% of all congenital malformations of the face and the neck in Ouagadougou [4]. In Burkina Faso, care of orofacial clefts is difficult, and to alleviate the governmental inadequacies, local, European and Canadian Non-Governmental Organizations (NGO) organize humanitarian campaigns to bring the specialized care of surgery to the patients. This study is aimed to describe the epidemiological, clinical aspects and management of CL/P among children seen within the framework of humanitarian missions of pediatric plastic surgery in Ouagadougou in Burkina Faso.

2. Materials and Method

2.1. Study Site

Burkina Faso is a landlocked country in the Sahelian region in western Africa which covers 272,967 km^2. It is populated with 14,017,262 inhabitants of whom more than 77% live in rural areas. The distribution of the population by age group shows that children 0 - 14 years, number 6,499,211. The population is in 49% under 15 years old. Economically, Burkina Faso is one of the poorest countries in the world, the gross national income is of US $1560; 44.46% of the population live with less than US $ 1/day. The sanitary statistics indicate a life expectancy at birth of 57 years; a rate of malformations of 4.1%; anemia has 88% prevalence in children under 5 years, 58% in pregnant women, and 50% in breast-feeding women [5]. The country is subdivided into 45 provinces including the Province of Kadiogo (12.3% of the population) situated in the center of the country in which the capital, Ouagadougou (10.5% of the population), is located. The public sanitary organization included three levels of care; the highest is constituted by the University Teaching Hospital (UTH) which is the reference level for specialized care. There are four UTHs in the country (3 in Ouagadougou and 1 in Bobo-Dioulasso, the 2nd largest city). This study took place at Clinique El Fateh-Suka (CFS) which is situated in Ouagadougou. It is a private hospital created by "Fondation Suka", a NGO the major objective of which is the improvement of the health of the mother and child in Burkina Faso. The partnership between "Fondation Suka", Canadian NGO "Missions Sourires d'Afrique", and international NGO "Smile Train", permits a Canadian medical and surgical team travelling to Ouagadougou to operate upon children presenting with oral or maxillofacial anomalies (*i.e.*, CL/P, aftereffects of Noma disease or burns), and to transfer the skills in the field of the pediatric plastic surgery to local surgeons. Burkina Faso still lacks a register of orofacial clefts.

2.2. Type, Population and Period of Study

It was a retrospective descriptive study of all the patients seen during the three missions of pediatric plastic surgery in November 2007, November 2010 and February 2014.

2.3. Criteria of Inclusion and Noninclusion in the Study

All patients aged 0 - 14 years at the time of the current surgical mission who consulted for a CL/P were included in the study. Patients, who were more than 14 years old, and those who did not have a CL/P, were excluded.

2.4. Procedures

Before the arrival of the Canadian team and the beginning of surgery, a national media campaign (radio, television, newspapers and posters) was held for publicity among the population. The children who lived in rural areas arrived with their guardians (generally the mothers) at Ouagadougou either by public transportation bus, or by the bus chartered by a local collaborator NGO. Upon their arrival, the children were accommodated in the premises of this NGO before being transported to CFS where the surgeries were performed. Before these surgeries, the patients were examined and blood analyses were performed. Then they were prioritized for surgery on the basis of the diagnosis, the operating risks (age, weight, health...) and expected functional results (e.g., capacity to re-educate the language). The medical files were completed; the consent forms filled up, and the photos of patients were taken.

For the surgical operations, the techniques used were those of Millard [6] for cleft lip repair and of Wardill [7] for cleft palate repair.

All the patients were examined again at the end of the campaign by the surgical team. After the departure of the Canadian team, the local team gave assurance for the follow-up of the patients.

2.5. Operational Definitions

As defined by Zandi and Heidari [8], we used the following abbreviations and criteria for cleft type classification: CL = isolated cleft lip (excludes isolated cleft palate and cleft lip with cleft palate), CP = isolated cleft palate (excludes isolated cleft lip and cleft lip with cleft palate), CLP = cleft lip with cleft palate associated (excludes CL, CP), CL +/− P = cleft lip with or without cleft palate (includes CL, CLP, excludes CP), and CL/P = cleft lip and/or cleft palate (includes CL, CP, CLP, no exclusions).

2.6. Data Collection and Analysis

We extracted data from the clinical files and from the anesthetics dossiers of the patients. A proforma allowed collecting demographic data (age, sex, residence), clinical presentation (type, side and seat of the cleft, associated anomalies), and surgery (type of surgery, peri- and postoperative outcome). Then data were entered and analyzed using Epi-info7^{TM} software (Center for Diseases Control, Atlanta, GA, USA).

2.7. Ethical Considerations

Prior to operation, the surgical procedure was explained to the responsible (father or mother or a legal guardian) of the child. In case of acceptance, a consent form was co-signed by this responsible and a member of the surgical team. This study was approved by the Ethics Committee of CFS.

3. Results

Three campaigns of pediatric plastic surgery allowed to examine 185 children aged 0 - 14 years presenting with CL/P, of whom 54 were seen in 2007, 65 were seen in 2010 and 66 were seen in 2014.

Among the children under 15 years old, the frequency of CL/P was 185/6,499,211 demonstrating a rate of 0.03/1000 population.

Table 1 shows the distribution of children by place of residence.

On the whole, there were 100 boys (54%) and 85 girls (46%), demonstrating a sex ratio of 1.18:1. Among 182 cases of CL +/− P, there were 98 boys and 84 girls, giving a sex ratio of 1.17:1. Among the 3 cases of CP, there were 2 boys and 1 girl.

The average age of children was 2.4 ± 3.2 years [0 - 12 years]; there were 6 newborns (8.7%). **Table 2** shows the distribution of the children by age group.

Table 1. Distribution of children presenting with cleft lip and/or palate by residence, Burkina Faso in 2007, 2010, 2014.

Residence	Frequency	Percentage (%)
Province of Kadiogo	62	33.5
Province of Séno	31	16.8
Province of Kouritenga	21	11.3
Province of Sanmatenga	18	9.7
Province of Yagha	15	8.1
Province of Oudalan	10	5.4
Province of Sanguié	7	3.8
Province of Gourma	5	2.7
Province of Yatenga	5	2.7
Province of Houet	4	2.2
Province of Kénédougou	4	2.2
Province of Comoé	2	1.1
Republic of Côte d'Ivoire	1	0.5
Total	**185**	**100.0**

Table 2. Distribution of children presenting with cleft lip and/or palate by age group; Burkina Faso in 2007, 2010, 2014.

Age group (years)	Frequency	Percentage (%)
<1	69	37.3
1 - 4	79	42.7
≥5	37	20.0
Total	**185**	**100.0**

Of the total number of clefts, 182 (98.4%) were CL +/− P of which 92 (49.7%) were CLP and 90 (48.7%) were CL. Unilateral CL +/− P frequency was 138 (74.6%), and involved the left side in 49.2% of cases and the right side in 25.4% of cases. Bilateral CL +/− P were 41 (22.2%) cases, while there were 3 (1.6%) cases of median CL +/− P. In this group of CL +/− P, there were 92 CLP; 63/92 (68.5%) were unilateral CLP of which 68.2% concerned the left side and 31.8% concerned the right side; there were 29/92 (31.5%) bilateral CLP. Among CL +/− P, there were 90 CL, unilateral CL represented 83.4% of cases of which 64.0% concerned the left side and 36.0% the right side; bilateral CL represented 12/90 (13.3%) of cases. There were three CP (1.6%).

According to the type, laterality and severity, the most frequent cleft was Unilateral Left Cleft Lip (ULCL) (25.9%) followed by ULCL and Palate (ULCLP) (23.2%) and Bilateral Cleft Lip and Palate (BCLP) (15.7%).

Among boys, ULCLP (28.0%) and ULCL (20.0%) were the most frequent clefts, whereas among girls, ULCL (33.0%) and Unilateral Right Cleft Lip (URCL) (18.8%) were the most frequent clefts.

Table 3 shows the distribution of the children by sex, type, laterality and severity of clefts.

Of the 185 CL/Ps, 146 (78.9%) were isolated clefts while 39 (21.1%) were associated with other congenital malformations.

A total of 160 surgeries were performed in 150 of 185 (81.1%) children consisting of 135 cheilorraphy and 25 palatorraphy. The postoperative period was uneventful. For the 35 nonoperated children (18.9%), the main reason for nonoperation was the young age and/or the small weight of the child; no newborns were operated upon. **Table 4** shows the distribution of the nonoperated children according to the reason for nonoperation.

Table 3. Distribution of children by sex and type, laterality and severity of clefts, Burkina Faso in 2007, 2010, 2014.

Sex	Type, laterality and severity of the cleft								Total
	BCL	MCL	BCLP	URCLP	ULCLP	URCL	ULCL	CP	
Girls	4	3	11	7	15	16	28	1	85
	(4.7)	(3.5)	(13.0)	(8.2)	(17.6)	(18.8)	(33.0)	(1.2)	(100.0)
	[33.3]	[100.0]	[37.9]	[35.0]	[34.9]	[59.3]	[58.3]	[33.3]	[45.9]
Boys	8	0	18	13	28	11	20	2	100
	(8.0)	(0.0)	(18.0)	(13.0)	(28.0)	(11,0)	(20.0)	(2.0)	(100.0)
	[66.7]	[0.0]	[62.1]	[65.0]	[65.1]	[40.7]	[41.7]	[66.7]	[54.1]
Total	12	3	29	20	43	27	48	3	185
	(6.5)	(1.6)	(15.7)	(10.8)	(23.2)	(14.6)	(25.9)	(1.6)	(100.0)
	[100.0]	[100.0]	[100.0]	[100.0]	[100.0]	[100.0]	[100.0]	[100.0]	[100.0]

The percentages in parenthesis refer to the lines; those in brackets refer to columns. BCL: Bilateral Cleft Lip; MCL: Median CL+/−P; BCLP: Bilateral CL+/−P; URCLP: Unilateral Right CL+/−P; ULCLP: Unilateral Left CL+/−P; URCL: Unilateral Right CL; ULCL: Unilateral Left CL; CP: Cleft Palate.

Table 4. Distribution by reason of 35 nonoperated cleft lip and/or palate cases, Burkina Faso in 2007, 2010, 2014.

Reason	Frequency	Percentage (%)*
Too young/low weight	20	57.1
Polymalformation/complexity of the cleft[†]	6	17.1
Severe anemia	5	14.3
Current infection	5	14.3
Severe malnutrition	2	5.7
Miscellaneous (cleft too short, lack of time)	2	5.7

*Total exceeds 100% because a child could combine several reasons for not being operated; [†]Tessier [#]3, 4, 7, 11.

4. Discussion

4.1. About Clefts Epidemiology

In this study, a low frequency of CL/P in children aged 0 - 14 years in Burkina Faso was observed. Unfortunately, given the limitations of the study, the prevalence of clefts could not be ascertained. If a registry existed, it would not only fill this gap but it would also constitute a database that would improve the level of knowledge available on birth prevalence of CL/P and the associated international, geographical, ethnic and cultural variations [9].

According to the residence, the province of Kadiogo was the most represented by one-third of the patients. The reason is that the population of this province had more easy access to the information about the surgical campaigns, besides having less distance to travel when compared with patients who came from other provinces. But overall, there were many more children who came from other provinces which are very distant from the capital, Ouagadougou, and in which the populations for a great part are rural and poor. This trend is also observes in other developing countries where the specialists hardly meet except in referral hospitals [10]-[12]. For all these reasons, many children usually do not have access to the specialized health services and they remain home. To receive benefits from the NGOs and avail of the humanitarian surgery, they can arrive up to the capital and receive adequate care.

On average, we have seen the children after their second anniversary. This finding is similar to that of Diakité in Mali a nearby country sharing the same climatic, social, demographic and economic characteristics as Burkina Faso. This author reported 133 children presenting with CL/P who had an average age of 2.5 years. He also found a distribution of the age at presentation which superimposed our results [13]. In developing countries, among the reasons that are put forward to explain the long time before consultation and/or surgery, we can quote the ignorance, the mystic and religious faiths, the social cultural heaviness, the inaccessibility, and the nonavailability of specialized health services; but also, and especially, the financial constraints, because most of the parents of the children presenting with clefts are poor [10] [14]. Where the children were seen earlier, it is the information of the populations on clefts and the free access of the treatment that explain the precocity of the diagnosis [15]. In Africa, the discovery of a CL/P is almost always a surprise for everybody including caregivers and parents, because the diagnosis is generally carried out in the delivery ward, with a malformed newborn. Contrary to the developed countries where prenatal diagnosis is possible [16], this is rarely (1%) made in Africa [13]. The causes of orofacial cleft underdiagnosis are, on one hand, the inaccessibility of the ultrasound facility for many pregnant women, and, on the other hand, the expertise of the technician, drawing attention to look for a cleft in the fetus is sometimes prompted only by a detail such as the presence of the anomaly in the mother [13]. In reality, in our context of a country with limited resources, these diagnostic limits do not, in particular, concern CL/P but generally all congenital malformations.

Our findings match the data of the literature relative to the predominance of males in overall CL/P and in CLP, in particular [2] [3] [13] [16]-[18]. However, other authors report a global ascendancy of girls compared with boys [19]. In our study, there were two boys and one girl presenting with CP, but the size of this sample was too small, as it did not allow discussing our results meaningfully with that of the other studies. According to certain authors, the difference of prevalence of clefts between the sexes would be due to the differences of sex hormones, speed of growth of tissues and organs, and mortality *in utero* between male and female fetuses [20]. However, considering that our statistics are based on patients who presented themselves for surgery rather than the number of children born with clefts, there may be a selection bias.

4.2. About Clefts Clinical Presentation

We noted ascendancy in CLP cases, followed by CL cases; CP cases were the least frequent. This distribution of the clefts in our study is in accordance with most of the data found in the literature [2] [3] [18] [21]. This order can, however, be upset and shows ascendancy in the CL [22] or CP cases [19] [23]. In this study, unilateral clefts were the most frequent compared with bilateral clefts, as well among CLP as CL; the left side was the most frequently affected, corresponding with the data in the literature [2] [16]-[18] [24]. According to the laterality and severity, ULCL were predominant followed by ULCLP, then BCLP, URCL, URCLP, BCL and, lastly, CP. Probably because of the different mode in recruitment of the patients, our findings are different from those of Franco *et al.* [12] in Brazil who found this sequence: ULCLP (27%)-CP (15.6%)-ULCL (13%)-URCL-URCLP-BCLP (each 7%)-BCL (2%). We found median clefts in the frequency of 1.6% closed to that of 1% found by Doray *et al.* [16], whereas, Aljohar *et al.* [23] found a threefold higher frequency of this type of cleft.

In this study, the frequency of 22.2% of bilateral clefts was higher than that found in the literature where it varies from less than 10% [12] [18] [25] to 17% - 19% [8] [13]. As previously mentioned, our data were based on patients who went for surgery encouraged in a certain way, and this could induce a selection bias. In addition, children with bilateral clefts present a most important surgical challenge, and it is possible that these children are not operated out of the humanitarian missions contrary to unilateral clefts which are frequently supported by local teams.

The frequency of 78.9% of isolated clefts found in this study was in compliance with the literature, which shows an ascendancy (more than 70%) of isolated CL/P [9] [17] [26]. However, in reality, this frequency of isolated clefts should be reviewed downward for the benefit of a more increased part of syndromic clefts because even seemingly isolated; 10% - 20% of the clefts are associated with other congenital malformations [9] [21].

4.3. About Care of Clefts

The majority of the children underwent surgery; cheilorraphy was frequently more practiced than palatorraphy which is in line with previous African studies [11] [15] [27]. As previously mentioned, the reasons for this may be the higher number of cleft lips than palates, as well as that cleft lip repair precedes palate repair [15]. In this study, all the interventions were successfully performed, and no peri- and postoperative negative outcomes were reported. This confirms that surgery of CL/P is satisfactory [15] [27] [28]; complications, such as desertion of suture, infection, keloid scars, narrowness of the mouth, are rarely reported [13], but oronasal fistulas can be tackled as postoperative complications [15] [22]. Factors which influence the surgical outcome of clefts are in relation to the severity of the cleft, the race and particular characteristics of the patient, the experience and expertise of the surgeon, the technique used, the time of the intervention, and the postoperative care [15] [29] [30]. In Burkina Faso, the care of children with CL/P constitutes a challenge for the patients and their families. Indeed, the services of otorhinolaryngology or maxillofacial surgery are concentrated in the four tertiary hospitals located in the two main cities which are far from the rural areas where the majority of patients live. We also know that in these referral hospitals, the specialists are in insufficient numbers and are underequipped. Furthermore, the poorest populations cannot financially support the surgical operation in the absence of free access to the care, or the absence of an affordable and attractive system of cost sharing for them. So, many clefts cases escape treatment, and the humanitarian surgery constitutes an opportunity for the patients to benefit from appropriate care. In such a context, we understand that the priority is in the surgery, the other components of the care (orthodontics, otorhinolaryngology, speech pathology, psychology…) being relegated back. Besides, at the moment, the recommendation for integrated CL/P care by a multidisciplinary healthcare team is a gamble in the African countries [31]; so much so, the specialists are too insufficient and are underequipped.

4.4. About Study Limitations

This study, however, presents limits which lie in its hospital-based and retrospective characteristics. Nevertheless, the results can be of use as a basis to investigations of higher scale at the hospital level than at the national level, to better assess the morbidity of CL/P, to approach their etiologies and risk factors, and to implement a specific program which addresses CL/P in Burkina Faso.

Acknowledgements

Authors thank "Missions Sourires d'Afrique", "Fondation Suka", and Clinique El Fateh-Suka staffs, and the children and their parents.

References

[1] Gorlin, R.J., Cohen, M.M. and Hennekam, R.C.M. (2001) Syndromes of the Head and Neck. Oxford University Press, New York.

[2] Gundlach, K.K. and Maus, C. (2006) Epidemiological Studies on the Frequency of Clefts in Europe and World-Wide. *Journal of Cranio-Maxillofacial Surgery*, **34**, 1-2. http://dx.doi.org/10.1016/s1010-5182(06)60001-2

[3] Butali, A., Adeyemo, W.L., Mosey, P.A., Olasoji, H.O., Onah, I.I., Adebola, A., *et al.* (2014) Prevalence of Orofacial Clefts in Nigeria. *The Cleft Palate-Craniofacial Journal*, **51**, 320-325. http://dx.doi.org/10.1597/12-135

[4] Ouédraogo, K.S. (2013) Congenital Malformations of the Face and Neck in Hospital Practice in Ouagadougou: Epidemiological, Anatomical, Clinical, and Therapeutic Aspects. Report of 170 Cases. M.D. Thesis, University of Ouagadougou, Ouagadougou.

[5] Burkina Faso, INSD (2006) General Census of the Population and of the Housing Conditions of Burkina Faso—Final Results. www.insd.bf/fr/IMG/pdf/Resultats_definitifs_RGPH_2006.pdf

[6] Millard Jr., D.R. (1964) Rotation-Advancement Principle in Cleft Lip Closure. *The Cleft Palate Journal*, **12**, 246-252.

[7] Wardill, W.E.M. (1937) The Technique of Operation for Cleft Palate. *British Journal of Surgery*, **25**, 117-130. http://dx.doi.org/10.1002/bjs.1800259715

[8] Zandi, M. and Heidari, A. (2011) An Epidemiologic Study of Orofacial Clefts in Hamedan City, Iran: A 15-Year Study. *The Cleft Palate-Craniofacial Journal*, **48**, 483-489. http://dx.doi.org/10.1597/09-035

[9] WHO (2003) Global Registry and Database on Craniofacial Anomalies: Report of a WHO Registry Meeting on Craniofacial Anomalies. In: Mossey, P.A. and Castilla, E.E., Eds., WHO, Geneva. http://apps.who.int/iris/handle/10665/42840

[10] Schwarz, R. and Bhai Khadka, S. (2004) Reasons for Late Presentations of Cleft Deformity in Nepal. *The Cleft Palate-Craniofacial Journal*, **41**, 199-201. http://dx.doi.org/10.1597/03-016

[11] Donkor, P., Plange-Rhule, G. and Amponsah, E.K. (2007) A Prospective Survey of Patients with Cleft Lip and Palate in Kumasi. *West African Journal of Medicine*, **26**, 14-16. http://dx.doi.org/10.4314/wajm.v26i1.28295

[12] Franco, D., Iani, M., Passalini, R., Demolinari, I., Arnaut, M. and Franco, T. (2012) Profile Evaluation of Patients with Cleft Lip and Palate Undergoing Surgery at a Reference Center in Rio de Janeiro, Brazil. *Plastic Surgery International*, **2012**, Article ID: 620302. http://dx.doi.org/10.1155/2012/620302

[13] Diakité, C.O. (2006) Oral Facial Clefts at Gabriel Touré Hospital and Mother and Child Hospital "Luxemburg". MD Thesis, University of Bamako, Bamako.

[14] Adeyemo, W.L., Ogunlewe, M.O., Desalu, I., Ladeinde, A.L., Mofikoya, B.O., Adeyemi, M.O., et al. (2009) Cleft Deformities in Adults and Children Aged over Six Years in Nigeria: Reasons for Late Presentation and Management Challenges. Clinical, Cosmetic and Investigational Dentistry, 1, 63-69. http://dx.doi.org/10.2147/CCIDEN.S6686

[15] Abdurrazaq, T.O., Micheal, A.O., Lanre, A.W., Olugbenga, O.M. and Akin, L.L. (2013) Surgical Outcome and Complications Following Cleft Lip and Palate Repair in a Teaching Hospital in Nigeria. African Journal of Paediatric Surgery, 10, 345-357. http://dx.doi.org/10.4103/0189-6725.125447

[16] Doray, B., Badila-Timbolschi, D., Schaefer, E., Fattori, D., Monga, B., Dott, B., et al. (2012) Epidemiology of Oral Clefts: Experience of the Register of Congenital Malformations of Alsace between 1995 and 2006. Archives de Pédiatrie, 19, 1021-1029. http://dx.doi.org/10.1016/j.arcped.2012.07.002

[17] Genisca, A.E., Frías, J.L., Broussard, C.S., Honein, M.A., Lammer, E.J., Moore, C.A., et al. (2009) Orofacial Clefts in the National Birth Defects Prevention Study, 1997-2004. American Journal of Medical Genetics Part A, 149A, 1149-1158. http://dx.doi.org/10.1002/ajmg.a.32854

[18] Jalili, D., Fathi, M. and Jalili, C. (2012) Frequency of Cleft Lip and Palate among Live Births in Akbar Abadi Hospital. Acta Medica Iranica, 50, 704-706.

[19] Shafi, T., Khan, M.R. and Atiq, M. (2003) Congenital Heart Disease and Associated Malformations in Children with Cleft Lip and Palate in Pakistan. British Journal of Plastic Surgery, 56, 106-109. http://dx.doi.org/10.1016/S0007-1226(03)00044-4

[20] Lary, J.M. and Paulozzi, L.J. (2001) Sex Differences in the Prevalence of Human Birth Defects: A Population-Based Study. Teratology, 64, 237-251. http://dx.doi.org/10.1002/tera.1070

[21] Rittler, M., Cosentino, V., Lopez-Camelo, J.S., Murray, J.C., Wehby, G. and Castilla, E.E. (2011) Associated Anomalies among Infants with Oral Clefts at Birth and during a 1-Year Follow-Up. American Journal of Medical Genetics Part A, 155A, 1588-1596. http://dx.doi.org/10.1002/ajmg.a.34046

[22] Buyu, Y., Manyama, M., Chandika, A. and Gilyoma, J. (2012) Orofacial Clefts at Bugando Medical Centre: Associated Factors and Postsurgical Complications. The Cleft Palate-Craniofacial Journal, 49, 736-740. http://dx.doi.org/10.1597/10-202

[23] Aljohar, A., Ravichandran, K. and Subhani, S. (2011) Pattern of Craniofacial Anomalies Seen in a Tertiary Care Hospital in Saudi Arabia. Annals of Saudi Medicine, 31, 488-493. http://dx.doi.org/10.4103/0256-4947.84626

[24] Sekhon, P.S., Ethunandan, M., Markus, A.F., Krishnan, G. and Rao, B. (2011) Congenital Anomalies with Cleft Lip and Palate—An Analysis of 1623 Consecutive Patients. The Cleft Palate-Craniofacial Journal, 48, 371-378. http://dx.doi.org/10.1597/09-264

[25] Al, Omari, F. and Al-Omari, I.K. (2004) Cleft Lip and Palate in Jordan: Birth Prevalence Rate. The Cleft Palate-Craniofacial Journal, 41, 609-612. http://dx.doi.org/10.1597/03-034.1

[26] IPDTOC Working Group (2011) Prevalence at Birth of Cleft Lip with or without Cleft Palate: Data from the International Perinatal Database of Typical Oral Clefts (IPDTOC). The Cleft Palate-Craniofacial Journal, 48, 66-78.

[27] Orkar, K.S., Ugwu, B.T. and Momoh, J.J. (2002) Cleft Lip and Palate: The Jos Experience. East African Medical Journal, 79, 510-513. http://dx.doi.org/10.4314/eamj.v79i10.8811

[28] Adeyemo, W.L., James, O., Adeyemi, M.O., Ogunlewe, M.O., Ladeinde, A.L., Butali, A., et al. (2013) An Evaluation of Surgical Outcome of Bilateral Cleft Lip Surgery Using a Modified Millard's (Fork Flap) Technique. African Journal of Paediatric Surgery, 10, 307-310. http://dx.doi.org/10.4103/0189-6725.125419

[29] Johnson, N. and Jonathan, S. (2003) An Aesthetic Index for Evaluation of Cleft Repair. The European Journal of Orthodontics, 25, 243-249. http://dx.doi.org/10.1093/ejo/25.3.243

[30] Semb, G., Brattstrom, V., Molsted, K., Prahl-Andersen, B., Zuurbier, P., Rumsey, N., et al. (2005) The Eurocleft Study: Intercenter Study of Treatment Outcome in Patients with Complete Cleft Lip and Palate. Part 4: Relationship among Treatment Outcome, Patient/Parent Satisfaction and the Burden of Care. The Cleft Palate-Craniofacial Journal, 42, 83-92. http://dx.doi.org/10.1597/02-119.4.1

[31] Akinmoladun, V.I., Obimakinde, O.S. and Okoje, V.N. (2013) Team Approach to Management of Oro-Facial Cleft among African Practitioners: A Survey. Nigerian Journal of Clinical Practice, 16, 86-90. http://dx.doi.org/10.4103/1119-3077.106773

8

Calcium Intake in Relation to Body Mass Index and Fatness in Thai School-Aged Children

Uruwan Yamborisut[1*], Wanphen Wimonpeerapattana[2], Nipa Rojroongwasinkul[2], Atitada Boonpraderm[3], Sayamon Senaprom[2], Wiyada Thasanasuwan[4], Ilse Khouw[5], Paul Deurenberg[6]

[1]Human Nutrition Unit, Institute of Nutrition, Mahidol University, Salaya, Thailand
[2]Biostatistics Unit, Institute of Nutrition, Mahidol University, Salaya, Thailand
[3]Community Nutrition Unit, Institute of Nutrition, Mahidol University, Salaya, Thailand
[4]Nutrition Physiology Unit, Institute of Nutrition, Mahidol University, Salaya, Thailand
[5]Friesland Campina, Amersfoort, The Netherlands
[6]Nutrition Consultant, Langkawi, Malaysia
Email: *uruwan.yam@mahidol.ac.th

Abstract

An emerging evidence suggests that dietary calcium may play a role in the regulation of body weight in humans. This study examined the relationship of calcium intake with body mass index and body fatness in Thai children. Methods: A cross-sectional study in 1570, 6 - 12 year-old children were conducted in representative provinces of Thailand. Body weight, height, sitting height and 4 sites skinfolds thickness were measured as well as the dietary intake using a 24 h recall and a food frequency questionnaire (FFQ). General linear model (GLM) analysis was used to determine the effect of calcium intake on body mass index (BMI) and body fatness of children. Results: There were no differences in parental education and family's socio-economic status between genders. Girls had significantly greater sitting height ($p = 0.035$), sitting height to height ratio ($p = 0.014$) and sum of four skinfold thickness ($p = 0.001$) than boys. Mean calcium intake was lower in girls than in boys. GLM analysis demonstrated that lower calcium intake among children was associated with higher body weight, BMI and sum 4-skinfold thickness. Conclusion: Lower calcium intake is associated with higher BMI and body fatness of Thai children. Further studies need to determine the optimal calcium intake to prevent overweight and obesity in children.

Keywords

Thai Children, Calcium Intake, Milk, Skinfold Thickness, Body Mass Index

---

*Corresponding author.

1. Introduction

The increasing prevalence of childhood obesity is a global public health problem [1] [2] as obesity is associated with increased risk of non-communicable chronic diseases such as diabetes, dyslipidemia, hypertension and cardiovascular disease in later life [3] [4]. The development of obesity is caused by multiple factors. Besides genetics, environmental factors affecting changes in dietary pattern and lifestyle appear to be important determinants for the increasing adiposity prevalence. It is known that excess energy intake for an extended period will lead to an increase in body weight. Additionally, emerging evidence suggests that dietary calcium may play a role in the regulation of body weight and body fat [5] [6]. Results from cross-sectional studies showed an inverse association between calcium and body mass index among adolescents and adults [7] [8]. Longitudinal studies in children and adolescents also indicated an inverse association between calcium intake and body fat or sum of skinfolds [9] [10] whilst randomized controlled trials revealed inconsistent results [11] [12]. In adults, high calcium intake was also found to be negatively correlated with plasma LDL-cholesterol and total cholesterol after adjustment for body fat and waist circumference [13]. In most diets, dairy contributes substantially to calcium intake. Regarding the role of dairy consumption on the development of obesity, a recent systematic review of 19 prospective studies has shown both positive and negative effects of dairy intake as well as no impact on weight gain in human subjects [14].

Thailand has experienced a rapid socio-economic development over the last few decades. This economic transformation included a process of urbanization and nutrition transition, thereby, bringing about an increasing prevalence of childhood obesity. When using weight-for-height as criteria, the prevalence of obesity increased from 5.8% to 7.9% for preschool children and from 5.8% to 6.7% for school-aged children from 1997 to 2001 [15]. A recent nutrition survey in 3119 Thai infants and children, aged 6 months - 12 years, from 4 regions of Thailand including Bangkok, showed an overall prevalence of childhood obesity of 11.8% for municipal and 5.9% for non-municipal areas and the highest proportion of obese children was found among the school-age group (6 to 12 years). The prevalence of underweight ranged between 6.4% - 10.2% and the stunting prevalence in non-municipal areas was twice as high as in municipal areas; 8.4% versus 4.1% [16]. Furthermore, results showed that calcium, iron and vitamin C intakes of children were relatively low compared to the recommendation [16]. Therefore, the aim of this study was to investigate the relationship between calcium intake and adiposity of Thai school-aged children.

2. Material and Methods

2.1. Study Design

This study was part of the South East Asian Nutrition Survey (SEANUTS) which aimed to examine nutritional status and nutrient intakes of infants and children, aged 6 months - 12 years, in Indonesia, Malaysia, Vietnam, and Thailand [16]. The survey in Thailand was carried out in four regions of the country during January-August 2011. The study was conducted according to the guidelines of the Declaration of Helsinki and approved by the Ethics Committee on Research involving Human Subjects of the Faculty of Medicine, Ramathibodi Hospital, Mahidol University (MURA 2010/467), Thailand. Written consent was obtained from parents or caretakers of the children. The study is registered in the Dutch trial register as NTR2462.

2.2. Study Population

Subjects were 1570, 6 - 12 year-old children whose families were residing in provinces located in 4 regions of Thailand. Multi-stage random sampling technique was applied to recruit the children. The representative province was sampled for each region, *i.e.*, Lop Buri province for the Central, Chiang Mai province for the North, Si SaKet and Kalasin provinces for the Northeast and Phang-nga province for the South region of Thailand. Bangkok (the Central region) was also chosen. Then each province was stratified according to proportion of municipal to non-municipal areas and subsequently villages were randomly selected as target groups. The target number of children was determined based on their proportion to the overall number of 6 - 12 year-old children in the specified regions.

2.3. Data Collection

Data collection was performed at health centers in each district. Information of demographic characteristics of the children's families was obtained by interviewing parents and/or care takers using structured questionnaires.

2.3.1. Anthropometric Measurements

Body weight was measured using a digital weighing scale (Seca Model 882, GmbH & Co., Hamburg, Germany) to the nearest 0.1 kg. Standing height was measured with a stadiometer (Microtoise, Stanley-Mabo®, Poissy, France) to the nearest 0.1 cm. Body mass index (BMI) was calculated as body weight divided by height squared (kg/m^2). Sitting height (SH) was measured with the subject sitting on a flat hard stool with the buttocks in contact with the backboard of the stadiometer while the legs were supported by a footrest so that the child's thighs were horizontal. The height of the stool was subtracted from the readings. Sitting height ratio (SHR) was calculated as SH/standing height × 100. Skinfold thickness was measured at four anatomical sites using a skinfold caliper (Holtain Ltd., Crymych, UK) to the nearest 0.2 mm. The triceps skinfold was measured on the left arm midway between the acromion process of the scapula and the olecranon process of the ulna. The biceps skinfold was measured at the same level as the triceps skinfold. The subscapular skinfold was measured just below and parallel to the medial border of the scapula at an angle of 45° and the supra-iliac skinfold was measured at the mid-axillary line, just above the left iliac crest and 45° towards the front of the body. Skinfold measurements were taken in triplicate and the average value was used in the statistics. The sum of four skinfolds was used as indicator of body fatness.

2.3.2. Dietary Assessment

Dietary assessment in children was performed using a semi-quantitative food frequency questionnaire covering the past month to estimate daily milk intake and the use of a 24-hour food recall to determine dietary calcium of children. For children aged <10 years, the information on food intakes and consumption frequency was obtained from children's mothers, whereas for children aged >10 years, food intake data were from interviews with the children. Household measuring cups and/or spoons and pictorial food models were used to estimate food portion size and the amount of cooked rice consumed by the children was also weighed. All food codes were converted and analyzed for nutrient intakes using the INMUCAL-N V2.0 (Institute of Nutrition, Mahidol University) program. Since only one 24 h recall was obtained, the estimating nutrient intake distributions of children were performed using external variance estimates to correct for day-to-day within person variation. The principle method has been described elsewhere [17] [18] and the Personal Computer Version of Software for Intake Distribution Estimation (PC-SIDE) was applied to determine the estimates of nutrient intakes of children [19].

2.4. Statistical Analysis

Data analysis was performed using Predictive Analytics Software Statistics (PASW) version 18 (SPSS Inc., Chicago, IL, USA). Results of anthropometric variables and nutrient intakes of children are presented as mean, standard deviation (SD) and median. The Kolmogorov Smirnov test was used to test normality of data and data that was not normally distributed were log-transformed and the transformed data were used in the statistics. Qualitative characteristics of children's families were compared using Chi-squared test. Mean differences in anthropometric indices and nutrient intakes between boys and girls were tested using Student's t-test and the Mann Whitney test. Calcium intake of children was categorized in tertiles and analysis of variance (ANOVA) was used to determine mean differences in variables between the three tertiles of calcium intake groups. General Linear Model (GLM) procedure was used to test the effect of calcium intake on body weight, body mass index and body fatness, after correcting for the confounding effects of gender, age, residential area, mother's education, family income, sitting height and energy intake. Statistical difference was set at $p < 0.05$.

3. Results

Table 1 shows the socio-demographic characteristics of the children's families. The proportion of children in non-municipal areas was twice as high as that of municipal areas but there was no significant difference in proportion between boys and girls. There was also no difference in the education background of the children's parents between the genders. It was found that about 50% of the parents completed primary education level. Around 40% of the families, earned 6000 - 14,000 Baht (approx. 183 - 427 USD, 1 USD = 32.7 THB) per month, whereas the proportion of families with an income of >14,000 baht per month was about 31% of the study group.

Table 1. Socio-demographic background variables of the study population.

Variables	Boys N (%)	Girls N (%)	p-value[c]
No. of subjects	789	781	
Residential area			
Municipal	258 (32.7)	253 (32.4)	0.897
Non-municipal	531 (67.3)	528 (67.6)	
Education of parents			
Child's father			
Primary school	372 (53.5)	362 (50.8)	0.398
Secondary school	268 (38.6)	282 (39.6)	
Bachelor and higher	55 (7.9)	69 (9.6)	
Child's mother			
Primary school	385 (52.1)	366 (49.1)	0.491
Secondary school	288 (39.0)	312 (41.9)	
Bachelor and higher	66 (8.9)	67 (9.0)	
Family income (baht/month)[a]			
<6000 (<183 USD)[b]	238 (30.4)	221 (28.7)	0.617
6000 - 14,000 (183 - 427 USD)	295 (37.8)	308 (40.1)	
>14,000 (>427 USD)	249 (31.8)	240 (31.2)	

[a]Family income is categorized in tertiles. There were 7 missing records for boy group and 12 missing records for girl group due to the participants did not specify their incomes; [b]1 USD = 32.7 baht; [c]P-value by Chi-square test.

Table 2 shows the results of anthropometry and nutrient intakes of children. Mean age was 9.4 ± 2.0 years for boys and girls, with no difference between the genders. Body weight, body height and BMI of boys were not different from that of girls. However, boys had significantly lower sitting height values ($p = 0.035$) and lower SHR ($p = 0.014$) than girls, meaning the boys' legs were relatively longer. The sum of four skinfolds of girls was significantly greater than that of boys ($p = 0.001$). Boys had significantly higher intakes of energy, protein, fat, carbohydrate ($p = 0.001$) and calcium ($p = 0.020$) than girls. Both boys and girls had noticeably higher protein but lower calcium intakes than the Thai Recommended Dietary Allowances (RDA).

Table 3 shows that children with calcium intakes of >253 mg/day (upper two calcium intake tertiles) had significantly lower body weight ($p < 0.05$) and sitting height ($p < 0.05$) than those with calcium intakes <253 mg/day (lower calcium intake tertile). Milk consumption was higher in the highest calcium intake tertile.

Table 4 shows that after correcting for confounding variables, children in the lowest two calcium intake tertiles had significantly higher body weight ($p = 0.01$) and BMI ($p = 0.025$) compared to those in the highest calcium intake tertile. Also, children in the lowest calcium intake tertile had significantly higher sum 4-SKF (p = 0.039) compared to those in the highest calcium intake tertile (Model I). Likewise, similar results were obtained when percentage ofcalcium intake from milk was the independent variable (Model II). But when milk intake from FFQ was used as independent variable, no effect of milk consumption on body weight, BMI or sum four skinfolds was found (Model III).

4. Discussion

Dietary calcium is known to be an essential nutrient for bone accretion and bone health. This study explored the relationship of calcium intake to adiposity in terms of body weight, BMI and subcutaneous body fat of Thai school-aged children. The study population was from low-to-middle socio-economic families in municipal and non-municipal areas. Although there were no differences in age and BMI between the genders, girls had significantly higher sitting height and SHR values than boys. Skeletal dimensions vary with age, gender and ethnicity and probably influence body composition. Children with greater SHR values have relatively short legs [20]. Furthermore, studies have shown that short leg length and SHR were associated with the risk of non-communicable chronic diseases, *i.e.*, hypertension and coronary heart disease [21] [22]. Girls also had a greater sum of skinfolds, thus had more subcutaneous fat than boys of similar age. Body fat is known to be associated with age and gender and a study has shown that female had greater sum of skinfold thicknesses than in males, with a larger increase with age [23].

Boys had significantly higher intakes of energy, protein, fat, carbohydrate and calcium than girls. However, the total calcium intake of both genders was relatively low; at only 42% and 39% of Thai RDA for boys and

Table 2. Anthropometric characteristics and nutrient intakes of the children.

Variables	Boys (N = 789)	Girls (N = 781)	p-value[g]
Age (years)	$9.4 \pm 2.0^a (9.4)^b$	$9.4 \pm 2.0 (9.5)$	0.853
Weight (kg)	$30.5 \pm 11.8 (27.7)$	$30.6 \pm 11.4 (28.1)$	0.805
Height (cm)	$131.7 \pm 12.3 (131.0)$	$132.7 \pm 13.3 (131.8)$	0.119
Sitting height (cm)	$70.5 \pm 5.8 (70.0)$	$71.4 \pm 6.7 (70.8)$	0.035
Sitting height ratio (%)	$53.6 \pm 1.9 (53.5)$	$53.8 \pm 2.0 (53.6)$	0.014
BMI (kg/m^2)	$17.1 \pm 4.0 (15.7)$	$16.9 \pm 3.7 (15.9)$	0.403
Sum 4-SKF[c] (mm)	$36.5 \pm 24.4 (26.0)$	$41.8 \pm 22.2 (34.4)$	0.001
Nutrient intake			
Energy (kcal/day)	$1425 \pm 281 (1417)$	$1302 \pm 241 (1293)$	0.001
Energy (% RDA)[d]	$91.1 \pm 18 (90)$	$86.1 \pm 16 (86)$	0.001
Protein (g/day)	$53.1 \pm 14.9 (51.1)$	$47.7 \pm 13.8 (47.4)$	0.001
Protein (% RDA)[d]	$155 \pm 45 (150)$	$142 \pm 44.0 (136)$	0.001
Fat (g/day)	$44.9 \pm 16.2 (43.0)$	$41.3 \pm 13.4 (40.1)$	0.001
Carbohydrate (g/day)	$202 \pm 44.5 (198.5)$	$184 \pm 45.3 (179.6)$	0.001
Total calcium intake (mg/day)	$377 \pm 199 (352)$	$351 \pm 183 (328)$	0.020
Total calcium intake (as% RDA)[d]	$42.0 \pm 23.2 (39)$	$39.2 \pm 20.9 (37)$	0.034
% Calcium from milk intake[e]	40.7 ± 33.0	39.2 ± 32.6	0.381
Milk intake from FFQ, ml/day[f]	$367 \pm 264 (320)$	$343 \pm 215 (309)$	0.146

[a]Mean ± SD; [b]Median values in the parentheses; [c]Sum 4-SKF, Sum of biceps + triceps + subscapular + supra-iliac skinfold thickness; [d]RDA, Thai Recommended Dietary Allowances; [e]Percentage of calcium from milk intake by 24 h-food recall; [f] Milk intake from food frequency questionnaire; [g]Significant mean difference between genders by Mann Whitney test for sitting height, sitting height ratio, sum 4-SKF, milk and nutrient intakes.

Table 3. Anthropometric and nutrient intakes of children in tertiles of calcium intake.

Variables	Calcium intake tertiles		
	<253 mg/day	253 - 417 mg/day	>417 mg/day
Boys: girls (N)	265:257	244:278	280:243
Age (years)	$9.8 \pm 2.0^a (9.9)^d$	$9.4 \pm 2.0^b (9.5)$	$9.2 \pm 2.0^b (9.0)$
Weight (kg)	$31.8 \pm 12.0^a (28.8)$	$30.2 \pm 11.8^b (27.1)$	$29.8 \pm 10.9^b (27.7)$
Height (cm)	$133.9 \pm 12.8^a (133.3)$	$132.0 \pm 12.8^b (131.0)$	$130.8 \pm 12.8^b (130.0)$
BMI (kg/m^2)	$17.2 \pm 4.0^a (15.9)$	$16.8 \pm 3.9^a (15.6)$	$16.9 \pm 3.7^a (15.9)$
Sitting height (cm)	$71.6 \pm 6.2^a (71.2)$	$70.8 \pm 6.2^b (70.2)$	$70.3 \pm 6.3^b (69.6)$
Sitting height ratio (%)	$53.6 \pm 1.6^a (53.5)$	$53.8 \pm 2.0^a (53.6)$	$53.8 \pm 2.1^a (53.7)$
Sum 4-SKF[e] (mm)	$40.0 \pm 23.6^a (30.5)$	$38.1 \pm 23.4^a (28.5)$	$39.3 \pm 23.5^a (30.6)$
Energy intake (kcal/day)	$1258 \pm 264^a (1223)$	$1355 \pm 254^b (1337)$	$1477 \pm 245^c (1462)$
Protein (g/day)	$45.5 \pm 14.0^a (43.8)$	$50.6 \pm 14.2^b (48.7)$	$56.7 \pm 13.0^c (55.1)$
Fat (g/day)	$37.3 \pm 14.2^a (35.2)$	$42.1 \pm 13.6^b (40.0)$	$50.0 \pm 14.4^b (48.3)$
Carbohydrate (g/day)	$181.7 \pm 47.1^a (175.0)$	$193.7 \pm 45.3^b (188.9)$	$203.7 \pm 42.4^c (201.2)$
Milk intake from FFQ (ml/day)	$312 \pm 202^a (283)$	$337 \pm 199^b (296)$	$415 \pm 298^c (341)$

Results are from total 1567 children (data of three girls were missing). [a,b,c]Significant mean difference between groups are denoted with different superscript letters by ANOVA, at $p < 0.05$; [d]Median values were in parentheses; [e]Sum 4-SKF, sum of biceps + triceps + subscapular + supra-iliac skinfolds.

Table 4. The effect of daily calcium intake on body weight, body mass index (BMI) and body fatness of children.

Variables	ln(Body weight)			ln(BMI)			ln(Sum 4-SKF)[i]		
	β	SE	*p*-value	β	SE	*p*-value	β	SE	*p*-value
Model I[a]									
Daily calcium intake[d]									
< 253 mg/day	1.05	1.02	0.002	1.04	1.01	0.003	1.07	1.03	0.039
253 - 417 mg/day	1.04	1.02	0.010	1.03	1.01	0.025	1.05	1.03	0.128
>417 mg/day[e]	-	-	-	-	-	-	-	-	-
Adjusted R^2		0.534			0.250			0.235	
Model II[b]									
Percentage calcium intake from milk[d]									
1st tertile	1.05	1.02	0.001	1.04	1.01	0.001	1.08	1.03	0.001
2nd tertile	1.02	1.02	0.219	1.01	1.01	0.342	1.02	1.03	0.543
3rd tertile[f]	-	-	-	-	-	-	-	-	-
Adjusted R^2		0.534			0.251			0.236	
Model III[c]									
Daily milk intake[g]									
<247 ml/day	−0.98	1.02	0.453	−1.00	1.01	0.674	−0.99	1.03	0.727
247 - 380 ml/day	−0.99	1.02	0.533	−0.99	1.01	0.582	−0.99	1.03	0.656
>380 ml/day[h]	-	-	-	-	-	-	-	-	-
Adjusted R^2		0.530			0.245			0.233	

ln, log transformations of the body weight, BMI and sum of 4-skinfolds. [a,b,c]GLM model is adjusted for gender, age, residential area, child's mother educational level, family income, sitting height ratio and energy intakes of children; [d]Calcium intake is from 24 hr food recall; [e]Reference group is calcium intake of >417 mg/day; [f]Reference group is percentage of calcium intake from milk as 3rd tertile; [g]Milk intake is from food frequency questionnaire; [h]Reference group is milk intake of >380 ml/day; [i]Sum 4-SKF, Sum of biceps + triceps + subscapular + supra-iliac skinfolds.

girls, respectively and about half of the children consumed less than 70% of the RDA of dietary calcium (data not shown). The contribution of percentage calcium from milk intake to children was 39.2% - 40.7% of total calcium from all food groups suggesting that milk was the main source of calcium. Average milk intakes of children as assessed by FFQ was relatively low with 367 and 343 ml/day in boys and girls respectively (**Table 2**). This reported milk intake by FFQ would result in a higher calcium intake of about 249 mg/day. It is well known that FFQ tends to overestimate intakes compared to 24h recall [24]. The reported milk intakes were slightly higher than that reported in the 2009 Thai National Health Examination Surveys which indicated that school-aged children consumed less than 250 ml milk and other dairy products per day [25]. Other potentially calcium sources in the Thai diet could be fish, anchovy and dried shrimp and some vegetables such as kale and amaranth. However, such food intakes were found to be relatively low in children; *i.e.*, average intake of fish and aquatic animal products was only about 11.4 g/day and the average intake of calcium-rich vegetables was less than 20 g/day, contributing to total calcium intake for 7.4% and 4.1% respectively (data not shown). Therefore, these foods did not substantially contribute to the calcium intake in these children.

The children did not achieve the RDA for calcium (**Table 2**), which is currently set for this age group at 800 - 1000 mg/day. Increasing milk consumption in the Thai diet to 400 ml/day (2 servings/day) as recommended by the Thai Food Based Dietary guideline [26] would increase the calcium intake to approximately 47% - 60% of RDA. Also other studies in the Asian region show that calcium intakes of children and adolescents are suboptimal with for example 59% - 64% of RDA in Taiwan [27] and 50% - 60% of RDA in Korea [28]. Factors affecting milk consumption included urbanization, which leads to changes in food consumption patterns, social and cultural norms and the relative prices of food commodities [29]. Results from nutrition surveys showed that inadequate calcium intake in children may also be related to the replacement of milk as beverage by sweetened soft drinks [30]. Moreover, family environment has been shown to be important for shaping children's eating behaviors. One study demonstrated that milk and soft drink consumption of the mothers predicted their daughters' intakes of such beverages [31]. Although our study did not deeply explore the influence of family environment on children's milk consumption, it has been suggested that parents are role models for their children's eating behaviors.

When children were categorized in three calcium intake levels, those who had high dietary calcium intakes had significantly lower body weight than children consuming less calcium although they were younger. As the fact that there will be the trend of increasing body weight according to the increasing child's age. However, results from **Table 4** indicated that when the child's age and other confounding variables were statistically adjusted in the GLM model, it was found that lower dietary calcium intake was associated with higher body weight, higher BMI and higher sum of skinfold thickness in children. Previous studies on the effect of dietary calcium on the regulation of body weight and body fat showed mixed results. Cross-sectional [7] [32] and longitudinal studies [9] [33] have shown an inverse association between calcium intake and BMI and between calcium intake and body fat among children and adolescents. However, a randomized controlled trial (RCT) study [34] and a review of evidence [35] showed inconsistent results. A possible explanation of the effect of calcium on body fat is, that higher dietary calcium can induce fecal fatty acid excretion [36]. At cellular level, studies in human adipocytes demonstrated that high calcium intake could be linked to decreased intracellular calcium, and thereby, decreased lipogenic gene expression and increased lipolysis [37].

In most diets, milk and dairy products are a major contributor to calcium intake. The fact that in this study no effect of milk intake from FFQ was found can have various reasons. First, it seems likely that the reported milk intake is an overestimation as in general FFQ tends to overestimate intakes [24]. Secondly, with the relatively low milk consumption pattern of the children, the contribution of milk to calcium intake is relatively low with on average 52%, thus a possible effect is more difficult to detect. This is also obvious from the results of model II in Table 4. Thirdly, depending on the type of milk consumed (skimmed or full cream), a possible positive effect of calcium in milk might be counterbalanced by a higher total fat consumption although total energy intake was corrected for in the analyses. A review of the literature showed either beneficial or neutral effects of dairy foods on body weight or body composition [38].

The strength of the present study is that the sample of children was obtained from multi-stage random sampling from all regions of Thailand, and therefore, the results can be seen as representative for the country. A limitation of this study is that food recall for each child were performed for only one day, which did not take into account the variation in nutrient intakes. In addition, body fat of the children was not directly measured, which might misclassify some children with a high BMI due to high lean body mass.

5. Conclusion

This study demonstrated that a lower calcium intake was associated with a higher body weight, BMI and skinfold thickness in Thai school-aged children. Future randomized controlled trial studies are needed to examine whether individual dairy food items, as main calcium contributors in the diet, may play a protective role on weight status, body proportion and/or body composition.

Acknowledgements

The study was funded by Royal Friesland Campina Innovation. The authors would like to thank Ms Jutatip-Wangsai and Ms Chumapa Deesudchit from Friesland Campina Thailand for their role in facilitating the research project. The authors are very grateful to all parents and children for their co-operation during data collection. Also, special thanks to all health care personnel at district health centers.

Conflict of Interest

The authors declared no conflict of interest.

References

[1]   de Onis, M., Blossner, M. and Borghi, E. (2010) Global Prevalence and Trends of Overweight and Obesity among Preschool Children. *American Journal of Clinical Nutrition*, **92**, 1257-1264. http://dx.doi.org/10.3945/ajcn.2010.29786

[2]   Rivera, J.A., de Cossío, T.G., Pedraza, L.S., Aburto, T.C., Sánchez, T.G. and Martorell, R. (2014) Childhood and Adolescent Overweight and Obesity in Latin America: A Systematic Review. *Lancet Diabetes Endocrinol*, **2**, 321-332. http://dx.doi.org/10.1016/S2213-8587(13)70173-6

[3]   Reilly, J.J. and Kelly, J. (2011) Long-Term Impact of Overweight and Obesity in Childhood and Adolescence on Morbidity and Premature Mortality in Adulthood: Systematic Review. *International Journal of Obesity*, **35**, 891-898.

http://dx.doi.org/10.1038/ijo.2010.222

[4]   Freedman, D.S., Mei, Z., Srinivasan, S.R., Berensen, G.S. and Dietz, W. (2007) Cardiovascular Risk Factors and
      Excess Adiposity among Overweight Children and Adolescents: The Bogalusa Heart Study. *Journal of Pediatrics*, **150**,
      12-17. http://dx.doi.org/10.1016/j.jpeds.2006.08.042

[5]   Heaney, R.P., Davies, K.M. and Barger-Lux, M.J. (2002) Calcium and Weight: Clinical Studies. *Journal of the American College of Nutrition*, **21**, S152-S155. http://dx.doi.org/10.1080/07315724.2002.10719213

[6]   Zemel, M.B., Shi, H., Greer, B., Dirienzo, D. and Zemel, P.C. (2000) Regulation of Adiposity by Dietary Calcium.
      FASEB Journal, **14**, 1132-1138.

[7]   Palacios, C., Benedetti, P. and Fonseca, S. (2007) Impact of Calcium Intake on Body Mass Index in Venezuelan Adolescents. *PR Health Sciences Journal*, **26**, 199-204.

[8]   Loos, R.J., Rankinen, T., Leon, A.S., Skinner, J.S., Wilmore, J.H., Rao, D.C., *et al.* (2004) Calcium Intake Is Associated with Adiposity in Black and White Men and White Women of the HERITAGE Family Study. *Journal of Nutrition*, **134**, 1772-1778.

[9]   Skinner, J.D., Bounds, W., Carruth, B.R. and Ziegler, P. (2003) Longitudinal Calcium Intake Is Negatively Related to
      Children's Body Fat Indexes. *Journal of the American Dietetic Association*, **103**, 1626-1631.
      http://dx.doi.org/10.1016/j.jada.2003.09.018

[10] Boon, N., Koppes, L.L., Saris, W.H. and Van Mechelen, W. (2005) The Relation between Calcium Intake and Body
      Composition in a Dutch Population: The Amsterdam Growth and Health Longitudinal Study. *American Journal of Epidemiology*, **162**, 27-32. http://dx.doi.org/10.1093/aje/kwi161

[11] Zemel, M.B., Thompson, W., Milstead, A., Morris, K. and Campbell, P. (2004) Calcium and Dairy Acceleration of
      Weight and Fat Loss during Energy Restriction in Obese Adults. *Obesity Research*, **12**, 582-590.
      http://dx.doi.org/10.1038/oby.2004.67

[12] Yanoski, J.A., Parikh, S.J., Yanoff, L.B., Denkinger, B.I., Calis, K.A., Reynolds, J.C., *et al.* (2009) Effect of Calcium
      Supplementation on Body Weight and Adiposity in Overweight and Obese Adults: A Randomized Trial. *Annals of Internal Medicine*, **150**, 821-829. http://dx.doi.org/10.7326/0003-4819-150-12-200906160-00005

[13] Jacqmain, M., Doucet, E., Despres, J.-P., Bouchard, C. and Tremblay, A. (2003) Calcium Intake, Body Composition
      and Lipoprotein-Lipid Concentrations in Adults. *The American Journal of Clinical Nutrition*, **77**, 1448-1452.

[14] Louie, J.C.Y., Flood, V.M., Hector, D.J., Rangan, A.M. and Gill, T.P. (2011) Dairy Consumption and Overweight and
      Obesity: A Systematic Review of Prospective Cohort Studies. *Obesity Reviews*, **12**, e582-e592.
      http://dx.doi.org/10.1111/j.1467-789X.2011.00881.x

[15] Aekplakorn, W. and Mo-Suwan, L. (2009) Prevalence of Obesity in Thailand. *Obesity Reviews*, **10**, 589-592.
      http://dx.doi.org/10.1111/j.1467-789X.2009.00626.x

[16] Rojroongwasinkul, N., Kijboonchoo, K., Wimonpeerapattana, W., Purttiponthanee, S., Yamborisut, U., Boonpraderm,
      A., *et al.* (2013) SEANUTS: The Nutritional Status and Dietary Intakes of 0.5-12 Year-Old Thai Children. *British Journal of Nutrition*, **110**, S36-S44. http://dx.doi.org/10.1017/S0007114513002110

[17] Guenther, P.M., Kott, P.S. and Carriquiry, A.L. (1997) Development of an Approach for Estimating Usual Nutrient Intake Distributions at the Population Level. *Journal of Nutrition*, **127**, 1106-1112.

[18] Jahns, L., Arab, L., Carriquiry, A. and Popkin, B.M. (2005) The Use of External Within-Person Variance Estimates to
      Adjust Nutrient Intake Distributions over Time and across Populations. *Public Health Nutrition*, **8**, 69-76.
      http://dx.doi.org/10.1079/PHN2005671

[19] Nusser, S.M., Carriquiry, A.L., Dodd, K.W., Fuller, W.A. and Jensen, H.H. (1996) A User's Guide to C-SIDE (Soft
      Ware for Intake Distribution Estimation). Version 1.0, Technical Report 96-TR31, Center for Agricultural and Rural
      Development Ames, Iowa State University, Ames.

[20] Varela-Silva, M.I. and Bogin, B. (2012) Leg Length and Anthropometric Applications: Effects on Health and Disease.
      In: Preedy, V.R., Ed., *Handbook of Anthropometry: Physical Measures of Human Form in Health and Disease*, Springer Science & Business Media, New York, 769-783. http://dx.doi.org/10.1007/978-1-4419-1788-1_43

[21] Langenberg, C., Hardy, R., Kuh, D. and Wadworht, M.E. (2003) Influence of Height, Leg and Trunk Length on Pulse
      Pressure, Systolic and Diastolic Blood Pressure. *Journal of Hypertension*, **21**, 537-543.
      http://dx.doi.org/10.1097/00004872-200303000-00019

[22] Lawlor, D.A., Davey Smith, G. and Ebrahim, S. (2003) Association between Leg Length and Offspring Birthweight:
      Partial Explanation for the Trans-Generational Association between Birthweight and Cardiovascular Disease: Findings
      from the British Women's Heart and Health Study. *Paediatric and Perinatal Epidemiology*, **17**, 148-155.
      http://dx.doi.org/10.1046/j.1365-3016.2003.00479.x

[23] Dekkers, C., Podolsky, R.H., Treiber, F.A., Barbeau, P., Gutin, B. and Snieder, H. (2004) Development of General and

Central Obesity from Childhood into Early Adulthood in African American and European American Males and Females with a Family History of Cardiovascular Disease. *The American Journal of Clinical Nutrition*, **79**, 661-668.

[24] Fumagalli, F., Monteiro, J.P., Sartorelli, D.S., Vieira, M.N.C.M. and Bianchi, M.L.P. (2008) Validation of a Food Frequency Questionnaire for Assessing Dietary Nutrients in Brazilian Children 5 to 10 Years of Age. *Nutrition*, **24**, 427-432. http://dx.doi.org/10.1016/j.nut.2008.01.008

[25] Health System Research Institute (2009) Survey of Food Consumption of Thai People. The 4th National Health Examination Survey, 2008-2009, National Health Examination Survey Office, Nonthaburi.

[26] Thai Food Based Dietary Guideline Working Group (2009) Nutrition Flag Manual. Ministry of Public Health, Department of Health.

[27] Wu, S.J., Pan, W.-H., Yeh, N.-H. and Chang, H.-Y. (2007) Dietary Nutrient Intake and Major Food Sources: The Nutrition and Health Survey of Taiwan Elementary School Children 2001-2002. *Asia Pacific Journal of Clinical Nutrition*, **16**, S518-S533.

[28] Im, J.G., Kim, S.H., Lee, G.-Y., Joung, H. and Park, M.-J. (2013) Inadequate Calcium Intake Is Highly Prevalent in Korean Children and Adolescents: The Korea National Health and Nutrition Examination Survey (KNHANES) 2007-2010. *Public Health Nutrition*, **17**, 2489-2495.

[29] Gerosa, S. and Skoet, J. (2013) Milk Availability: Current Production and Demand and Medium-Term Outlook. In: Muehlhoff, E., Bennett, A. and McMahon, D., Eds., *Milk and Dairy Products in Human Nutrition*, Food Agricultural Organization, Rome, 11-40.

[30] Rampersaud, G.C., Bailey, L.B. and Kauwell, G.P. (2003) National Survey Beverage Consumption Data for Children and Adolescents Indicate the Need to Encourage a Shift toward More Nutritive Beverages. *Journal of the American Dietetic Association*, **103**, 97-100. http://dx.doi.org/10.1053/jada.2003.50006

[31] Fisher, J.O., Mitchell, D.C., Smicklas-Wright, H. and Birch, L.L. (2001) Maternal Milk Consumption Predicts the Trade-Off between Milk and Soft Drinks in Young Girls' Diets. *Journal of Nutrition*, **131**, 246-250.

[32] dos Santos, L.C., de Padua Cintra, I., Fisberg, M. and Martini, L.A. (2008) Calcium Intake and Its Relationship with Adiposity and Insulin Resistance in Post-Pubertal Adolescents. *Journal of Human Nutrition and Dietetics*, **21**, 109-116. http://dx.doi.org/10.1111/j.1365-277X.2008.00848.x

[33] Carruth, B.R. and Skinner, J.D. (2001) The Role of Dietary Calcium and Other Nutrients in Moderating Body Fat in Preschool Children. *International Journal of Obesity*, **25**, 559-566. http://dx.doi.org/10.1038/sj.ijo.0801562

[34] Lappe, J.M., Rafferty, K.A., Davies, K.M. and Lypaczewski, G. (2004) Girls on a High-Calcium Diet Gain Weight at the Same Rate as Girls on a Normal Diet: A Pilot Study. *Journal of the American Dietetic Association*, **104**, 1361-1367. http://dx.doi.org/10.1016/j.jada.2004.06.025

[35] Barba, G. and Russo, P. (2006) Dairy Foods, Dietary Calcium and Obesity: A Short Review of Evidence. *Nutrition, Metabolism and Cardiovascular Diseases*, **16**, 445-451. http://dx.doi.org/10.1016/j.numecd.2006.04.004

[36] Parikh, S.J. and Yanovski, J.A. (2003) Calcium Intake and Adiposity. *The American Journal of Clinical Nutrition*, **77**, 281-287.

[37] Zemel, M.B. (2004) Role of Calcium and Dairy Products in Energy Partitioning and Weight Management. *The American Journal of Clinical Nutrition*, **79**, S907-S912.

[38] Spence, L.A., Cifelli, C.J. and Miller, G.D. (2011) The Role of Dairy Products in Healthy Weight and Body Composition in Children and Adolescents. *Current Nutrition & Food Science*, **7**, 40-49. http://dx.doi.org/10.2174/157340111794941111

Verbal Autopsy of Stillbirths and Neonatal Deaths in a Rural Area of Burkina Faso

Fla Koueta[1,2,3], Kisito Nagalo[1,2,4*], Leatitia Ouedraogo[2], François Housseini Tall[1], Diarra Ye[1,2,3]

[1]The Burkinabe Pediatrics Society, Ouagadougou, Burkina Faso
[2]Training and Research Unit of Health Sciences, University of Ouagadougou, Ouagadougou, Burkina Faso
[3]Service of Medical Pediatrics, Charles De Gaulle Pediatric University Teaching Hospital, Ouagadougou, Burkina Faso
[4]Service of Pediatrics, Clinique El Fateh-Suka, Ouagadougou, Burkina Faso
Email: *kiki_nagalo@yahoo.fr

Abstract

Introduction: In developing countries, many neonatal deaths still occur at home and the causes of these deaths are not ascertained. Objective: To identify the causes of stillbirths and neonatal deaths that occur at home and the factors that have contributed to these deaths. Materials and Method: We have used the method of verbal autopsy to investigate the stillbirths and neonatal deaths in nine villages in the health area of Namsiguia, health district of Ouahigouya, Burkina Faso, during the period January 1, 2007 to December 8, 2012. Results: Over these six years, we have recorded 19 stillbirths and 36 neonatal deaths among 1507 live births, demonstrating a neonatal mortality rate of 28.8 per1000 and a rate of stillbirths of 12.6 per 1000. The average age of newborns at death was 5.6 days and the sex-ratio was 1.6. The major cause of stillbirths was antenatal hypoxia and birth asphyxia (42.1%). The direct causes of neonatal deaths were neonatal sepsis (41.7%), preterm birth (19.4%) and hypoxia and birth asphyxia (11.1%). There were 42.1% deliveries and 58.3% neonatal deaths, which occurred at home. We have noted 89.5% fresh stillbirths. Death occurred more often during the early neonatal period (55.5%). Factors significantly associated with neonatal death were, lack of school education of mothers (OR = 4), precocious marriage of the mother (OR = 8), poor follow-up of pregnancies (OR = 3), birth at home (OR = 4), low socioeconomic level (OR = 6), and low geographical access to the health facility (OR = 4). Conclusions: Strengthening of the health infrastructure and improving their accessibility, reinforcement of the staff for high quality care, and communication for a change in behavior in rural communities, will contribute toward reducing neonatal mortality in the area of health of Namsiguia.

Keywords

Verbal Autopsy, Neonatal Deaths, Stillbirths, Cause of Death

---

*Corresponding author.

1. Introduction

Of the 130 million annual births worldwide, there are approximately four million neonatal deaths, an equivalent of stillbirths is counted, and more than 98% of these deaths occur in developing countries [1]-[3]. Furthermore, most of these neonatal deaths occur at the community level and are, therefore, not recorded and their exact causes not elucidated. Verbal autopsy is a method that aims to identify the causes and factors that contribute to these deaths when they occur outside a health facility [4]. This method is an alternative to medical audit, in the context of low accessibility to health services, in order to determine the avoidable factors of death and take appropriate corrective measures. It is, therefore, particularly suitable for poor countries like Burkina Faso, where the neonatal mortality rate is estimated at 28 per 1000, where more than 77% of the population live in rural areas, and where 45% live under the threshold of poverty, with a low attendance of health services [3]. This verbal autopsy, which was carried out in a rural area was designed to determine the causes of stillbirths and neonatal deaths, as well as the factors leading to the deaths. Taking account of the identified modifiable factors should enable the reduction of neonatal mortality and contribute to the achievement of the Fourth Millennium Development Goal (MDG4), whose target is to reduce the under-five mortality rate by two-thirds, by 2015.

2. Materials and Method

2.1. Setting

The study was carried out in the rural area of the health and social promotion center (CSPS) of Namsiguia. The CSPS depends on the health district of Ouahigouya, which is a town located 200 km north off Ouagadougou, the capital of Burkina Faso. The infrastructure of the CSPS included a dispensary, a repository of essential generic medicines and a maternity ward, which was under construction. The CSPS team comprised of two nurses and an auxiliary midwife. Two community health workers served as community relays. The CSPS covered nine villages, with a population estimated at approximately 9000 inhabitants. Accessibility to the CSPS was difficult during the rainy season owing to flooding in the lowland situated between the villages and the health center.

2.2. Method and Study Population

A descriptive and analytic study allowed inclusion of all cases of stillbirths and neonatal deaths that occurred in the health area of the CSPS of Namsiguia between January 2007 and December 2012, or a six year period. The method of the verbal autopsy was used. A proforma, adapted by the World Health Organization (WHO) standard No. 1 questionnaire of verbal autopsy, was designed for this study [5]. The interview respondents were the mother and/or the father of the stillborn or deceased newborn. Close family members who were present at the time of the death were also interviewed.

2.3. Data Collection and Management

Data collection unwound from February 1 to March 31, 2014. The main technique of data collection was a direct interview with individual or collective respondents, with their consent. If necessary, this technique was complemented by the review of files and records of the patients at the CSPS or at the regional hospital. Four health personnel and six investigators, who conducted the data collection, had been previously trained on the verbal autopsy technique and filling investigation proforma. The questionnaire was pretested, which allowed its revision. Births and neonatal deaths were identified before the beginning of the investigation by the two community health workers, who were well informed of these events in the villages. This allowed the investigators to go directly to the families where the death took place. Two doctors insured the supervision of the survey. After collection of the data, the audit was conducted by a team consisting of two pediatricians, two medical practitioners, and a nurse during a staff meeting. This allowed determination of the direct and indirect causes of the deaths and identified the factors associated with these deaths. Each sheet was reviewed and the causes of the death were set, depending on the algorithm used by Manandhar *et al.* [6]. A single cause of death and stillbirth was assigned per child. Causes of neonatal deaths were classified using the international classification of diseases of the WHO, tenth edition (ICD 10) [7]. The socioeconomic level of the surveyed family was classified as low, medium or high, according to the WHO classification [8]. To find the existence of a statistical significance associated with the studied factors, each deceased newborn was matched to a control, who was a living newborn. The matching was made on date of birth, sex, and the village of birth of the deceased infants, with a ratio equal to 1. The matching on the date of birth was obtained more or less to a 15-day extent. Data were entered using the Sphinx^{TM} version 5 software (the Sphinx development, 27, rue Cassiopée, Parc Atlais, Chavanod, France) and then analyzed using SPSS 16.0 (IBM SPSS Inc., Chicago, Illinois, USA). Chi-square and Fisher's tests were used for comparisons between proportions. The odds ratio (OR) was computed to determine the significance of the association between variables, and the 95% confidence interval (CI) was calculated. Statistical tests yielding p-values < 0.05 were considered significant.

2.4. Ethical Considerations

During the preparatory phase of the investigation, we first obtained permission from the Ministry of Health. Furthermore, during a seminar, the community leaders (heads customary and religious, village development advisers) and the administrative authorities (mayor, prefect) of the study area were informed and sensitized on the verbal autopsy of neonatal deaths and its objectives. Populations that were the subject of the study were also informed on the project of study and it was with their consent that we conducted this investigation.

3. Results

3.1. Frequency of Stillbirths and Neonatal Deaths

Over the period of the study, a total of 55 stillbirths and neonatal deaths were identified consisting of 19 stillbirths and 36 neonatal deaths. During the same period, 1507 births were identified, demonstrating a rate of stillbirth of 12.6 per 1000 and a neonatal mortality rate of 28.8 per 1000. The state of stillbirths was specified in 16 cases and fresh stillbirths were 14 (87.5%), the other two (12.5%) were macerated stillborns. The sex ratio of the deceased newborns was 1.6 and the average age at death was 5.6 days.

3.2. Causes of Stillbirths and Neonatal Deaths

The direct causes of stillbirths were antenatal hypoxia and asphyxia at birth (eight cases), preterm birth (one case), and low birth weight (one case). The indirect causes found were related to maternal illness during pregnancy consisting of malaria (five cases), anemia (three cases), and hypertension (one case). The main direct causes of neonatal deaths were sepsis (41.7%), preterm birth (19.4%), and antenatal hypoxia and asphyxia at birth (11.1%). Sepsis was the most common cause of death in the late neonatal period (75.0%), whereas, antenatal hypoxia and asphyxia at birth (20.0%) and preterm birth (25.0%) were the most common causes of death in the early neonatal period, as shown in **Table 1**.

The indirect causes of neonatal deaths were maternal causes that were found in 19 cases out of 36 (52.8%). It was sepsis in 13 cases (68.5%) of which nine cases were of fever of unknown origin, three cases were of possible urinary tract infection, and one case was of malaria. Hypertension, prolonged labor, and anemia (two cases each) were the other maternal causes of neonatal deaths.

Table 1. Distribution of neonatal deaths by cause and timing of death, Namsiguia, Burkina Faso, 2012.

Cause of death	Timing of death		
	ENNP[*] No. of deaths (%)	LNNP[†] No. of deaths (%)	Total No. of deaths (%)
Neonatal sepsis	3 (15.0)	12 (75.0)	15 (41.7)
Preterm birth	5 (25.0)	2 (12.5)	7 (19.4)
Birth asphyxia	4 (20.0)	0 (0.0)	4 (11.1)
Congenital anomalies	0 (0.0)	1 (6.25)	1 (2.8)
Unspecified	8 (40.0)	1 (6.25)	9 (25.0)
Total	20 (100.0)	16 (100.0)	36 (100.0)

[*]ENNP: Early Neonatal Period (0 - 6 days); [†]LNNP: Late Neonatal Period (7 - 28 days).

Table 2. Factors associated with neonatal deaths, Namsiguia, Burkina Faso, 2012.

Putative risk factor for death	Newborn			
	Deceased (n = 36)	Alive (n = 36)	OR [95% CI]*	p-value
Lack of maternal education				
Yes	30	20	4 [1.2 - 13.9]	0.01
No	6	16	1.0	
Precocious marriage (mother < 18 years)				
Yes	25	8	8 [2.8 - 22.9]	0.00006
No	11	28	1.0	
Large multiparous mother (>= 5 para)				
Yes	9	3	4 [0.8 - 2.0]	0.5
No	27	33	1.0	
Poor follow-up of pregnancy (No. of ANC†s < 3)				
Yes	16	7	3 [1.0 - 10.9]	0.02
No	20	29	1.0	
Birth at home				
Yes	15	5	4 [1.2 - 16.6]	0.01
No	21	31	1.0	
Socioeconomic level of parents				
Low	32	20	6 [1.7 - 26.8]	0.001
Medium	4	16	1.0	
Lack of geographical access to the health center				
Yes	30	20	4 [1.2 - 13.9]	0.01
No	6	16	1.0	

*Odds ratio [95% Confident interval]; †Antenatal cares.

3.3. Factors Related to Neonatal Deaths

Deaths were early (55.5%) and more often occurred at home (58.3%). Factors significantly associated with neonatal deaths were, lack of maternal education (OR = 4), precocious marriage (OR = 8), poor follow-up of pregnancies (OR = 3), birth at home (OR = 4), low socioeconomic level (OR = 6), and lack of geographical access to the health center (OR = 4) (**Table 2**).

4. Discussion

Verbal autopsy aims at reduction of mortality. When it is implemented as a participatory process in a community, it can provide awareness of the factors that lead to deaths and can stimulate collective action. Despite the memory potential bias, owing to the retrospective collection of painful memories, questioning the mothers allowed us to obtain sufficient reliable information about stillbirths and neonatal deaths, which we have compared with data from the literature.

4.1. Stillbirths

With 12.6 per1000, the rate of stillbirths in our study was lower than the national rate, which is estimated to be 26 per 1000 [9]. This lower rate in our study is probably because of the small size of our sample, in a well-circumscribed health area, while the national rate is global and masks the disparity between regions. Antenatal hypoxia and asphyxia at birth were the main causes of stillbirths in this study. The discovery of a fresh stillbirth suggests that the child was viable during labor [6] and death dates back to less than 12 hours before birth [10]. In this study, as in those of other authors from countries with limited resources [11]-[13], the observed proportions of fresh stillbirths may reflect that women in labor had a delay in receiving care or there was lack of monitoring of the delivery by the care providers. This low capacity of the health care centers to provide quality rural perinatal care in Burkina Faso was already noted by Nikiema et al. [14], in the North East of the country. This high level of stillbirths is compounded by the fact that there are no skilled care providers in the community to take over deliveries or give neonatal care at home in accordance with our current national health policy. However, according to several authors, community health workers do exist, who are trained to recognize the signs of danger and practice basic neonatal resuscitation to reduce deaths from asphyxia during labor [6] [15] [16].

4.2. Neonatal Deaths

The rate of 28.8 per 1000 of neonatal mortality in this study is comparable to the national neonatal mortality of 28 per 1000 [3]. Neonatal mortality remains a factor of worry in our country despite the efforts of giving a grant for obstetric and neonatal emergency care [17]. The causes of neonatal deaths were dominated by neonatal sepsis (41.7%) in this study and these deaths by sepsis were most frequent in the late neonatal period (75%). The high rate of deaths by sepsis after the first week was especially on account of the many deliveries that took place at home, which occurred in poor conditions of hygiene and traditional practices, harmful to the health of the newborn child during the section and the care of umbilical cord. These poor conditions of delivery and umbilical cord care had already been reported by Bagui *et al.* in India [11] and Manandhar *et al.* in the Nepal [6]. To reduce neonatal sepsis, awareness messages should be addressed to women and their families, to encourage deliveries at the health center and to abandon the traditional practices harmful to the health of the newborn.

This study has identified preterm birth (19.4%) as the second cause of neonatal death. Sombie [18] in the West of Burkina Faso, Edmond *et al.* [13] in Ghana, and Turnbull *et al.* [12] in Zambia had made the same observation, with the respective preterm death rates of 15%, 19.7%, and 34%. Poverty, hardship of field work and chores, the long walks on foot to look for firewood and water are situations experienced daily by women in the area of this study, which encourage preterm deliveries. In this study, preterm deaths were mainly related to the inadequacy of their management in a health center, however precarious this may be in a rural area of a developing country like Burkina Faso. However, the implementation of low-cost methods that have proven their effectiveness and that are adopted by poor countries, such as the Kangaroo method, can reduce neonatal mortality linked to preterm birth and low birth weight [19]. Actions that are aimed at improving the social economic status of women in developing countries, as well as the promotion of essential neonatal care in the context of a community health policy will reduce preterm-related morbidity and neonatal mortality.

Antenatal hypoxia and asphyxia at birth was the third cause of neonatal deaths in our study with a mortality rate of 11.1%; which is three times lesser than in the study of Manandhar *et al.* [6] in the Nepal and Edmond *et al.* [13] in Ghana. In sub-Saharan Africa, asphyxia at birth is responsible for 280,000 deaths per year, especially on the first day of life [9]. Poor quality of care, inadequate fetal monitoring, and lack of skills of the health personnel are frequently associated with asphyxia at birth [20]. The training and equipment of community health workers for basic neonatal resuscitation can combat neonatal asphyxia and death which are linked [6] [16].

4.3. Factors Associated with Neonatal Deaths

The occurrence of the death of a newborn is often the result of several factors, some of which are preventable. In this study, the factors associated with neonatal deaths were the social, cultural, economic, and environmental factors. The analysis of these factors allows us to classify them in three delays according to the conceptual model proposed by Thaddeus [21] and used by other authors [22] [23] to trace the path that leads to the death of a newborn. The first delay is relative to the decision to go to a health facility. It follows from a persistence of the harmful social cultural constraints to health, lack of knowledge of the signs of danger, and the weakness of the decision-making power of the woman, who is yet the center of care of the children. In this study the risk of neonatal death was multiplied four times in the absence of mother's school education, five times in the event of precocious marriage, three times if pregnancy was poorly followed, and four times in the event of delivering at home. The second delay deals with access to the health facility. In this study, the risk of death was significantly associated with lack of geographical access to the health center (OR = 4) and the low socioeconomic level of parents (OR = 6). The third delay relates to the quality of care received once the newborn arrives in the health center. In this study, we observed the failing in the care of the newborn and the ignorance of pregnancies at risk by the health personnel. Beyond the social cultural constraints, delays seem to be interdependent. Indeed, going by the challenges for the transport and the cost of care in health facilities, the population often resigns to stay at home, abandoning themselves to fatalism. With the optimal implementation of a subsidy policy of obstetric and neonatal care emergency care, which has begun in Burkina Faso, since 2006, in particular in its section on transport and medical care, it is expected to accelerate the reduction of neonatal mortality.

5. Conclusion

Verbal autopsy permitted the identification of preventable causes of stillbirths and neonatal deaths in the health area of Namsiguia, Burkina Faso. The associated factors, in particular, were economic and social cultural. Improving school education, especially for women, reduction of extreme poverty, improvement of accessibility to high quality health services, promotion of essential newborn care, and adoption and implementation of a community health policy are essential for the reduction in neonatal mortality and for improving newborn survival in Burkina Faso, especially in the rural area.

Acknowledgements

The authors thank the staff of the Regional Directorate of Health of the North and the Regional Directorate of the Health District of Ouahigouya. They express their gratitude to the members of the bereaved families who have accepted to talk about an event as painful as the loss of one of their own.

Funding

This study was conducted with financial support from the West African Health Organization (WAHO), Bobo-Dioulasso, Burkina Faso.

References

[1] Lawn, J.E., Cousens, S., Bhutta, J.A., Darmstadt, G.L., Martines, J., Pual, V., *et al.* (2005) 4 Millions Neonatal Deaths: When? Where? Why? *The Lancet*, **365**, 891-900. http://dx.doi.org/10.1016/S0140-6736(05)71048-5

[2] Labie, D. (2005) Le scandale des 4 millions de morts néonatales chaque année: Bilan et actions possibles. *Médecine/Sciences*, **21**, 768-771. http://dx.doi.org/10.1051/medsci/2005218-9768

[3] Institut national de la statistique et de la démographie (Burkina Faso) (2010) Enquête Démographique et de Santé et à Indicateurs Multiples (EDSBF-MICS IV). http://www.insd.bf

[4] Patel, Z., Kumar, V., Singh, P., Singh, V., Yadav, R., Baqui, A.H., *et al.* (2007) Feasibility of Community Neonatal Death Audits in Rural Uttar Pradesh, India. *Journal of Perinatology*, **27**, 556-564. http://dx.doi.org/10.1038/sj.jp.7211788

[5] WHO (2012) Verbal Autopsy Standards: 2012 WHO Verbal Autopsy Instrument. http://www.who.int/healthinfo/statistics/WHO_VA_2012_RC1_Instrument.pdf?ua=1

[6] Manandhar, S., Ojha, A., Manandhar, D.S., Shrestha, B., Shrestha, D., Saville, N., *et al.* (2010) Causes of Stillbirths and Neonatal Deaths in Dhanusha District, Nepal: A Verbal Autopsy Study. *Kathmandu University Medical Journal*, **29**, 62-72. http://dx.doi.org/10.3126/kumj.v8i1.3224

[7] WHO (2012) International Statistical Classification of Diseases and Related Health Problems 10th Revision. http://apps.who.int/classifications/icd10/browse/2010/en

[8] Yach, D., Mathews, A.C. and Buch, E. (1990) Urbanisation and Health: Methodological Difficulties in Undertaking Epidemiological Research in Developing Countries. *Social Science & Medicine*, **31**, 507-514. http://dx.doi.org/10.1016/0277-9536(90)90047-V

[9] Lawn, J. and Kerber, K. (2006) Opportunities for Africa's Newborns: Practical Data, Policy and Programmatic Support for Newborn Care in Africa. PMNCH, Cape Town. http://www.who.int/pmnch/media/publications/opportunitiesfr.pdf

[10] Lawn, J., Shibuya, K. and Stein, C. (2005) No Cry at Birth: Global Estimates of Intrapartum Stillbirths and Intrapartum-Related Neonatal Deaths. *Bulletin of the World Health Organization*, **83**, 409-417.

[11] Baqui, A.H., Darmstadt, G.L., Williams, E.K., Kumar, V., Kiran, T.U., Panwar, D., *et al.* (2006) Rates, Timing and Causes of Neonatal Deaths in Rural India: Implications for Neonatal Health Programs. *Bulletin of the World Health Organization*, **84**, 706-713. http://dx.doi.org/10.2471/BLT.05.026443

[12] Turnbull, E., Lembalemba, M.K., Guffey, M.B., Bolton-Moore, C., Mubiana-Mbewe, M., Chintu, N., *et al.* (2011) Causes of Stillbirth, Neonatal Death and Early Childhood Death in Rural Zambia by Verbal Autopsy Assessments. *Tropical Medicine & International Health*, **16**, 894-901. http://dx.doi.org/10.1111/j.1365-3156.2011.02776.x

[13] Edmond, K.M., Quigley, M.A., Zandoh, C., Danso, S., Hurt, C., Agyei, S.O., *et al.* (2008) Aetiology of Stillbirths and Early Neonatal Deaths in Rural Ghana: Implications for Health Programming in Developing Countries. *Paediatric and Perinatal Epidemiology*, **22**, 430-437. http://dx.doi.org/10.1111/j.1365-3016.2008.00961.x

[14] Nikiema, L., Kameli, Y., Capon, G., Sondo, B. and Martin-Prevel, Y. (2010) Quality of Antenatal Care and Obstetrical Coverage in Rural Burkina Faso. *Journal of Health, Population and Nutrition*, **28**, 67-75.

http://dx.doi.org/10.3329/jhpn.v28i1.4525

[15] Carlo, W.A., Goudar, S.S., Jehan, I., Chomba, E., Tshefu, A., Garces, A., *et al.* (2010) Newborn-Care Training and Perinatal Mortality in Developing Countries. *New England Journal of Medicine*, **362**, 614-623. http://dx.doi.org/10.1056/NEJMsa0806033

[16] Sangho, H., Doumbia, S., Dembélé-Kéïta, H., Sidibé-Kéïta, A., Coulibaly, L., Diakité, B., *et al.* (2010) Intervention Communautaire Pour réduire au Mali la mortalité néonatale due à l'asphyxie. *Sante Publique*, **22**, 471-479.

[17] Ministère de la santé (Burkina Faso) (2006) Plan d'accélération de réduction de la mortalité maternelle et néonatale au Burkina Faso (Feuille de Route). Direction de la Santé de la Famille, Ouagadougou. http://www.unfpa.org/sowmy/resources/docs/library/R061_MOHBURKINAFASO_2006_Plan_daccelerationMMR_Octobre_2006.pdf

[18] Sombié, I. (2002) Mortalité néonatale et maternelle en milieu rural au Burkina Faso. Université Libre de Bruxelles, Bruxelles. http://www.memoireonline.com/a/fr/cart/download/t4mBNXRPO8Z8

[19] Lawn, J.E., Mwansa-Kambafwile, J., Horta, B.L., Barros, F.C. and Cousens, S. (2010) "Kangaroo Mother Care" to Prevent Neonatal Deaths Due to Preterm Birth Complications. *International Journal of Epidemiology*, **39**, i144-i154. http://dx.doi.org/10.1093/ije/dyq03

[20] Andreasen, S., Backe, B. and Oian, P. (2013) Claims for Compensation after Alleged Birth Asphyxia: A Nationwide Study Covering 15 Years. *Acta Obstetricia et Gynecologia Scandinavia*, **93**, 152-158.

[21] Thaddeus, S. and Maine, D. (1994) Too Far to Walk: Maternal Mortality in Context. *Social Science & Medicine*, **38**, 1091-1110. http://dx.doi.org/10.1016/0277-9536(94)90226-7

[22] Waiswa, P., Kallander, K., Peterson, S., Tomson, G. and Pariyo, G.W. (2010) Using the Three Delays Model to Understand Why Newborn Babies Die in Eastern Uganda. *Tropical Medicine & International Health*, **15**, 964-972. http://dx.doi.org/10.1111/j.1365-3156.2010.02557.x

[23] Kouéta, F., Yugbaré-Ouédraogo, S.O., Dao, L., Dao, F., Yé, D. and Kam, K.L. (2011) Audit médical des décès néonatals selon le modèle des trois retards, en milieu hospitalier pédiatrique de Ouagadougou. *Santé*, **21**, 209-214.

Correlation between Vitamin C Deficiency and Hydroxyproline Amino Acid in Young Children of Northern Part in Palestine

Maen Mahfouz[1], Ismail Masri[2], Haneen Mahfouz[3], Yara Mahfouz[4]

[1]Department of Orthodontics and Pediatric Dentistry, Dental School, Arab American University, Jenin, Palestine
[2]Department of Basic Biomedical Sciences, Dental School, Arab American University, Jenin, Palestine
[3]Biomedical Department, Central Public Health Lab, Palestinian Ministry of Health, Ramallah, Palestine
[4]Dental Department, Al Zafer Hospital, Najran, Saudi Arabia
Email: maenmahfouz@gmail.com, ismailmmasri@yahoo.com, haneen_medlab@yahoo.com, dr_cuteee@yahoo.com

Abstract

Vitamin C is a water soluble vitamin found in many natural sources, citric fruits, vegetables, particularly as antioxidants and as a factor to catabolism and metabolism. The aim of this article is to correlate the level of vitamin C and the hydroxyproline level in urine samples among young palestinian children from age 5 - 14 years. Materials and Methods: Urine samples of 34 individuals of both sexes, their ages ranged from 5 - 14 years were collected and analyzed for determination of Urinary Hydroxyproline by using Modified Neuman and Logan Method. The result of this study shows a significant correlation between Vitamin C and Hydroxyproline at level 0.01. The conclusion of this study was that low vitamin C intake was found among young palestinian children from age 5 - 14 years, Vitamin C should be supplemented in the drinks taken by young palestinian children from age 5 - 14 years as well as further research and investigation with large samples required to include all children from middle and southern Palestine.

Keywords

Vitamin C, Hydroxyproline, Palestinian Children

1. Introduction

Vitamin C is a water soluble vitamin found in many natural sources, citric fruits, vegetables a particularly as antioxidants and as a factor to catabolism and metabolism [1].

From the earliest descriptions of scurvy, the disease caused by vitamin C deficiency, it was evident that there were effects on connective tissues, especially in healing wounds [2]. The history of experiments that led to the conclusion that collagen metabolism was affected by the disease and that formation of hydroxyproline, animino acid found almost uniquely in collagen, might be involved was reviewed extensively [3] [4].

Many of the clinical problems associated with ascorbic acid deficiency, such as abnormalities of the skeleton seen in infantile scurvy [5], the lesions of the gingiva [6] [7], as well as the impairment of wound healing and faulty healing of bony fractures [5] [8] [9], are related to alterations in collagen metabolism.

The relationship between vitamin C and collagen is well established and lies in the hydroxylation of proline and lysine residues in the preformed protocollagen molecule [10] [11].

The aim of this article is to correlate the level of vitamin C and the hydroxyproline level in urine samples among young palestinian children from age 5 - 14 years.

2. Materials & Methodology

This study has been carried out on 34 individuals of both sexes their ages ranged from 5 - 14 years between 2013 and 2014. The sample randomly selected from out patients attending department of orthodontics and pediatric Dentistry at the faculty of dentistry—Arab American university—jenin in northern part of Palestine.

Inclusions criteria were healthy patients older than 5 years till 14 years, with ASA class I and no supplemental vitamin C intake. Unhealthy patients with ASA class II, III, IV, V and using supplemental vitamin c drugs were considered as exclusion criteria.

Ethical approval, this study registered and approved by the biomedical department at dental faculty of Arab American university in which all records of the samples were examined. Parental informed consent was carried out for each subject involved in this study by using a written form.

Case history had been taken for each subject and Clinical Examination carried out on dental chair for each subject who seated in reclining position. Plain mirrors, blunt probes (0.6 - 0.7 mm in diameter). Arab American university-jenin Assessment forms (2010) used.

The collected Urine samples were analyzed as the following:

Determination of Urinary Hydroxyproline:

Method Modified Neuman and Logan [12].

Principle: Hydroxyproline is treated with $CuSO_4$ and H_2O_2 in alkaline solution, this results in the formation of pyrroline-4-carboxylic acid.

Acidification is converted to pyyrole-2-carboxylic acid.

The later condenses with P-dimethylaminobenzaldehyde to give a coloured complex which is measured at 540 nm (**Table 1**).

Reagents:

1) Copper sulphate (0.01 M): Dissolve 0.159 g of it in 100 ml Distilled water.

Table 1. Procedure.

S.N	Reagent/Sample	Blank	Standard	Test
1	Urine			1 ml
2	Standard		1 ml	
3	Distilled Water	1 ml		
4	$CuSO_4$ (0.01) M	1 ml	1 ml	1 ml
5	NaOH (2.5) M	1 ml	1 ml	1 ml
6	6.6% H_2O_2	1 ml	1 ml	1 ml
7	3N H_2SO_4 (with agitation)	4 ml	4 ml	4 ml
8	5% P-dimethylamionbenzaldehyde	2 ml	2 ml	2 ml

2) Sodium Hydroxide (2.5 N): Dissolve 10 g of it in 100 ml distilled water.

3) 6% hydohen peoxide

4) Sulpharic acid (6 N).

5) P-dimethylaminobenzaldehyde (5% solution in n-propanol).

6) Hydroxyproline standard: A series of it corresponding to 5, 10, 15, 20, 25, 30, 35, 40, 45 microgram of it are prepared.

The solution are mixed and shaken occasionally during a period of 5 minutes, and then placed in water bath at 80°C for 5 minutes with frequent vigrous shaking. The heating and shaking destroys the excess of peroxide. Traces of peroxide, which remain, will decrease color formation and produce an orange-red hue. The tubes are chilled in an ice water bath and then added.

The tubes are placed in water bath at 70°C for 16 minutes and then placed in tap water. Read the color at 540 nm.

1) Hydroxyproline is estimated in ug/dl of urine and creatinine is estimated in mg/dl of urine.

2) Urine creatinine is estimated in micro cuvette by Jeff's reaction.

Statistical assessment was carried out using SPSS software version 20.0 (SPSS Inc., Chicago, IL, USA). Pearson Correlation test was used to define the correlation between vitamin C and hydroxyproline amino acid.

3. Results

This study aimed to correlate the level of vitamin C and the hydroxyproline level in urine samples among young palestinian children from age 5 - 14 years.

The lab value measurements of vitamin C and Hydroxyproline among children from 5 - 14 years of both sexes were taken as shown in **Table 2**.

The mean value of urine hydroxyproline: creatinine ratio in 35 healthy children of both sexes aged 5 - 14 years old was 0.01 ± 0.004.

The findings of this study show a significant correlation between Vitamin C and Hydroxyproline at level 0.01 as shown in **Table 3**.

4. Discussion

The study reported here represents the first comprehensive analysis that correlate the level of vitamin C and the hydroxyproline level in urine samples among young palestinian children from age 5 - 14 years.

Vitamin C has many vital functions in the body. Humans cannot make vitamin C (ascorbic acid or ascorbate) and must obtain it through the diet or as supplements [13].

A low vitamin C intake agrees with the observation of direct relationship between vitamin C and the hydroxyproline which the results of this study confirmed and ascertained as the results of other studies [10] [11].

Modern life from high technology to fast food among young generation health diet raising children from age 5 - 14 years who suffering vitamin C deficiency, most probably due to the artificial flavor and coloring had been supplemented to different types of snacks which had been consumed in large quantities by children in school and playing games on TV.

In addition this particular age group of people from 5 to 14 year old has longer outdoors stay at this age leading to greater consumption of in between meals snack food full of fillers, artificial flavor and colors and consequently to be considered at high risk in terms of Vitamin C deficiency.

The extent of the generalisability of the findings from a reasonable small sample is considered to be as a potential limitation and which will lead to further investigations in the future.

This paper is important for pediatric dentists for the following reasons:

1) Dietary advice is an essential part of oral care of children.

2) As our children constantly drinking and snacking, it is very important to be able to give sensible practical advice regarding drinks.

The basic advice is straight forward Vitamin C should be supplemented in the drinks taken by young children.

5. Conclusions

1) A low vitamin C intake was found among young palestinian children from age 5 - 14 years, so there should be increase intake of Vitamin C.

Table 2. Lab value measurements of vitamin C and OH-PR among children from 5 - 14 years of both sexes.

Paient No.	Age years	Gender	Vitamin C N-R 20 - 30 mg/dl	OH-PR N-R 0.01 ± 0.004	Diseases
1	5	M	22	0.03	
2	8	F	35	0.03	G6PD
3	35	M	18	0.012	
4	10	F	20	0.015	
5	10	F	32	0.021	
6	9	M	18	0.01	
7	6	M	27	0.02	
8	13	M	24	0.015	
9	9	M	32	0.012	
10	9	M	29	0.032	
11	10	M	25	0.032	
12	12	F	20	0.0145	
13	10	M	22	0.021	
14	7	F	25	0.033	
15	14	M	25	0.025	
16	7	M	21	0.015	
17	9	F	29	0.0135	
18	8.5	F	31	0.021	
19	3.5	M	31	0.012	
20	9	M	33	0.013	
21	13	F	25	0.015	
22	11	F	29	0.0135	
23	8.5	M	38	0.044	
24	7	M	27	0.02	
25	10	M	25	0.016	
26	8	F	5	0.003	Vitamin C Deficiency
27	11	F	15	0.008	Vitamin C Deficiency
28	9	F	2	0.002	Vitamin C Deficiency
29	12	M	10	0.02	Vitamin C Deficiency
30	13	F	5	0.0015	Vitamin C Deficiency
31	13	M	7	0.0091	Vitamin C Deficiency
32	9	M	3	0.005	Vitamin C Deficiency
33	7	F	8	0.004	Vitamin C Deficiency
34	5	M	5	0.002	Vitamin C Deficiency

Table 3. Correlation between Vitamin C and hydroxyproline amino acid.

		Vitamin C	OH-PR
Vitamin C	Pearson Correlation	1	0.696**
	Sig. (2-tailed)		0.000
	N	34	34
OH-PR	Pearson Correlation	0.696**	1
	Sig. (2-tailed)	0.000	
	N	34	34

**Correlation is significant at the 0.01 level (2-tailed).

2) Vitamin C should be supplemented in the drinks taken by young palestinian children from age 5 - 14 years as drinks highly consumed among young palestinian children.

3) Further research and investigation with large samples required to include all children from middle and southern Palestine.

Acknowledgements

Special thanks to Dr. Ismail Masri for his insights, feedback, and perspectives in hydroxyproline amino acid, as well as special Thanks for 2014 and 2015 graduating Class of faculty of dentistry—Arab American university for their valuable great cooperation and support.

References

[1]   Jacob, R.A. (1990) Assessment of Human Vitamin C Status. American Institute of Nutrition.

[2]   Lind, J. (1980) Treatise on the Scurvy. 3rd Edition, Classics of Medicine Library, Birmingham.

[3]   Chatterjee, G.C. (1967) Effects of Ascorbic Acid Deficiency in Animals. In: Sebrell Jr., W.H. and Harris, R.S., Eds., *The Vitamins*, Academic Press, New York, 407-457.

[4]   Gould, B.S. (1968) The Role of Certain Vitamins in Collagen Formation. In: Ramachandran, G.N. and Gould, B.S., Eds., *Treatise on Collagen*, Vol. 2A, Academic Press, New York, 323-365.

[5]   Watson, R.C., Grossman, H. and Meyers, M.A. (1980) Radiological Findings in Nutritional Disturbances. In: Goodhart, R.S., Shils, M.E., Eds., *Modern Nutrition in Health and Disease*, 6th Edition, Lea & Febiger, Philadelphia, 641-666.

[6]   Leggott, P.J., Robertson, P.B., Rothman, D.L., Murray, P.A. and Jacob, R.A. (1986) The Effect of Controlled Ascorbic Acid Depletion and Suppbementation on Periodontal Health. *Journal of Periodontology*, 7, 480-485. http://dx.doi.org/10.1902/jop.1986.57.8.480

[7]   Buzina, R., Aurer-Kozelj, J., Srdak-Jorgic, K., Buhler, E. and Gey, K.F. (1986) Increase of Gingival Hydroxyproline and Proline by Improvement of Ascorbic Acid in Man. *International Journal for Vitamin and Nutrition Research*, 56, 367-372.

[8]   Wolfer, J.A., Farmer, C.I., Carroll, W.W. and Manshardt, D.O. (1947) An Experimental Study of Wound Healing in Vitamin C Depleted Human Subjects. *Surgery, Gynecology, and Obstetrics*, 84, 1-15.

[9]   Hodges, R.E. (1980) Ascorbic Acid. In: Goodhart, R.S. and Shils, M.E., Eds., *Modem Nutrition in Health and Disease*, 6th Edition, Lea & Febiger, Philadelphia, 259-273.

[10] Barnes, M.J. and Kodicek, E. (1972) Biological Hydroxylation Sand Ascorbic Acid with Special Regard to Collagen Metabolism. *Vitamins Hormones*, 30, 1-43.

[11] Barnes, M.J., Constable, B.J., Morton, L.F. and Kodicek, E. (1970) Studies *in Vivo* on the Biosynthesis of Collagen and Elastin in Ascorbic Acid Deficient Guinea Pigs. Evidence for the Formation and Degradation of a Partially Hydroxylated Collagen. *Biochemical Journal*, 19, 575-585.

[12] Neuman, R.E. and Logan, M.A. (1950) The Determination of Hydroxyproline. *Journal of Biological Chemistry*, 184, 299.

[13] Levine, M. (1986) New Concepts in the Biology and Biochemistry of Ascorbic acid. *New England Journal of Medicine*, 314, 892-901. http://dx.doi.org/10.1056/NEJM198604033141407

Education of Parents When a Child Born with an Imperforate Anus; Does It Improve the Health of the Child?

Thi Hoa Chu[1], Thi Hoa Duong[1,2]*

[1]National Hospital of Pediatrics, Hanoi, Vietnam
[2]Centre for Person-Centred Care (GPCC), Institute of Health and Care Sciences, Sahlgrenska Academy, University of Gothenburg, Gothenburg, Sweden
Email: hoa_nhpa5@yahoo.com, *hoadt_nhp@yahoo.com

Abstract

Objectives: To describe and investigate the value of an education program for parents of children born with an imperforate anus in order to help them cope with the new situation of having a stoma. A comparison is made with a group of parents following routine hospital. A secondary aim was to illuminate the parents' feelings and concerns in the first month after the birth of the child. Subjects and methods: The program was tested in 20 Vietnamese mothers of babies born with an imperforate anus; 10 followed an intervention comprising an education program and 10 the ordinary routine hospital. The study design is both qualitative and quantitative. The mothers were interviewed, using open-ended questions, within a week of their child's birth and then repeatedly for up to one month. Finally, the conditions of children were accessed on their return to the hospital for the second operation after one month of care at home. The qualitative data were subjected to content analysis. Results: All mothers felt sad and worried in the beginning, but this quickly changed to confidence, particularly among mothers in the intervention group who received education. While at home, mothers in both groups had financial concerns, as they were unable to work as much as expected and also had to buy equipment for colostomy care. The mothers in the control group complained about a lack of knowledge and how it affected the care of their child. The mothers in the intervention group, however, felt confident in their caring even at home. When the families returned for the second operation, the children in the intervention group were significantly healthier, had increased more in weight, and had fewer complications and emergency return visits to hospital compared to the control group. In the control group skin problems around the stoma, diarrhea, bleeding or constipation while at home were reported ($p < 0.01$). Conclusion: The education improved the care at home resulting in healthier children and more confident parents.

---

*Corresponding author.

Keywords

Imperforate Anus, Participation, Education for Parents

1. Introduction

Becoming a parent for most of people implies a transition to something new and important in life. If the child is born with a malformation, it is usually very stressful for the parents. In order to offer the best treatment for the child, guidelines based on scientific results and recommendations are created and followed. Involving parents in decisions, and the treatment and care of their child are highly recommended in order to increase attachment and encourage parenthood [1]-[5]. The present study investigates the value of such guidelines for parents of children born with an imperforate anus living in Vietnam.

Imperforate anus is a malformation affecting 1 in 5000 babies and is slightly more common in males [6]. Its exact cause is unknown. Environmental factors or drug exposure during pregnancy may play a role in some cases, but have remained unclear. Imperforate anus may occur at a high or low level; in the high level the rectum is too short and ends above the levatorani muscle while in low level the rectum ends below the levatorani. Treatment depends on the type of abnormality present, but the first measure that has to be taken is to ensure fecal drain age [6]-[8]. All infants with imperforate anus need to have same surgery in order to correct the problem. At the National Hospital of Pediatrics (NHP) Hanoi, for most of children stool drainage is ensured by means of a colostomy as a first step to enabling recovery from delivery and growth.

When a child is diagnosed with anal malformation, it usually results in a traumatic period for a family, especially if the parents are new and young and it can be difficult for them to accept or comprehend the information [3] [9]. Information and support from health care personnel need to be ongoing as open communication between caregivers and parents is an important factor in pediatric care [10] [11]. Once discharged from hospital after the colostomy operation, the parents are responsible for the care of their child's stoma. In the hospital the parents are shown in general how to carry out the care, but in Vietnamese hospitals there are nospecific guidelines for stoma care in infants at home. This means that parents may often go home without sufficient experience of changing bags or knowledge about aids or where to buy them. In the present study such guidelines were created and tested. The aim was to describe and investigate the value of an education program for parents to a child born with an imperforate anus in order to help them cope with the new situation of caring for a child with a stoma. A comparison is done with a group of parents following the routine of the hospital. A secondary aim was to illuminate the parents' feelings and concerns during the first month after the child was born.

2. Participants

Twenty consecutive parents of newborn infants with anorectic malformations waiting colostomy operations (within 2 - 3 days after birth) at the surgical department of NHP were informed about the study design and invited to participate.

They were selected to either the intervention or the control group in consecutive order.

3. Method

The study was qualitative in design. Interviews with the parents followed an interview guide and asked open-ended question. In addition, an infant health protocol was used and analyzed in quantitative terms. The parents' experience of being the parent of a child born with an anal malformation was investigated continuously over one month. The usefulness of the intervention was investigated by comparing findings from the infant health protocol together with the interviews of parents who received the education program with a control group of parents followed the routines of the hospital. The interviews were tape recorded and then transcribed verbatim [12].

The interview guide was developed and tested before being used in the field for appropriateness and completeness with reference to the aim of the study. Supporting questions were used such as, Please tell me more; What exactly did you mean? Please explain?

The parents were interviewed four times. The first time was at the point of inclusion in the study, after delivery. They were asked about their experience of being the parents of a baby with special needs. After congratulating them to their beautiful baby the opening question was, *"How do you feel after the delivery? Would you like to tell me about your feelings concerning your child's illness?*

The second interview took place after the surgery and they were again asked about their feelings, *"How do you feel now?"* The third interviews, for the intervention group, was after they have received the education program and just before discharge when they were asked about the program *"What is your opinion about participating in your child's care from the beginning? Can you tell about it?"* The control group was asked about has they felt when they were discharged from hospital, *"How do you feel now that you are going home?"*

The final interviews took place approximately one month later when the families returned to hospital for the next planned surgery on their child. An open question was used, *"Can you tell me how things have been at home? Did you have any problems when caring for the child at home?"* The interviews were conducted by the study nurse in the ward's meeting room, and each parent was interviewed for about 20 - 30 minutes. The child was also examined with reference to health status, skin, weight and height, following the health protocol.

4. Intervention

The guidelines for the education program for parents included oral and written information about the malformation disease and care based on the child's health and wellbeing, as well as how to clean and dress the colostomy to prevent complications and should these occur, how to treat them at home. The doctor informed the parents about the malformation and they were invited to participate in the care of their child, including practicing cleaning and changing the colostomy appliance. They were able to practice step-by-step supported by the staff, so that before leaving the hospital they were able to perform the whole procedure for their child. During this learning period, an experienced nurse supported them with the aim of making them feel confident and they were encouraged to ask about anything they wanted to. The parents were also informed about nutrition and breast-feeding practical aids that could be used. The control group, treated according to the routine at NHP, had the ability to give the child basic care. The doctor gave them information about the malformation. Before discharge from hospital they was given oral information about stoma and shown how to clean the colostomy and how to apply the bandage.

5. Ethics

Permission to carry out the study was obtained from the head of NHP and the Ethics Committee of the hospital approved it. After informed consent was given and participation was voluntary and participants were aware that they could withdraw from the study at anytime. All information about subjects has been kept confidential. Data were reported in such a way that no one outside the study would be able to recognize who had said what.

6. Analysis

Content analysis was applied to the data [12]. The transcription was checked against the audio-recorded data for accuracy and to gain a holistic overview of the material. The analytic technique was based on reviewing data from all the interviews and from field notes in order to determine the essential meanings in relation to the aims of the study. The main author, in collaboration, carried out the initial search for meaning units and coded the interview text with the co-worker on the project. The primary themes were classified into sub-categories and then divided into categories. The findings were translated into English with the help of a professional Vietnamese-English translator to ensure that the original meaning in Vietnamese was not lost. Validity and reliability are ensured by describing the analysis process, and using quotations but also by independent analysis and discussion back and forth until agreement within the research group was reached. The infant health protocols were analyzed and compared using non-parametric statistics. Mann-Whitney was used for continuous variables (weight, height) and Fisher's exact test for categorical variables. The limit for statistical significance was set at $p < 0.05$.

7. Results/Findings

All the 20 parents invited gave their informed consent, however; only the mothers participated despite both parents being invited. Eight children in the intervention group were born with a high anal malformation and 2 with a low malformation. In the control group 7 had high malformation and 3 low malformations. Both groups had the same colostomy operation. The educational intervention following the guidelines, took place in the hospital after surgery. The mothers in the control group participated in the basic care of their child during their stay in hospital, but did not participate in the care of the stoma. The intervention and control groups were similar with no significant differences between them regarding demographic conditions (**Table 1**). In order to avoid affecting the result they had no opportunity to meet each other during the study period.

8. Parents' Feelings about the Situation before and after the First Operation

The findings from the analysis of the first interviews, which took place within 2 - 3 days after delivery, and the second interview, on the day after the first surgery, are presented in two categories, "Sadness" and "Worries", derived from the 5 subcategories; disappointed, sad, why, poorness and uncertainty. Both groups of mothers revealed similar feelings. Examples of the analysis process are given in **Table 2**. When they were informed that their newborn child had an anal malformation they felt sadness, disappointment and guilt, and had problems accepting the situation. Some mothers said they thought it was their fault, that they had been born with bad luck or that they had made mistakes and were being punished.

"I was doing very well during pregnancy" "I haven't used drugs and my first child was healthy, so I and my family can't accept this malformation in the baby...". "I think I always have bad luck, my first child had a heart disease and this child has malformation of the anus".

When the child had colostomy surgery the mothers were more or less in a state of acceptance and their feelings changed. They started to worry about the health of the child, his/her future life and how they could afford to care for the child at home: *"I'm worried.... because he's weak after the operation and has a fever"*. When they were interviewed concerning their knowledge about anal malformation, they revealed uncertainty; the condition was new for them as was how to care for a colostomy. *"I don't know about this illness, the first and second children are healthy. I think caring at home will be very difficult for me. Can you help me?"*

9. Knowledge of Parents and Education, Following Guidelines, before Discharge from Hospital

The mothers in the intervention group felt confident and were satisfied with the education. They knew what an anal rectal malformation meant and how to care for the child at home. They knew about feeding, colostomy care, prevention of complication and how to treat them if they occurred.

Onecategory, "Confidence" emerged from interview text, derived from four subcategories; better mood, abil-

Table 1. Demographic data from 20 mothers who participated in interviews.

	Intervention group	Control group	P value
	n = 10	n = 10	
Age of the mother			0.23
<20 years old	2	2	
20 - 30 years old	5	6	
>30 years old	3	2	
Occupation			0.61
Farmer	5	4	
Worker	3	4	
Official	2	2	
Standard of living			0.08
Low	2	1	
Middle	6	7	
High	2	2	
Number of children			
Range	1 - 3	1 - 4	

Table 2. Demographic data from 20 mothers who participated in interviews.

Meaning units	Codes	Sub-categories	Categories
I'm very sad, I wanted a son but now this is a girl with imperforate anus.	Sad Disappointed	Disappointed	Sadness
Everything around me Is very bad. Don't understand the reason for the malformation	Feels bad Doesn't understand why	Why	Sadness
The baby is weak after the operation don't know what happened	Weak baby Worried	Uncertainty	Worries
My family hasn't enough money to care for a sick child. I haven't any knowledge about this condition	Lack of money, Lack of knowledge about care	Poverty Uncertainty	Worries

ity, not damaging life and useful education. After the education the mothers' emotion had changed emotions from worries and sadness to feeling confident. They felt they could take care for their child by themselves and they were also were able to show other parents what to do: "*I'm fine now, I feel better having received information about this disease and how to manage the care… now I think this disease has not damaged the life of the baby.*" "*I am prepared enough to care for him at home. I am not worried now*". The education was useful and important for the caregiver: *… is necessary for all parents.*

The parents who followed the general routines received information about how to change the colostomy bag but had less knowledge and skill regarding prevention and treatment of complications. On the day they were discharged from the hospital they still felt worried about caring for the baby at home: "*I still worry a lot, although I know how to change and clean the colostomy. But I haven't got enough knowledge about this disease, so I think caring at home will be difficult for me*".

10. Factors Affecting the Wellbeing of the Child at Home

When they returned to hospital for the next operation both groups of mothers were asked how things had been at home and if they had had any problems concerning the care. From the analysis of this interview text the category "Concern" emerged, derived from five subcategories; uncertainty, need to work, accessibility to medical and social help, lack of knowledge. The concern now had its origin in their experiences at home. Some first-time mothers lacked experience in taking care of a newborn child and this, together with their baby's special needs, led to them having difficulties in caring for their babies at home. Mothers from both the control and the intervention groups felt uncertain and uncomfortable because of the child´s frequent bowel management. All day and at any time it was about stools, they felt dirty and afraid. "*… bowel movements anytime and anywhere, I'm always busy dealing with it and feel dirty. Sometime I don't want go to crowded places*" (CG).

A lot of the parents were farmers (see **Table 1**) and both parents needed to work in order to earn enough money to run the household. They had problems providing for the child's special needs.

Some were poor and also had problems feeding the child when out working. They could not buy high quality bandages and colostomy bags or medicine when the child developed complication: "*My family is small and nobody can help to take care of him, we need to work to earn money to live, … so my child can't gain weight, he is weak, easily gets other diseases and complications. I think these things affect the result of the treatment*" (IG). These concerns were present in both groups but the babies in the IG had fewer complications including fewer costs, see **Table 3**.

Accessibility to medical and social help was important factors for the CG. "*My home is far from a medical centre….. I can't go to hospital so my child usually has irritated skin around the colostomy*" (CG). Belonging to a social organization could be helpful but only some parents lived in a city and could benefit from such help. "*At home, I received money from the social organization and health care centre; immunization, special food for my child, examinations and check ups… my child is developing well and has a good immune defense*" (CG).

Table 3. Condition of the children after one month's participation in the study .The first ten are children in the intervention group (IG) and the following ten are children following routine case, the control group (CG). The p value shows the difference between IG and CG groups.

	Birth Weight (kg)	Weight after 1 month (increase in kg)	Birth Height (cm)	Height after 1 month (increase in cm)	Skin around stoma	Character stool	Diarrhea number	Bleeding stoma	Vomiting	Acute return to hospital
IG1	3	1.1	43	3.5	Soft healthy	Normal	0	0	0	0
IG2	3	1.3	44	3	Soft healthy	Normal	0	0	0	0
IG3	3	1.3	43	5	Soft healthy	Normal	0	0	0	0
IG4	2.5	1.2	40	5	Soft healthy	Liquid	1	0	1	1
IG5	2.2	0.8	40	3	Soft healthy	Normal	1	0	0	0
IG6	2.5	0.9	42	3	Soft healthy	Normal	0	0	0	0
IG7	3	0.9	42	3	Soft healthy	Liquid	1	0	0	0
IG8	2.5	1.1	42	3	Soft healthy	Normal	0	0	0	0
IG9	3	1.3	43	4	Soft healthy	Normal	0	0	0	0
IG10	2	1	40	3	Red	Normal	0	1	0	0
CG1	2.5	0.5	43	3	Red wet	Liquid	0	1	0	0
CG2	2.5	0.7	43	2	Irritated	Normal	1	0	1	0
CG3	3	0.5	42	3	Soft healthy	Liquid	2	0	0	1
CG4	3	0.6	40	3	Irritated	Liquid	1	0	0	0
CG5	2.8	0.5	43	3	Irritated	Liquid	1	0	0	0
CG6	3.2	0.8	43	3	Soft healthy	Normal	0	0	1	1
CG7	3.4	0.6	42	3	Irritated	Normal	1	1	0	0
CG8	3	1.1	43	3	Irritated	Normal	0	0	1	1
CG9	2.7	0.8	42	3	Irritated	Liquid	1	0	0	1
CG10	3.1	0.6	42	3	Soft healthy	Liquid	0	0	1	1
P value	0.19	0.001	0.18	0.02	0.01	0.08	0.1	0.5	0.1	0.07

Centimeters (cm), kilograms (kg).

11. Does Education Affect the Complications with the Child at Home?

All the mothers in the intervention group changed regarding how they felt about the colostomy after the education; they felt competent and confident about their knowledge of the malformation and the care of the colostomy when back home. This is shown by the results of the examination of the children and interviews with the mothers. **Table 3** shows the condition of the child on return to the hospital for the next surgery.

The assessment included: general condition (weigh, height), the condition of the colostomy (skin color, irritated or not), and complication that occurred while the child was at home (**Table 3**). The differences in findings show that children in the IG might be healthier. The mean weight at birth was 2.6 kg in the IG and 2.9 kg in the CG, a slight but not significant different. However, after 1 month there was a significant difference; the IG had gained weight by a mean 3.7 kg, range 0.8 - 1.3 kg (increase in weight 1.090 kg). The corresponding values for the CG were 3.5 kg, range 0.4 - 1.1 kg (increase in weight 0.067 kg). The difference in increased weight amounts to more than 1 kg ($p \leq 0.001$, Fisher's exact test).

According to the interviews the mothers in the IG were happy about breast feeding and said that their child had hardly any complications and therefore was able to eat and grow. However, the mothers in the CG said that their child was not exclusively breast-fed despite them having enough milk. Their child had complications caused by the stoma: diarrhea, fever, sometimes bleeding. They felt they lacked suitable knowledge about how to care for their child and the colostomy and thought that this had the effected of the child getting complications. This is also shown in **Table 3**.

All except one child in the IG had soft and healthy skin around the colostomy, normal stool movement and no bleeding or vomiting, just one had had diarrhea, while seven children in CG had had irritated skin, six had had diarrhea, four had had vomiting and constipation to such an extent that they had had to return to the hospital for help. The differences between the groups were significant ($p \leq 0.05$, Fisher's exact test).

12. Discussion

The results of this paper agree with those of other authors: parents of a child with anal malformation need a lot of attention [10] [13]. The present study follows the parents from 2 - 3 days after delivery, to after colostomy surgery and education and ultimately to one month after surgery. The findings show that their emotions change over, even within the short perspective of one month. Participation, education and taking part in the child´s care made the parents feel confident, resulting in a child who was healthy despite the colostomy.

The present study, which has both a qualitative and quantitative design, investigates 20 parents of children born with an imperforate anus, all of them underwent colostomy surgery. Both parents were invited to participate but traditional thinking and practical circumstances meant that only mothers were involved.

Comparison were made between a control group' which followed hospital's normally routines and an intervention group, who were trained in caring for the colostomy at home, preventing complications and, if they occurred treating them. They also received nutrition advice. These mothers had been given the opportunity to discuss matters with the staff and to practice under observation at the hospital. The control group had not practised at the hospital and was given only basic information about care of the colostomy.

The interviews reveal that for all the mothers the initial feeling about the situation was sadness. They experienced feelings of guilt, were disappointed and looked for reasons why this had happened to them. Their feelings were in the beginning overwhelming but soon changed to worries about their child's health and their economy. The mothers in the intervention group gained a more optimistic view of their situation earlier than those in the CG. Similar findings have been reported from other studies concerning colostomy care in children [3] [9] [10].

Vietnam is a developing country and many of the participating families were poor. In Vietnamese culture old traditions dictate how should act being a good mother. We have shown earlier how mothers potty train infants with good outcomes from when they are newborn, even in infants born with posterior urethra valves [14] [15]. The mothers in the present study knew they needed to work to earn money to cover family costs; there was no money to meet extra costs. In Vietnamese society a healthy child principally a son, is a guarantee that the parents will be cared for in their old age. Despite the differences in living standards and wealth between countries people in Western countries also worry and feel sad [3] [9] [10].

Stressful factors and uncertainty about their child's illness and recovery, disrupt the parental role, and this is exacerbated by being in an unfamiliar environment. These were the findings from Kristensson-Hallström's study in a surgical ward and could also be seen in our study [1]. In recent years, pediatric health care has shifted toward family-centered care based on the close and continuous involvement of the child's family members. Parental participation is beneficial for children, parents, and healthcare facilities, based on communication among all parts. To achieve this goal ongoing quality control of routines and outcomes is mandatory [16].

In order to be responsible for the care at home the parents need confidence. In earlier studies children and parents have described how they were insufficiently informed and prepared for the necessary procedures at home and how they felt excluded from decision making regarding themselves or their children which resulted in anxiety, indignation, anger and fear [17] [18]. In the intervention studied, the staff tried to respect and meet the parents' needs, when they invited them to participate in the care and in decisions making; they tried to listen to them and support them. This is in accordance with the United Nations Convention of the Rights of the Child [19]. However, the actual process of person-centered care was not investigated in the present study. The mothers were satisfied with the education and support they received and the outcomes were good but the study did not reveal much about the interaction between the nurses and the parents.

When parents returned for the second surgery, parents in both groups had concerns arising from their experiences of daily life at home. According to the findings almost all the mothers in the IG could change the colostomy bag satisfactorily. They could prevent and treat complications at home, such as bleeding, diarrhea, irritated skin and they knew when it was necessary to take the child to hospital. Mothers from the CG felt uncertain due to insufficient knowledge and skill regarding caring for their child in the best way and they complained about extra costs.

Some families had been offered help from a social centre, which had helped. Money was a major factor concerning treatment. The farmers and families living in the mountains were often poor and their incomes come from the agriculture. If the mothers did not work in the fields there was less to eat, and they could not buy proper colostomy bags or other equipment necessary for the care. The health care centre was usually far from their homes so when the children developed problems it was difficult to take them to the hospital. The families in the cities had easier access to medical or social help. Our findings show that the parents' ability to overcome obstacles depended largely on their knowledge and confidence. In this case, the education program in the intervention led to the parents feeling well prepared for caring for the child at home.

In the assessment of the children when they returned to the hospital for the second surgery we found significant differences between the groups (**Table 3**). The children in the IG had had fewer complications than those in the CG. The intervention group children were healthier and had grown more quickly. The children in the CG often returned to hospital before time because of diarrhea, bleeding or absence of stool movement.

These complications could probably have all been prevented if the mothers had had enough knowledge and skill to manage the care of the colostomy successfully. Many studies have shown that parents play an important role in the care of the child [2] [4] [13] [20]. In children with anal malformation this is particularly true, as the parents have to take a lot of responsibility for the follow-up treatment [3] [13].

Our findings show that the mothers' ability to overcome problems and obstacles depended largely on their knowledge and confidence. The results of this study illuminate the importance of attention, education and participation, in agreement between the care provider and the mother, for improving health outcomes related to person-centered care (PCC) [16] [21] [22]. The families living with a child who has a long-term illness need care and support which addresses their own researches and need. The education program in the intervention was a useful tool in making parents feel well prepared before leaving hospital.

This study had a small number of mothers, but the findings were significant and clear. In order to help families with a child born with an imperforate anus to cope with the new situation, we still need more research on this topic, particularly about the education process and the interaction between the nurses and the parent.

13. Conclusions

Education of parents when a child is born with an imperforate anus improves the health of the child.

Worries and feelings of sadness about their child and the future are common among mothers.

The emotions of the mothers in the intervention group changed and became more positive earlier than the case for mother in the control group.

All mothers had concerns regarding the care for economic reasons.

Education and practice, step by step, supported by the staff resulted in a confident mother with the competence to take care of her child and a healthier child with significantly fewer complications and emergency return visits to the hospital compared to the situation in a control group. Ultimately this meant lower costs for both the family and the healthcare system.

References

[1]   Kristensson-Hallstrom, I. (2000) Parental Participation in Pediatric Surgical Care. *AORN Journal*, **71**, 1021-1024, 1026-1029. http://dx.doi.org/10.1016/S0001-2092(06)61551-2

[2]   Lam, L.W., Chang, A.M. and Morrissey, J. (2006) Parents' Experiences of Participation in the Care of Hospitalised Children: A Qualitative Study. *International Journal of Nursing Studies*, **43**, 535-545. http://dx.doi.org/10.1016/j.ijnurstu.2005.07.009

[3]   Ojmyr-Joelsson, M., *et al.* (2006) Parental Experiences: Care of Children with High and Intermediate Imperforate Anus. *Clinical Nursing Research*, **15**, 290-305. http://dx.doi.org/10.1177/1054773806291856

[4]   Ygge, B.M. and Arnetz, J.E. (2004) A Study of Parental Involvement in Pediatric Hospital Care: Implications for Clinical Practice. *Journal of Pediatric Nursing*, **19**, 217-223. http://dx.doi.org/10.1016/j.pedn.2004.02.005

[5]   Wigert, H., *et al.* (2006) Mothers' Experiences of Having Their Newborn Child in a Neonatal Intensive Care Unit.

Scandinavian Journal of Caring Sciences, **20**, 35-41. http://dx.doi.org/10.1111/j.1471-6712.2006.00377.x

[6] Mo, R., Kim, J.H., Zhang, J., Chiang, C., Hui, C.C. and Kim, P.C. (2001) Anorectal Malformations Caused by Defects in Sonic Hedgehog Signaling. *American Journal of Pathology*, **159**, 765-774.

[7] Ozturk, H., *et al.* (2007) A Comprehensive Analysis of 51 Neonates with Congenital Intestinal Atresia. *Saudi Medical Journal*, **28**, 1050-1054.

[8] Pena, A., Grasshoff, S. and Levitt, M. (2007) Reoperations in Anorectal Malformations. *Journal of Pediatric Surgery*, **42**, 318-325. http://dx.doi.org/10.1016/j.jpedsurg.2006.10.034

[9] Searles, J.M., Nour, S. and MacKinnon, A.E. (1995) Mitrofanoff Stoma—An Iceberg of Problems? *European Journal of Pediatric Surgery*, **5**, 19-20. http://dx.doi.org/10.1055/s-2008-1066256

[10] Ameh, E.A., Mshelbwala, P.M., Sabiu, L. and Chirdan, L.B. (2006) Colostomy in Children—An Evaluation of Acceptance among Mothers and Caregivers in a Developing Country. *South African Journal of Surgery*, **44**, 138-139.

[11] Polit, E.P. and Beck, C.T. (2006) Essentials of Nursing Research. 6th Edition, Lippincott Williams & Wilkins, Philadelphia.

[12] Krippendorf, K. (2004) Content Analysis: An Introduction to Its Methodology. Sage Publications, Thousands Oakes.

[13] Nisell, M., Öjmyr-Joelsson, M., Frenckner, B., Rydelius, P.A. and Christensson, K. (2003) How a Family Is Affected When a Child Is Born with Anorectal Malformation. Interviews with Three Patients and Their Parents. *Journal of Pediatric Nursing*, **18**, 423-432. http://dx.doi.org/10.1016/S0882-5963(03)00029-0

[14] Duong, T.H., Jansson, U.B. and Hellstrom, A.L. (2012) Vietnamese Mothers' Experiences with Potty Training Procedure for Children from Birth to 2 Years of Age. *Journal of Pediatric Urology*, **9**, 808-814.

[15] Duong, T.H., Holmdahl, G., Viet Nguyen, D., Sillén, U., Jansson, U.-B. and Hellström, A.L. (2013) Micturition Pattern in Young Boys with Posterior Urethral Valves—A Pilot Study in Small Boys Who Are Potty-Trained from Infancy. *Open Journal of Pediatrics*, **3**, 358-363. http://dx.doi.org/10.4236/ojped.2013.34064

[16] Ekman, I., Swedberg, K., Taft, C., Lindseth, A., Norberg, A., Brink, E., *et al.* (2011) Person-Centered Care—Ready for Prime Time. *European Journal of Cardiovascular Nursing*, **10**, 248-251. http://dx.doi.org/10.1016/j.ejcnurse.2011.06.008

[17] Noyes, J. (2000) Enabling Young "Ventilator-Dependent" People to Express Their Views and Experiences of Their Care in Hospital. *Journal of Advanced Nursing*, **31**, 1206-1215. http://dx.doi.org/10.1046/j.1365-2648.2000.01376.x

[18] Bray, L., Callery, P. and Kirk, S. (2012) A Qualitative Study of the Pre-Operative Preparation of Children, Young People and Their Parents' for Planned Continence Surgery: Experiences and Expectations. *Journal of Clinical Nursing*, **21**, 1964-1973. http://dx.doi.org/10.1111/j.1365-2702.2011.03996.x

[19] Nations, U. (1989) UN Convention of the Rights of the Child. United Nations, Geneva.

[20] Nisell, M., Öjmyr-Joelsson, M., Frenckner, B., Rydelius P.A. and Christensson, K. (2008) Views on Psychosocial Functioning: Responses from Children with Imperforate Anus and Their Parents. *Journal of Pediatric Health Care*, **22**, 166-174. http://dx.doi.org/10.1016/j.pedhc.2007.04.016

[21] Josefsson, U., Berg, M., Koinberg, I., Hellström, A.L., Nolbris, M.J., Ranerup, A., *et al.* (2013) Person-Centred Web-Based Support—Development through a Swedish Multi-Case Study. *BMC Medical Informatics and Decision Making*, **13**, 119. http://dx.doi.org/10.1186/1472-6947-13-119

[22] Hellstrom, A.L., Svensson, A.S., Samuelsson, I.P. and Nolbris, M.J. (2012) A Web-Based Programme for Person-Centred Learning and Support Designed for Preschool Children with Long-Term Illness: A Pilot Study of a New Intervention. *Nursing Research and Practice*, **2012**, Article ID: 326506.

12

Allergies in Children: What's New?
—A Cross-Sectional
Descriptive Study

Daniela Simoncini[1*], Anna Peirolo[1], Alberto Macchi[2], Stefania Porcu[1], Daniela Graziani[1], Luigi Nespoli[1]

[1]Department of Clinical and Experimental Medicine, University of Insubria c/o Ospedale Filippo del Ponte, Varese, Italy
[2]Otorhinolaringology Clinic University of Insubria Varese, AICNA, c/o Ospedale di Circolo, Varese, Italy
Email: *daniela_simoncini@libero.it, anna.peirolo@hotmail.it

Abstract

Background: The prevalence of respiratory allergies is increasing worldwide, with important consequences especially for little children. Objective: The aim of this study was to assess the prevalence of respiratory allergies, such as rhinitis and asthma, and to point out the risk factors and their relationship with allergic diseases in a specific area of Northern Italy. Methods: 110 children, male and female, from our outpatient service for allergic children, between 3 and 17 years old, were examined. After a skin prick test and a nasal cytology, the written questionnaire of the International Study of Asthma and Allergies in Childhood was filled by parents together with their children. Results: 110 children were examined. 74% of children had rhinitis and 71% asthma. 88 patients were allergic, grass pollen and house dust mite was the most frequent allergens. A family history of atopy, family background, geographic area, active and passive smoking and home pets were associated to allergies. Older children (6 - 15 years old) had more often rhinitis associated with asthma and conjunctivitis as compared to younger. 21 Children were also affected by non allergic rhinitis. Conclusions: Respiratory allergies are widespread and associated to a low quality of life among little children. Sensitization to Ragweed is increasing with important consequences. Rhinitis precedes the onset of asthmatic symptoms. Moreover non allergic rhinitis is increasing and frequently underdiagnosed.

Keywords

Allergies, Environment, Asthma, Rhinitis

---

*Corresponding author.

1. Introduction

More than 150 million European Union citizens suffer from chronic allergic diseases and they will be 250 million in the next ten years; moreover allergic diseases are increasing especially among young children [1]-[3].

Allergic diseases are the first leading cause of loss of productivity, low quality of life, and reduction of school performance followed by cardiovascular diseases. They must be considered a major global public health issue and a real epidemic in the European Union [1] [4] [5].

Despite this data they are underdiagnosed, in fact 45% of patients have never received a diagnosis [4] [6].

Allergic rhinitis has a prevalence of 0.8% to 14.9% in the 6 - 7 years old group and of 1.4% to 39.7% in the 13 - 14 years old, till 20% - 30% among teenagers and young adults.

These data are underestimated because especially young children do not present sufficiently severe symptoms to require medical attention, in fact they often have rhinorrea, coughing and sneezing; 19% - 38% of patients have also asthma associated with rhinitis which may lead to a worsening of their clinical condition [6].

The aim of this study was to investigate the prevalence and the risk factor of allergic diseases, such as rhinitis and asthma, in a specific area of Northern Italy, Varese and surroundings (an area of 1.199 km²), with particular characteristics possibly affecting the spread of these diseases (presence of urban, mountain, and lake areas; rainfall: more than 1500 mm of annual average, wetness: 75.2% of annual average). It could be considered a little model of the different conditions that can be found everywhere.

Although primarily descriptive this study allows us to have an analysis of the epidemiological situation in the pediatric population.

2. Methods

This was a cross-sectional, descriptive study. 110 children, 70 males and 40 females, aged 3 to 17 (15% aged 3 - 5, 8 males and 8 females, 47% aged 6 - 10, 36 males and 16 females, 32% aged 11 - 15, 22 males and 13 females, and 6% aged 15 - 17, 4 males and 3 females) from our outpatient service for allergic children, were examined from November 2013 to March 2014. Children with asthma, rhinitis or dermatitis, who came for the first time or were already followed by our service, were eligible to participate.

First each child underwent an ear, nose, throat, lung examination, a skin prick test and a nasal cytology. We tested a panel of allergens: grasses, birch, nut tree, olive tree, ragweed, lichwort, dog, cat, house dust mite (Dermatophagoides pteronyssinus, DPP, and Dermatophagoides farinae, DPF), mould (alternaria) and foods (cow lactalbumin, cow casein, egg white and yolk, peanuts), according to the European society guidelines [7] and to Gelardi recommendation for the nasal cytology [8].

Then each child with his/her parents was asked to fill a questionnaire. The questionnaire used in this study was primarily adapted from the reliable, written questionnaire of the International Study of Asthma and Allergies in Childhood (ISAAC), the largest worldwide epidemiological collaborative research project ever undertaken [9]. Questions (84) included socioeconomic status, parental atopy, presence of cigarette smokers and furred pets at home, therapy. Additional questions were about the presence of wheezing, rhinorrea, coughing, and sneezing.

3. Results

Of children evaluated 88 showed positive skin prick tests (60 males, 28 females), 22 negative (12 females, 10 males) and they were affected by asthma or rhinitis as shown in **Figure 1**. Of children between 3 and 5, 4% presented only rhinitis; among children from 6 to 10, 9% had asthma, 8% rhinitis, 9% rhinitis associated with asthma and/or rhinoconjunctivitis; 10% of patients from 11 to 15 presented rhinoconjunctivitis and asthma. According to the nasal cytology, 21 non allergic children were affected by non allergic rhinitis (20 non-allergic rhinitis with eosinophils, NARES, 1 non-allergic rhinitis with eosinophils and mast cells, NARESMA).

Of allergic patients 56% was polyallergic both to perennial and seasonal allergens, 9% was polysensitized but only to perennial allergens, 15% was sensitized to only one allergen (10% grasses, 6% DPP, 2% mould). 16 children were allergic to grasses and to another allergen (13% DPP, 3% animals, 1% food). The most common sensitizing allergens are shown in **Figure 2**. According to the age, 98% of allergic children was more than 6 years old, only 2 children were aged 3 - 5, most of them were polyallergic: 26 children aged 6 - 10, 17 aged 11 - 15 and 5 older than 15 years. Positivity to specific allergens according to age is shown in **Figure 3(a)**. In 13 children a variation of allergens over time was seen: positivity to allergens increased through the years, especially to grasses and DPP. Positivity to ragweed is more common when the child grows up (**Figure 3(b)**).

We also evaluated the treatments followed by the children as shown in **Figure 4**. Each child received treatments with Montelukast or Fluticasone dipropionate and 13 children were under SLIT (Sublingual Immunotherapy), 2 for grasses and 11 for DPP.

4. Risk Factors

Family History and Socioeconomic Status

Of patients evaluated 68% reported a family history of diagnosed allergy (17% both parents, 26% mother only, 25% father only). Allergies were more common among children whose parents had high school education: 47% mother, 40% father.

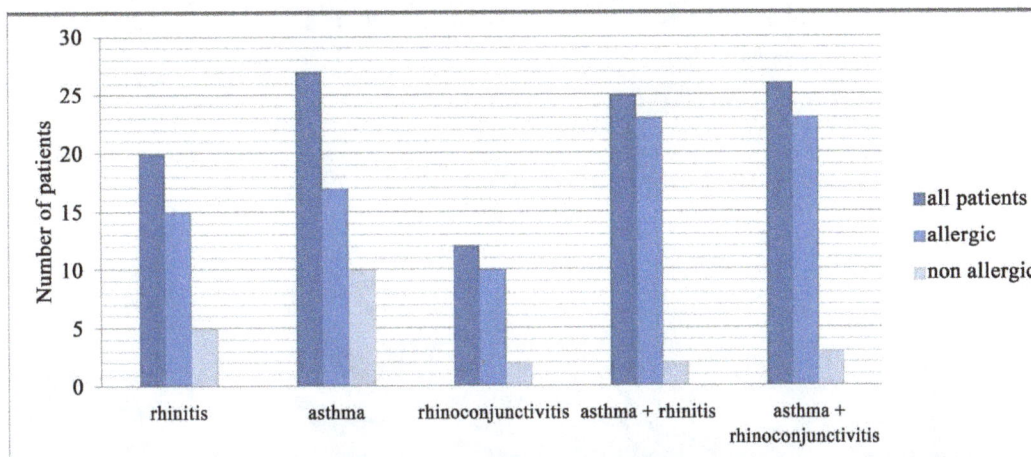

Figure 1. Prevalence of respiratory diseases: Among allergic children there was a prevalence of asthma associated with rhinitis (26%) or rhinoconjunctivitis (26%). Among non allergic children 5 had only rhinitis, 10 asthma and 2 rhinoconjunctivitis, 5 asthma with rhinitis or rhinoconjunctivitis.

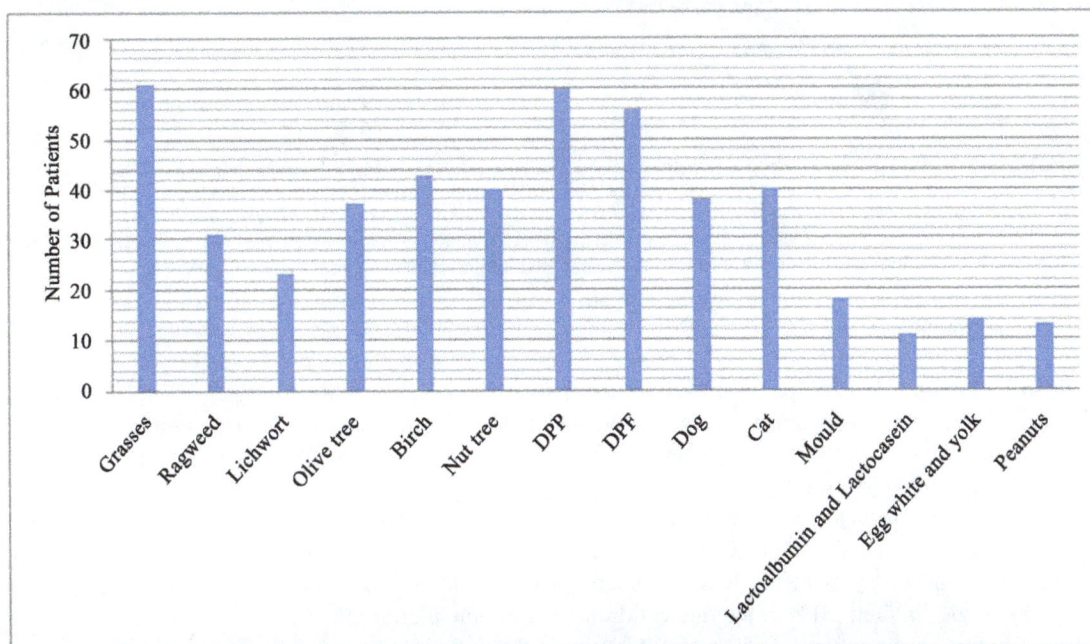

Figure 2. Prevalence of sensitization to different allergens: The most common sensitizing allergens in children were grasses 69%, DPP 68%, DPF 64%, Birch 49%, Cat 45%.

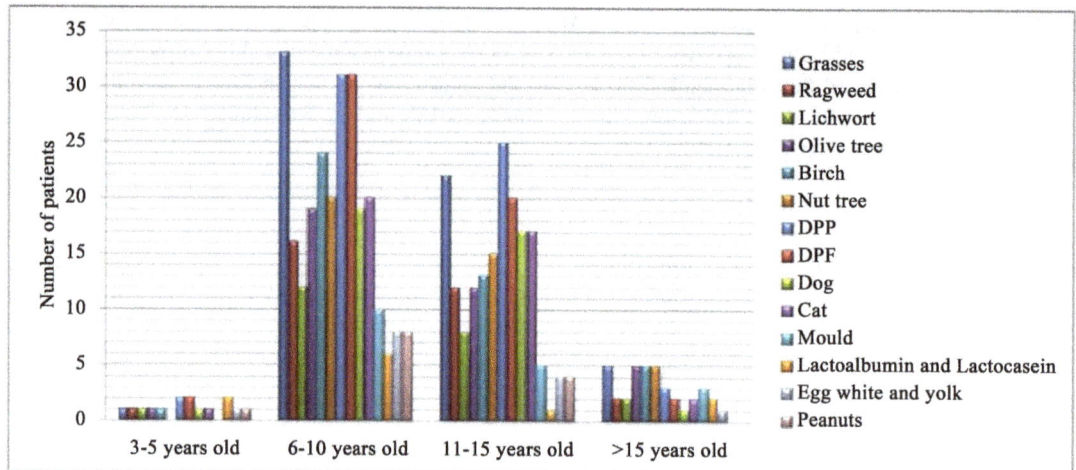

(a)

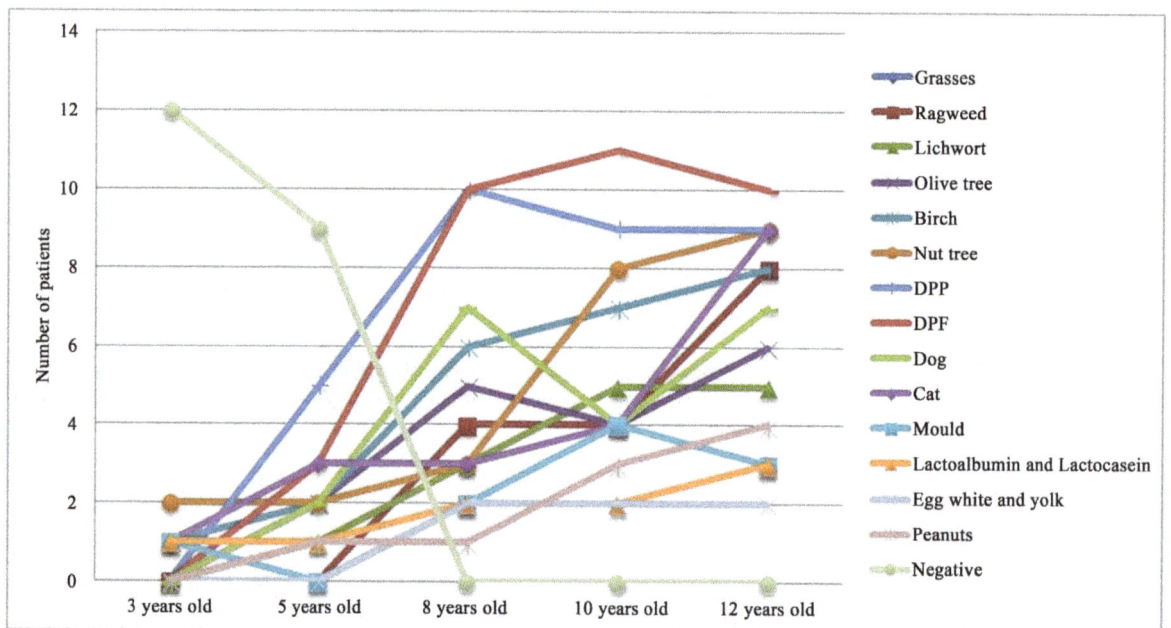

(b)

Figure 3. (a) Prevalence of sensitization to different allergens according to the age of patients; (b) variation of the positivity to allergens in 13 patients followed through the years: each child underwent skin prick test at 3, 5, 8, 10, 12 years old.

Geographic Area

The children living areas were examined. Varese and surroundings were divided into: urban, lake and mountain (>1000 m) areas: 61 patients lived in urban areas (53 allergic, 8 non allergic), 33 in lake areas (23 allergic, 10 non allergic), 5 in mountain areas (4 allergic, 1 non allergic). Among allergic children 60% lives in urban areas and only 5% in the mountains; among non allergic children 45% lives near a lake, 36% in urban areas.

Presence of Animals at Home, Smoking Exposure, Antibiotics Use

Of children evaluated 57 have animals at home, (47 allergic, 10 non allergic), 47 have no animals, (35 allergic, 12 non allergic). Of allergic patients 53% has pets, while 55% of non allergic children has no pets. The presence of pets in the first year of life was examined: allergic children hadn't more often pets at home as compared to non allergic children (51% of allergic children, 36% of non allergic).

Among allergic patients, 86% used antibiotics in the first years of life, 73% of non allergic.

Of all children 44%, allergic and non allergic (32% only one, 12% both) and 44% of allergic children (33% only one, 11% both) have smoking parents.

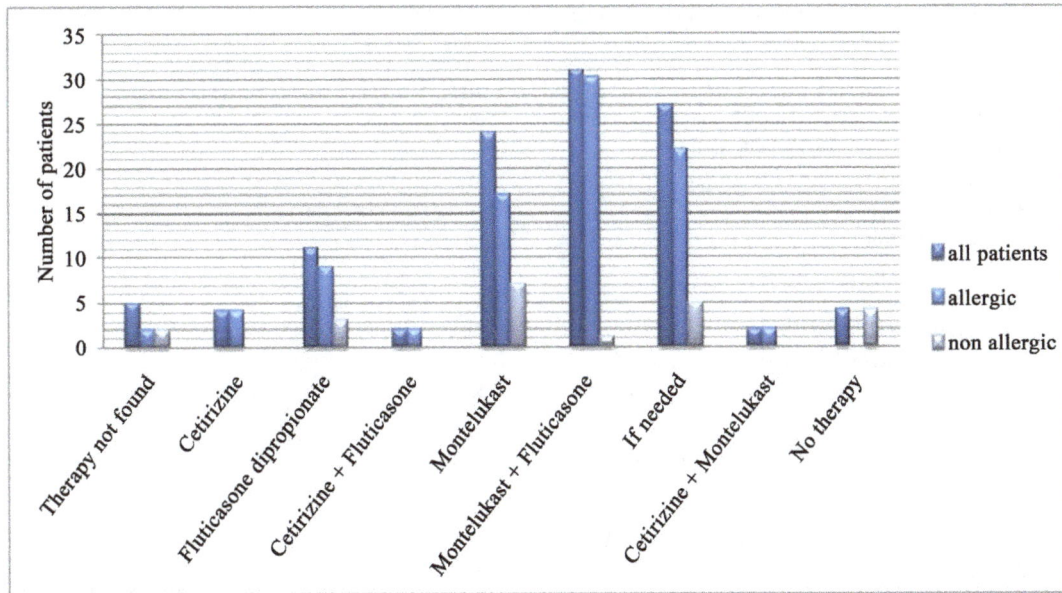

Figure 4. Patients' treatments of the patients studied 74 received treatment with montelukast and fluticasone dipropionate (85% allergic, 15% non allergic), 27 patients used treatments only when symptoms appeared, (81% allergic, 16% non allergic), 4 didn't follow any treatment, all non allergic; of allergic children 34% received a current treatment with Montelukast and Fluticasone, 32% of non allergic children only with montelukast.

Symptoms and Diseases

Of all children 89% reported to have sneezing, running and blocked nose in the past 12 months, both allergic and non allergic (91% allergic, 82% non allergic). However in 38% of allergic children symptoms didn't affect day-to-day routine; on the contrary in 36% of non allergic children "a little" was the answer. Children reported also the loss of school days for asthma and rhinitis, 23% 1 to 5 days, 11% 6 to 10, 7% more than 10. Both allergic and non allergic children reported that colds and flu are the first condition that make wheezing worse, followed by pollen and dust for allergic patients and weather for non allergic (**Table 1**).

5. Discussion

The study design allowed us to investigate the epidemiological situation of children affected by asthma and rhinitis and to point out the issues on which to focus the attention.

Despite the sample group analyzed is recruited from a single specialty clinic, it was heterogeneous as to age, diagnosis and living areas; this allowed us to examine the different spread of allergies and allergens and to compare our results with other centres.

Polyallergic children, affected by respiratory diseases and who underwent different treatments, were examined. This type of child is common in pediatric clinical practice. The majority of children was male and allergic, in fact boys are more likely to develop allergies than girls [4].

Children were more often polyallergic and the most common sensitizing allergens were grass pollen and DPP along with other Italian studies, as D.P. Peroni's [6]. Moreover allergies increased with the increasing of children age; 3 - 5 years old children were more often monosensitized or had negative skin prick test than older children and at this age skin prick test were positive to DPP and food; on the contrary when children grew up, sensitization to grass pollen and tree (birch, olive tree, nut tree) appeared.

In the last years Ragweed is spreading invasively in many countries, also in Northern Italy. In the north-west region of Italy, where Varese is situated, ragweed started to colonise the area in the 1930s and nowadays is widely widespread. It takes some years of exposure to high pollen concentration to develop an allergy [10] and therefore previous studies showed that the age of onset of ragweed allergy is adult age, around 35, and only 10% of the subjects is younger than 20 [11]. Despite this, in our study the prevalence of Ragweed sensitization is higher with an important prevalence, in fact 35% of children is positive; probably because of the increased diffusion of Ragweed and because of its allergenic potency, children will be exposed to this allergen at early ages

Table 1. Prevalence of symptoms and interference with children daily life.

	All patients (110)		Allergic (88)		Non allergic (22)	
	n	%	n	%	n	%
Sneezing, runny or blocked nose in the last 12 months	98	89	80	91	18	82
Symptoms interference with daily activities						
Not at all	38	35	33	38	5	23
A little	40	36	32	36	8	36
A moderate amount	13	12	11	13	2	9
A lot	4	4	2	2	2	9
No answer	15	14	10	11	5	23
Use of medication for rhinitis	51	46	42	48	9	41
Loss of school days for respiratory diseases						
None	55	50	48	55	7	32
1 to 5	25	23	20	23	5	23
6 to 10	12	11	10	11	2	9
More than 10	8	7	4	5	4	18
No answer	10	9	6	7	4	5
Presence of wheezing and asthma in the last 12 months	77	70	63	74	12	55
What makes child wheezing worse						
Weather	24	22	20	23	4	18
Pollen	34	31	33	38	1	5
Emotion	10	9	10	11	0	0
Fume	6	5	5	6	1	5
Dust	30	27	30	34	0	0
Pets	9	8	8	9	1	5
Wool clothing	3	3	3	3	0	0
Colds or flu	47	43	37	42	10	45
Cigarette smoke	7	6	6	7	1	5
Food or drinks	3	3	3	3	0	0
Soap, sprays, detergents	5	5	4	5	1	5
Other things/nothing	9	8	6	7	3	14

and so they are going to develop sensitization earlier and more and more children will show this allergy. It might be important to monitor the situation, because the exposure to Ragweed has serious consequences.

Allergy is more common in children whose parents had high school education, as shown also in other studies where this result was interpreted as an easier access to physicians [12].

Although the number of our patients is low for this type of study, it looks like that environmental factors have an influence on respiratory diseases. According to other studies, most of allergic children lived in an urban area. The ISAAC study has shown an increase of asthma and allergy in urban areas because children are exposed to higher levels of outdoor and indoor allergens and pollutants [12]-[16]. On the other hand, most of non allergic children (45%) lived near lakes, an increase of rhinitis in these patients may be associated to the wetter environment.

Also in our study a family history of allergic disorders and the presence of pets at home are associated with the development of allergies. Pets kept at home are more common in allergic children than in non allergic. Even if cats are more often a risk factor for atopy, Anne L. Wright at all. found that atopic rhinitis was associated more with the presence at home of dogs rather than cats; in our study we obtain the same results, possibly because more families kept dogs as opposed to cats. Furthermore, in our study we observed these data because of a higher presence of dogs at home. On the contrary, in the first year of life the situation was different: allergic children weren't exposed to pets, this fact was already observed by Strachan, Von Mutius and Vercelli: early contact with multiple animal species is a protective factor for atopy because there is a modulation of the human immune system [17]-[19].

Although in another study, always adopting the ISAAC questionnaire, it was found an association between antibiotic use in the first year of life and the presence of rhinitis and wheezing in the next years [20], we didn't find this correlation; as it is said in other studies it is difficult to make this correlation because there are too many biases [20]-[22].

Of children studied 44% was exposed to parental smoking, this datum is alarming because environmental tobacco smoke exposure makes rhinitis and especially asthma symptoms worse [23]-[26].

Our data show that sneezing, rhinorrea and blocked nose are more common than the real diagnosis of rhinitis. This was observed in another epidemiological study were nasal symptoms were reported in 16.8% of children while diagnosis of allergic rhinitis was present only in the 4% of the study population. This confirms the fact that allergic rhinitis are underestimated because physicians think more often of a viral cause [6].

We found also an early onset of allergic rhinitis, and after the development of other allergic manifestations. In fact patients between 11 and 15 years old have more often rhinoconjunctivitis and asthma. Rhinitis may be considered a risk factor for the development of asthma, this is important to offer an appropriate treatment to the patient [5]. Moreover rhinitis is frequently associated with rhinoconjunctivitis as it was also shown in phase three of the ISAAC study, where it was reported that rhinoconjunctivitis is increasing in European children especially among children aged 13 - 14 [19].

We also made the diagnosis of non allergic rhinitis in 21 children. Non allergic rhinitis are increasing worldwide, NAR:AR is 1:4, but they are usually underdiagnosed [27].

Most of children received a current treatment, especially allergic patients and subjects with asthma, probably because of the strict follow up undergone in these children. Allergic children are usually treated with Fluticasone and Montelukast, non allergic patients only with Montelukast. On the other hand 25% of children used treatments only when there were symptoms. 23% of patients reported a 1 to 5 school days loss for allergic symptoms, these data support what stated in the European Federation of Allergy and Airways Diseases Patients' Association (EFA) book and by the European Academy of Allergy and Clinical Immunology (EAACI) [1] [4].

6. Conclusion

Our study confirms that allergies are constantly increasing; family history of atopy, pet and smoke exposure, and urban area are risk factors for them. An important raising of positivity to Ragweed was also found. As children are exposed to this allergen since early ages, these data are going to increase in the next years. It is important to pay attention to this fact because it could have important consequences. Rhinitis is more often associated with rhinoconjunctivitis and asthma, especially when the child grows up, and this makes children quality of life worse. Moreover non allergic rhinitis is widespread but underdiagnosed, and so they must be taken into account. All these situations should be considered in order to offer appropriate diagnosis, correct treatments and to give children a better life quality.

References

[1]   A European Declaration on Allergen Immunotherapy. The European Academy of Allergy and Clinical Immunology (EAACI) 2011. http://www.eaaci.org/372-resources/immunotherapy-declaration.html

[2]   Ring, J. (2012) Davos Declaration: Allergy as a Global Problem. *Allergy*, **67**, 141-143. http://dx.doi.org/10.1111/j.1398-9995.2011.02770.x

[3]   Bousquet, J., Schünemann, H.J., Samolinski, B., *et al.* (2012) Allergic Rhinitis and Its Impact on Asthma (ARIA): Achievements in 10 Years and Future Needs. *Journal of Allergy and Clinical Immunology*, **130**, 1049-1062. http://dx.doi.org/10.1016/j.jaci.2012.07.053

[4]   Valovirta, E. (2011) EFA Book on Respiratory Allergies: Raise Awareness, Relieve the Burden. http://www.efanet.org

[5]   Keil, T., Bockelbronk, A., Reich, A., *et al.* (2010) The Natural History of Allergic Rhinitis in Childhood. *Pediatric Allergy and Immunology*, **21**, 962-969. http://dx.doi.org/10.1111/j.1399-3038.2010.01046.x

[6]   Peroni, D.G., Piacentini, G.L., Alfonsi, L., *et al.* (2003) Rhinitis in Pre-School Children: Prevalence, Association with Allergic Diseases and Risk Factors. *Clinical & Experimental Allergy*, **33**, 1349-1354. http://dx.doi.org/10.1046/j.1365-2222.2003.01766.x

[7]   Bousquet, J., Heinzerling, L., Bachert, C., *et al.* (2012) Practical Guide to Skin Prick Tests in Allergy to Aeroallergens. *Allergy*, **67**, 18-24. http://dx.doi.org/10.1111/j.1398-9995.2011.02728.x

[8]   Gelardi, M., Fiorella, M.L., Leo, G. and Incorvaia, C. (2007) Cytology in the Diagnosis of Rhinosinusitis. *Pediatric Allergy and Immunology*, **18**, 50-52. http://dx.doi.org/10.1111/j.1399-3038.2007.00634.x

[9]   The International Study of Asthma and Allergies in Childhood, 2012. http://isaac.auckland.ac.nz/

[10] Tosi, A., Wüthrich, B., Bonini, M. and Pietragalla-Köhler, B. (2011) Time Lag between Ambrosia Sensitisation and Ambrosia Allergy: A 20-Year Study (1989-2008) in Legnano, Northern Italy. *Swiss Medical Weekly*, 9 October 2011, 141:w13253.

[11] Asero, R. (2012) Ragweed Allergy in Northern Italy: Are Patterns of Sensitization Changing? *European Annals of Allergy and Clinical Immunology*, **44**, 157-159.

[12] Morais-Almeida, M., Santos, N., Pereira, A.M., Branco-Ferreira, M., Nunes, C., Bousquet, J. and Fonseca, J.A. (2013) Prevalence and Classification of Rhinitis in Preschool Children in Portugal: A Nationwide Study. *Allergy*, **68**, 1278-1288. http://dx.doi.org/10.1111/all.12221

[13] Wright, A.L., Holberg, C.J., Martinez, F.D., Halonen, M., Morgan, W. and Taussig, L.M. (1994) Epidemiology of Physician-Diagnosed Allergic Rhinitis in Childhood. *Pediatrics*, **94**, 895-901.

[14] Fuertes, E., Butland, B.K., Ross Anderson, H., Carlsten, C., Strachan, D.P. and Brauer, M., ISAAC Phase Three Study Group (2014) Childhood Intermittent and Persistent Rhinitis Prevalence and Climate and Vegetation: A Global Ecologic Analysis. *Annals of Allergy, Asthma & Immunology*, **113**, 386-392.e9. http://dx.doi.org/10.1016/j.anai.2014.06.021

[15] Stafoggia, M., Cesaroni, G., Galassi, C., Badaloni, C. and Forastiere, F. (2014) Long-Term Health Effects of Air Pollution: Results of the European Project ESCAPE. *Recenti Progressi in Medicina*, **105**, 450-453.

[16] Di Menno di Bucchianico, A., Cattani, G., Gaeta, A., Caricchia, A.M., Troiano, F., Sozzi, R., *et al.* (2014) Air Pollution in an Urban Area nearby the Rome-Ciampino City Airport. *Epidemiologia & Prevenzione*, **38**, 244-253.

[17] Genuneit, J. (2012) Exposure to Farming Environments in Childhood and Asthma and Wheeze in Rural Populations: A Systematic Review with Meta-Analysis. *Pediatric Allergy and Immunology*, **23**, 509-518. http://dx.doi.org/10.1111/j.1399-3038.2012.01312.x

[18] Von Mutius, E. and Vercelli, D. (2010) Farm Living: Effects on Childhood Asthma and Allergy. *Nature Reviews Immunology*, **10**, 861-868. http://dx.doi.org/10.1038/nri2871

[19] Genuneit, J., Strachan, D.P., Büchele, G., Weber, J., Loss, G., Sozanska, B., *et al.* (2013) The Combined Effects of Family Size and Farm Exposure on Childhood Hay Fever and Atopy. *Pediatric Allergy and Immunology*, **24**, 293-298. http://dx.doi.org/10.1111/pai.12053

[20] Foliaki, S., Pearce, N., Björksten, B., Mallol, J., Montefort, S., von Mutius, E. and the International Study of Asthma and Allergies in Childhood Phase III Study Group (2009) Antibiotics Use in Infancy and Symptoms of Asthma, Rhinoconjunctivitis, and Eczema in Children 6 and 7 Years Old: International Study of Asthma and Allergies in Childhood Phase III. *Journal of Allergy and Clinical Immunology*, **124**, 982-989. http://dx.doi.org/10.1016/j.jaci.2009.08.017

[21] Gagliardi, L., Rusconi, F., Galassi, C. and Forastiere, F. (2011) Re.: "Antibiotic Exposure by 6 Months and Asthma and Allergy at 6 Years: Findings in a Cohort of 1,401 US Children". *American Journal of Epidemiology*, **173**, 1343. http://dx.doi.org/10.1093/aje/kwr082

[22] Rusconi, F., Gagliardi, L., Galassi, C., Forastiere, F., Brunetti, L., La Grutta, S., Piffer, S. and Talassi, F., SIDRIA-2 Collaborative Group (2011) Paracetamol and Antibiotics in Childhood and Subsequent Development of Wheezing/Asthma: Association or Causation? *International Journal of Epidemiology*, **40**, 662-667. http://dx.doi.org/10.1093/ije/dyq263

[23] Agabiti, N., Mallone, S., Forastiere, F., Corbo, G.M., Ferro, S., Renzoni, E., *et al.* (1999) The Impact of Parental Smoking on Asthma and Wheezing. SIDRIA Collaborative Group. Studi Italiani sui Disturbi Respiratori nell'Infanzia e l'Ambiente. *Epidemiology*, **10**, 692-698. http://dx.doi.org/10.1097/00001648-199911000-00008

[24] Virkkula, P., Liukkonen, K., Suomalainen, A.K., Aronen, E.T., Kirjavainen, T. and Pitkaranta, A. (2011) Parental Smoking Nasal Resistance and Rhinitis in Children. *Acta Paediatrica*, **100**, 1234-1238. http://dx.doi.org/10.1111/j.1651-2227.2011.02240.x

[25] Landau, L.I. (2001) Parental Smoking: Asthma and Wheezing Illnesses in Infants and Children. *Paediatric Respiratory Reviews*, **2**, 202-206. http://dx.doi.org/10.1053/prrv.2001.0141

[26] Silvestri, M., Franchi, S., Pistorio, A., Petecchia, L. and Rusconi, F. (2015) Smoke Exposure, Wheezing, and Asthma Development: A Systematic Review and Meta-Analysis in Unselected Birth Cohorts. *Pediatric Pulmonology*, **50**, 353-362. http://dx.doi.org/10.1002/ppul.23037

[27] Mølgaard, E., Thomsen, S.F., Lund, T., Pedersen, L., Nolte, H. and Backer, V. (2007) Differences between Allergic and Nonallergic Rhinitis in a Large Sample of Adolescents and Adults. *Allergy*, **62**, 1033-1037. http://dx.doi.org/10.1111/j.1398-9995.2007.01355.x

13

Prevalence of Neural Tube Defects: Moroccan Study 2008-2011

Mohammed Amine Radouani[1,2]*, Naima Chahid[1,2]*, Loubna Benmiloud[1,2], Leila El Ammari[3], Aicha Kharbach[1,2], Larbi Rjimati[3], Laila Acharrai[3], Khalid Lahlou[3], Hassan Aguenaou[4], Amina Barkat[1,2]

[1]Department of Medicine and Neonatal Resuscitation, National Center for Neonatology and Nutrition, Rabat, Morocco
[2]Faculté de Medicine et de Pharmacie de Rabat, Université Mohammed V de Rabat, Rabat, Morocco
[3]Population Department, Ministry of Health, Rabat, Morocco
[4]Joint Research Unit in Nutrition and Food URAC 39, (Ibn Tofaïl University—CNESTEN), Regional Designated Center of Nutrition Associated with AFRA/IAEA, Kénitra, Morocco
Email: barakatamina@yahoo.fr, dr.med.radouani@gmail.com

Abstract

Background: Neural tube defects have a considerable importance because they can be prevented by supplementing Folic acid & Vitamin B12 during periconceptional period and fortification of staple foods. In Morocco, the Ministry of Health launched a national program for fortification of flour with folic acid. Our goal should be to evaluate the prevalence of neural tube defects after fortification. Description: This is a retrospective descriptive at the National Reference Centre for Nutrition and Neonatology of the Children's Hospital of Rabat over 4 years. Data were identified from the registry of congenital malformations held at the perinatology unit. Results: During the 4 years, 674 congenital malformations were identified. The neural tube defects NTDs account for 11.9%. Their annual prevalence decreased significantly from 21.78 in 2008 to 12.1 per 10,000 total births in 2011. The most common form was anencephaly (60%). Neural tube defects were isolated in 85% of cases and associated with other malformations in 15% of cases. 49.4% of infants with neural tube defects were female and 50.6% were male. Perinatal mortality in newborns with neural tube defects was 63.8% versus 25.2% in malformed newborns without neural tube defects. Conclusions: The neural tube defects seem to be common in our context. Permanent epidemiological surveillance is needed to determine the true prevalence at the national as well as its temporal trends level.

Keywords

Neural Tube Defects, Anencephaly, Spina Bifida, Folic Acid, Prevalence

---

*These two authors have equal contribution.

1. Background

The term "Neural tube defects" means a group of birth defects resulting from defective closure of the neural tube during embryogenesis, about 25 - 27 days after conception [1]. This accident can occur at any level of the neural plate, the cephalic end to the caudal end, and to a variable extent. This results in abnormalities of the meninges, the bony structures (vertebrae or skull), and integument compared with a variable impact on the nervous tissue [2]. These malformations are usually divided into cephalic and spinal forms. They include anencephaly, spina bifida and encephalocele [3]. The importance of this type of malformations due to both morbidity and mortality they cause and the opportunities that exist to control the appearance by means of primary prevention. There are two possibilities for this prevention: systematic drug supplementation and fortification of staple foods. Means neither is sufficient in itself and it is probably a combination of the two that will prevent the neural tube defects [4].

Reddi Rani, Manjula in their clinical and USG study of evaluation of 100 cases of polyhydramnios observed 40 babies with congenital anomalies, and 21 cases had craniospinal CNS anomalies [52.5%]. NTDs were 14 3 [14%] [5]. Balakumar K. studied 30,030 singleton 9 41 weeks gestation, ultrasonography done and the analysis reported as 2.59% had major foetal anomalies, 336 cases [39.20%] had CNS anomalies, NTDs were 250 [0.83%] [6]. Sania Tanveer *et al.* reported study of 3310 deliveries and 46 cases with NTDs giving incidence of 1.39%. Ghanashyam Das *et al.* [7] reported a rare occurence of a case of Dizygotic twin with meningomyelocele in both the 7 babies.

Ministry of Health in Morrocco, with the support of its partners, has launched a national flour fortification with folic acid and conducted a pilot experience at 20 public health centers and 4 hospital departments. The results reported an estimated 33.6 per 10,000 live births before starting the fortification program in Morocco [4].

The purpose of this study was to evaluate the prevalence of NTDs changes at the National Reference Centre for Nutrition and Neonatology of the Children's Hospital of Rabat during the years 2008, 2009, 2010 and 2011, during which the fortified flour with folic acid is on the Moroccan market.

2. Construction and Content

2.1. Data Source

This is a unicentric retrospective descriptive study at the National Reference Centre for Nutrition and Neonatology of the Children's Hospital of Rabat over a period of 4 years between 1 January 2008 and 31 December 2011 data were recorded from the register of Congenital Malformations held at the perinatology unit. The sex of the newborn, its viability at birth and the type of malformation.

Case definition: All defects were taken into account whether single or multiple. Malformations were classified according to the categories proposed by the standardized classification of European surveillance of congenital anomalies. These categories are: nervous system, eye, ear, face, neck, heart, respiratory system, oral facial clefts, the digestive system, abdominal wall, the urogenital system, members and anomalies chromosome (EUROCAT: www.eurocat-network.eu).

Newborn with malformation syndromes were classified polymalformation. Newborns whose specific type of malformation was not mentioned on the record or having a defect that is not part of the categories listed above were classified in the category unspecified malformation or other. NTDs are classified in the category of malformations of the nervous system and include cases of anencephaly, spina bifida and isolated or associated with other malformations of the nervous system malformations classified in other categories encephalocele.

The prevalence of congenital malformations of all types refers to the number of newborns with malformations among births (live births and stillbirths), divided by the total number of births. The prevalence of NTDs in turn refers to the number of newborns with NTDs among births (live births and stillbirths), divided by the total number of births.

Immediate perinatal mortality in infants malformed corresponds to the number of stillbirths and deaths in the delivery room with a malformation based on the total number of malformed newborns.

2.2. Statistical Analysis

The statistical study was performed using SPSS Version 17.0 software. Data were expressed as percentages and comparisons were performed by the Chi^2 test (χ^2) of Pearson. A p value less than 0.05 was used as the threshold for statistical significance.

3. Results

- Birth defects of all types

The number of total births registered during the 4 years was 60,017: 13,768 in 2008, 14,569 in 2009, 15,152 in 2010 and 16,528 in 2011; 492 malformed infants were identified.

The annual prevalence decreased from 98.77 per 10,000 total births in 2008 to 80.46 in 2011. This decrease is not statistically significant (p = 0.07) (**Figure 1**). 54.5% of infants were male, 42.1% female and 3.4% of unknown sex. 13.4% of infants were stillborn. Early neonatal deaths were recorded in 18.1% of cases. The most common malformations were neurological malformations (20%) and first NTDs (11.9%) (**Table 1**).

- NTDs

3.1. Prevalence

The annual prevalence of NTDs has declined significantly between 2008 and 2011 (p = 0.01) (**Figure 2**). That of anencephaly increased from 15.25 in 2008 to 7.86 per 10,000 total births in 2011 (**Figure 3**). This decrease was statistically significant (p < 0.01). About spina bifida, prevalence decreased non significantly between 2008 and 2011 (p = 0.7) (**Figure 4**). A single case of encephalocele was recorded in 2008.

3.2. Distribution of NTDs by Type

Eighty neural tube defects were identified. The most common form was anencephaly (60%). Spina bifida was found in 38.8% of cases.

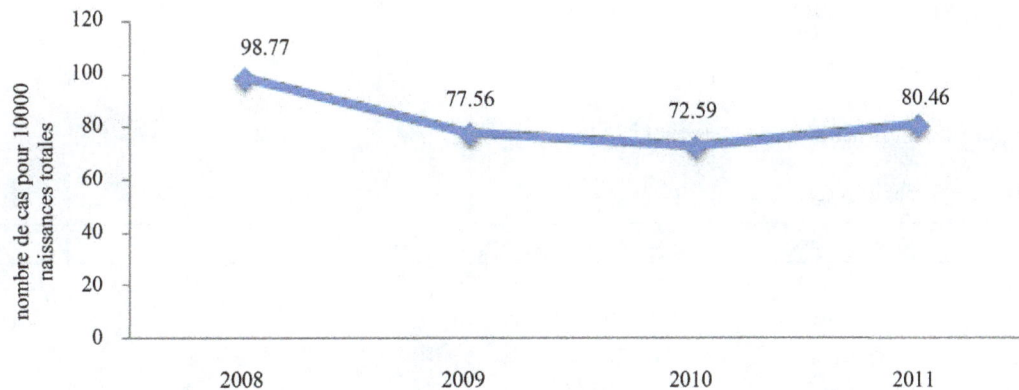

Figure 1. Prevalence of congenital malformations 2008-2011.

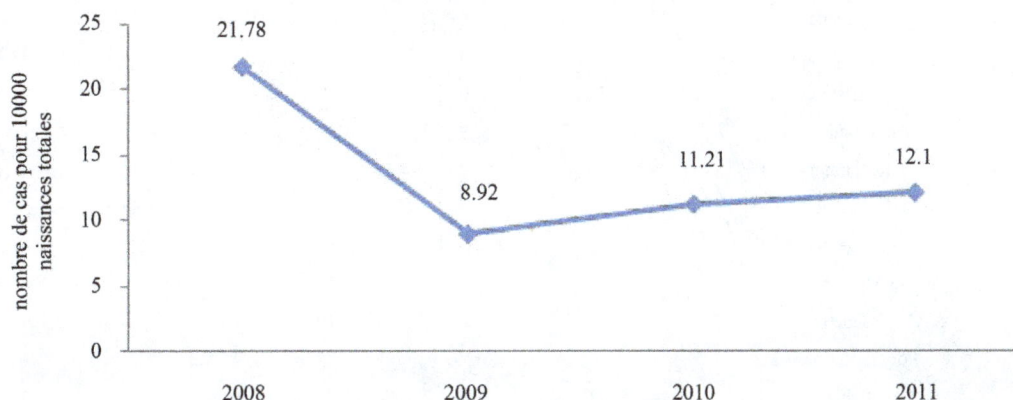

Figure 2. Prevalence of NTDs 2008-2011.

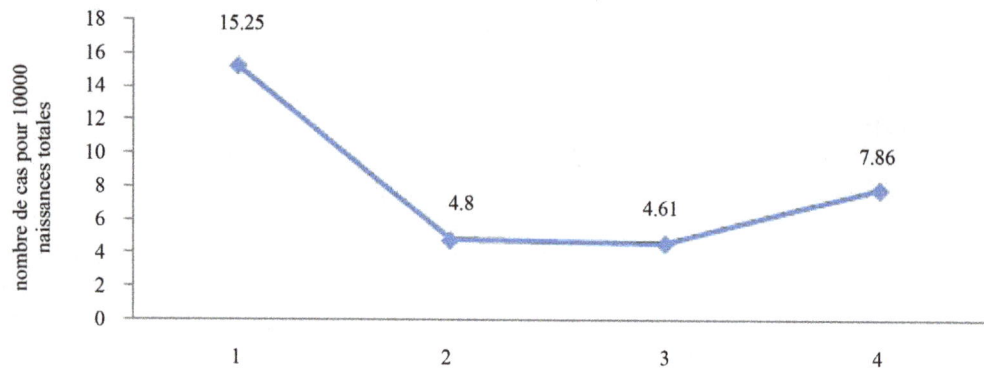

Figure 3. Prevalence of anencephaly 2008-2011.

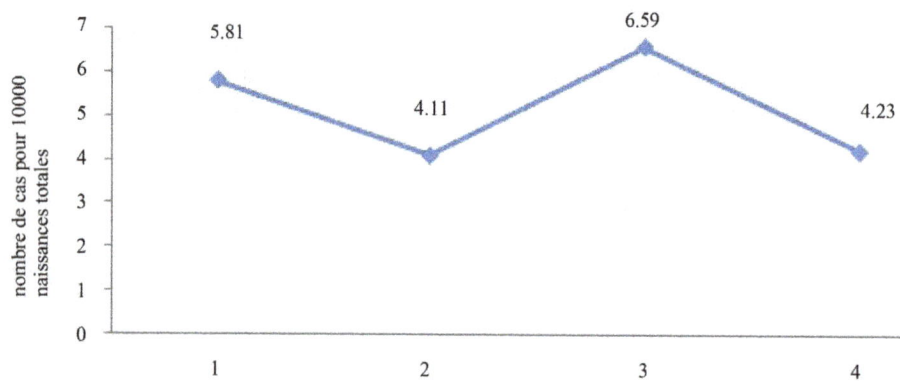

Figure 4. Prevalence of spina bifida 2008-2011.

Table 1. Types of NTDs.

Malformation	2008	2009	2010	2011	Total
Neurological	50	19	31	33	133 (19.7%)
Neural tube	30	13	17	20	80 (11.9%)
Microcephaly	0	1	1	0	2 (0.3%)
Hydrocephaly	17	4	11	12	44 (6.5%)
Others	3	1	2	1	7 (1%)
Eye	1	1	1	0	3 (0.4%)
Ear, face	4	4	3	3	14 (2%)
Orofacial clefts	9	3	9	12	33 (4.9%)
Digestive	5	0	3	0	8 (1.2%)
Abdominal wall	8	3	5	2	18 (2.7%)
Respiratory	1	0	2	0	3 (0.4%)
Cardiac	1	0	1	0	2 (0.3%)
Urogenital	14	14	10	14	52 (7.7%)
Membres	24	28	22	25	99 (14.7%)
Genetic	16	17	10	16	59 (8.8%)
Polymalformation	17	19	23	28	87 (13%)
Others	8	10	1	11	30 (4.5%)
Total	208	137	152	177	674

3.3. Distribution of NTDs by Isolated or Associated Character with Other Abnormalities

NTDs were isolated in 85% of cases and associated with other malformations in 15% of cases. Of the 48 children with anencephaly, 3 had other malformations polymalformation in 2 children and ambiguity and clubfoot in children. Spina bifida was isolated from 22 newborns and associated with other malformations in 9 neonates (**Table 2**).

3.4. Sex Distribution

49.4% of infants with neural tube defects were female and 50.6% male. The difference is not significant (p = 0.26). 54.3% of anencephalic infants were female and 45.7% male. Statistically, the difference was not significant (p = 0.12). 43.9% of newborns with spina bifida were female and 56.7% male. The difference is not significant (p = 0.97). The only patient with an encephalocele is a boy.

3.5. Immediate Perinatal Mortality

Perinatal mortality in newborns with neural tube defects was 63.8% against 25.2% in newborns without malformed neural tube defects. The difference is statistically significant (p < 0.01).

4. Utility and Discussion

Birth defects are the leading cause of infant mortality in developed countries [8] and they are among the five leading causes in many developing countries [9].

Malformations of the central nervous system are the most common birth defects and NTDs constitute the greater part [2]. In our work, malformations of the nervous system are the most frequent and the first neural tube defects. NTDs are the result of a combination of environmental and genetic factors. Only nutritional factors are risk factors on which it is possible to influence [10].

Folate (vitamin B9) and vitamin B12 are very important in reducing the occurrences of NTDs [11]. Folate is required for the production and maintenance of new cells, for DNA synthesis and RNA synthesis. Folate is needed to carry one carbon groups for methylation and nucleic acid synthesis. It has been hypothesized that the early human embryo may be particularly vulnerable to folate deficiency due to differences of the functional enzymes in this pathway during embryogenesis combined with high demand for post translational methylations

Table 2. Distribution of NTDs based on single or associated character.

Anomalies	Number of cases
Isolated NTD	68 (85%)
Anencephaly	45
Spina bifida	22
Encephalocele	1
Associeted NTD	12 (15%)
Spina bifida + hydrocephaly	4
Spina bifida + macrocrania	1
Spina bifida, cleft lip and palate, malformation of members, cardiopathy	1
Spina bifida, club foot, trisomic facies	1
Spina bifida + club foot	1
Anencephaly + polymalformation	2
Anencephaly, trouble of sex differences, club foot	1
Spina bifida + polymalformation	1

Neural tube defects (NTDs).

of the cytoskeleton in neural cells during neural tube closure [11].

The association seen between reduced neural tube defects and folic acid supplementation is due to a gene-environment interaction such as venerability caused by the C677T Methylenetetrahydro folate reductase (MTHFR) variant. Supplementing folic acid during pregnancy reduces the prevalence of NTDs by not exposing this otherwise sub-clinical mutation to aggravating conditions [12].

Other potential causes can include folate antimetabolites (such as methotrexate), maternal diabetes, maternal obesity, mycotoxins in contaminated corn meal, arsenic, hyperthermia in early development, and radiation [13]. Studies have shown that both maternal cigarette smoking and maternal exposure to secondhand smoke increased the risk for neural tube defects in offspring. A mechanism by which maternal exposure to cigarette smoke could increase NTD risk in offspring is suggested by several studies that show an association between cigarette smoking and elevations of homocysteine levels. The study suggests that cigarette smoke, including secondhand exposure, is not only hazardous to the mother, but may also interfere with neural tube closure in the developing embryo [14].

All of the above may act by interference with some aspect of normal folic acid metabolism and folate linked methylation related cellular processes as there are multiple genes of this type associated with neural tube defects.

Our cohort allowed having an annual incidence of occurrence of TND based solely on the parturients s prenatal care regardless of other known risk factors in the literature.

Many interventional and observational studies have shown that 50% to 70% of NTDs can be prevented by supplementing Folic acid & Vitamin B12 during periconceptional period [15]. These data led, in 1992, health authorities in several countries to advocate routine supplementation for all women in the periconceptional period, using synthetic folic acid at a daily dose of 400 mcg orally in the general population and 4 mg in women who have had one child with NTD [16]. Today, approximately 40 countries have mandated the fortification of flour with folic acid [9]. More recently several studies on the effects of folic acid fortification have been published [16].

The protective effect was confirmed in several countries and regions studied and ranged from 16% to 78% [17]. Trough these data, Morocco has adopted a national program of fortification of flour with folic acid since 2007. Nevertheless, this strategy has not yet been assessed nationally.

At maternity care Souissi, the prevalence of neural tube defects has declined between 2008 and 2011 in a meaningful way. This decrease is mainly attributed to the decrease in prevalence of anencephaly which decreased 15.25 2008 7.86 in 2011. Although the relationship of cause and effect can not be inferred, the decrease prevalence of NTDs could be explained by the effect of fortification but also by improving prenatal diagnosis. However, the observed prevalence of NTDs remains high compared to other countries which have decided the systematic fortification of flour with folic acid as Chile 8.6 per 10,000 births [18] and Costa Rica 5.04 per 10,000 births [9]. This little be explained by geographic and ethnic variations that have been reported in the literature [2]-[19].

Anencephaly is the most common neural tube defects form. It represents 50% to 65% [20]. In our series, it was found in 60% of cases reported during the 4 years. NTDs are more common in newborns female [20]. This predominance is more pronounced for anencephalic infants [20]. In our series, a female predominance was observed in newborns with NTDs and in anencephalic infants, but the difference with malformed infants not having a neural tube defect is not significant.

The association of neural tube defects with other malformations has been reported in the literature in 20% of cases [8]. This was found in 15% of neonates in our series.

5. Conclusion

The TNDs are purveyors of high mortality and morbidity. They seem to be common in our context from the data of this work. Permanent epidemiological surveillance is needed to determine the true prevalence at the national as well as its time trend. It will also enable to evaluate strategies of health authorities concerning such defects. For this, the establishment of a national registry of NTDs is necessary. The participation of health actors whether it be general practitioners, gynecology obstetricians, paediatricians and midwives is essential.

Acknowledgements

To all the mothers and babies who contributed to the study.

Competing Interests

The authors declare that there are no conflicts of interest and shall disclose any potential conflicts of interest in the future.

Authors' Contributions

Hajar Rhouda, N. Chahid, M.A. Radouani: Writing. L. Elammari, Aicha Kharbach, A. Rjimati, L. Acharaai, K. Lahlou: Collect data. Amina Barkat: Reading and correcting.

Ethical Approval Statement

Read and approved by the Ethics Committee of the Faculty of Medicine and Pharmacy of Rabat.

References

[1]   Moore, K.L. and Persaud, T.V.N. (1998) The Developing Human. Clinically Oriented Embryology. WB Saunders Company, Toronto.

[2]   Cabaret, A.S. (2004) Les malformations du tube neural: Ethiopathogénie et facteurs pronostiques: A partir de 83 cas du centre pluridisciplinaire du diagnostic prénatal de Rennes [Thèse]. Université de Rennes, Rennes.

[3]   Elwood, M., Elwood, H. and Little, J. (1992) Epidemiology and Control of Neural Tube Defects. Oxford University Press, Oxford.

[4]   Barkat, A., Elammari, L., Acharai, L., Rjimati, L., Mahfoudi, M., Zerrari, A., *et al.* (2009) Malformations en rapport avec un déficit en acide folique: De la notification à la prévention. *Biosanté*, **2**, 13-17.

[5]   Reddi Rani, M. (2003) Clinical and Ultrasonographic Evaluation of Polyhydramnios. *The Journal of Obstetrics and Gynecology of India*, **53**, 145-148.

[6]   Balakumar, K. (2007) Major Anatomical Fetal Anomalies in Northern Kerala. *The Journal of Obstetrics and Gynecology of India*, **57**, 311-315.

[7]   Das, G., Aggarwal, A. and Faridi. M.M.A. (2003) Dizygotic Twins with Myelomeningocele. *Indian Journal of Paediatrics*, **70**, 265-267. http://dx.doi.org/10.1007/BF02725595

[8]   Stevenson, R.E., Allen, W.P., Pai, G.S., Best, R., Seaver, L.H., Dean, J., *et al.* (2000) Decline in Prevalence of Neural Tube Defects in a High-Risk Region of the United States. *Pediatrics*, **106**, 677-683. http://dx.doi.org/10.1542/peds.106.4.677

[9]   Barboza Argüello, M.L. and Umaña Solís, L.M. (2011) Impacto de la fortificación de alimentos con ácido fólico en los defectos del tubo neural en Costa Rica. *American Journal of Public Health*, **30**, 1-6.

[10] Wanat, S., Brazier, M., Boitte, F. and Lemay, C. (2005) Serum Levels of Vitamin B9 and B12 in Women with a Pregnancy Complicated by Neural Tube Defects. *Immunology & Cell Biology*, **20**, 28-31.

[11] Molloy, A.M., Kirke, P.N., Troendle, J.F., Burke, H., Sutton, M., Brody, L.C., Scott, J.M. and Mills, J.L. (2009) Maternal Vitamin B-12 Status and Risk of Neural Tube Defects in a Population with High Neural Tube Defect Prevalence and No Folic Acid Fortification. *Pediatrics*, **123**, 917-923. http://dx.doi.org/10.1542/peds.2008-1173

[12] Yan, L.F., Zhao, L., Long, Y., Zou, P., Ji, G.X., Gu, A.H. and Zhao, P. (2012) Association of the Maternal MTHFR C677T Polymorphism with Susceptibility to Neural Tube Defects in Offsprings: Evidence from 25 Case-Control Studies. *PLoS ONE*, **7**, e41689. http://dx.doi.org/10.1371/journal.pone.0041689

[13] Neural Tube Defects at eMedicine.

[14] Suarez, L., Felkner, M., Brender, J.D., Canfield, M. and Hendricks, K. (2008) Maternal Exposures to Cigarette Smoke, Alcohol, and Street Drugs and Neural Tube Defect Occurrence in Offspring. *Maternal and Child Health Journal*, **12**, 394-401. http://dx.doi.org/10.1007/s10995-007-0251-y

[15] De Wals, P., Tairou, F., Ouakki, M. and Six, M. (2007) Impact de la politique d'enrichissement des farines par l'acide folique sur la fréquence des malformations congénitales au Québec. Direction des risques biologiques, environnementaux et occupationnels. Institut national de santé publique du Québec.

[16] Vidailhet, M., Bocquet, A., Bresson, J.L., Briend, A., Chouraqui, J.P., Dupont, C., *et al.* (2008) Prévention par l'acide folique des défauts de fermeture du tube neural: La question n'est toujours pas réglée. *Archives de Pédiatrie*, **15**, 1223-1231. http://dx.doi.org/10.1016/j.arcped.2008.04.012

[17] Santos, L.M.P. and Pereira, M.Z. (2007) Efeito da fortifi cação com ácido fólico na redução dos defeitos do tubo neural. *Cadernos de Saúde Pública*, **23**, 17-24. http://dx.doi.org/10.1590/S0102-311X2007000100003

[18] Cortés, F., Mellado, C., Pardo, R.A., Villarroel, L.A. and Hertrampf, E. (2012) Wheat Flour Fortification with Folic Acid: Changes in Neural Tube Defects Rates in Chile. *American Journal of Medical Genetics Part A*, **158**, 1885-1890. http://dx.doi.org/10.1002/ajmg.a.35430

[19] Zhu, J., Li, X.H., Wang, Y.P., Mu, D.Z., Dai, L., Zhou, G.X., *et al.* (2012) Prevalence of Neural Tube Defect Pregnancies in China and the Impact of Gestational Age of the Births from 2006 to 2008: A Hospital-Based Study. *Journal of Maternal-Fetal and Neonatal Medicine*, **25**, 1730-1734. http://dx.doi.org/10.3109/14767058.2012.663022

[20] Himmetoglu, O., Tiras, M.B., Gursoy, R., Karabacak, O., Sahin, I. and Onan, A. (1996) The Incidence of Congenital Malformations in a Turkish Population. *International Journal of Gynecology & Obstetrics*, **55**, 117-121. http://dx.doi.org/10.1016/S0020-7292(96)02743-9

List of Abbreviations

NTDs: Neural tube defects

14

On Relationship between Pediatric Shi Ji and Fever

Xiangyu Hu*, Lina Hu

Pingdingshang City Hospital of Traditional Chinese Medicine, Pingdingshan, China
Email: *pds-hxy025@163.com

Abstract

Based on the clinical effect of the treatment on 546 Pediatric Shi Ji fever cases, the thesis tries to explore the effectiveness of Traditional Chinese Medicine(TCM) treatment on Pediatric Shi Ji and the relationship between Pediatric Shi Ji and fever. The methodology applied is a retrospective analysis on the clinical curative effect of TCM treatment on Shi Ji fever cases in our hospital from January 2008 to December 2012. And the results show that a total effective rate of 96.3% could be guaranteed through either oral Chinese Medicinal Herbs, Chinese Medicine Enema, Massage Therapy, or navel administration with TCM. The thesis holds that Pediatric Shi Ji may cause fever, which could be cured simply by applying TCM treatment (promoting digestion to eliminate stagnation) with less or no use of antibiotics.

Keywords

TCM, Pediatric Shi Ji, Fever, Retrospective Analysis

1. Introduction

Similar to digestive function disorder in western medicine, Shi Ji (Indigestion with Food Retention) is a common kind of pediatric symptom, which can result in poor appetite, dyspepsia, diarrhea, constipation, even fever and sometimes multiple organ function damage such as respiratory system, cardiovascular system, nervous system, etc. For the last six years, as high as 546 fever cases caused by Pediatric Shi Ji have been diagnosed in our Hospital as follows:

2. Materials and Methods

2.1. Source

566 pediatric cases from our hospital in-patient department (233 cases) and outpatient department (312 cases)

---
*Corresponding author.

from January 2008 to December 2012; Within which, 73 cases aged from 1 to 6 months, 186 cases aged from 7 to 36 months, 148 cases aged from 4 to 7 years, and 49 cases from 8 to 14 years old; Temperature: about 368 cases between 37.5°C and 38.5°C, 246 cases between 38.5°C and 38.9°C, 50 cases above 40°C.

2.2. Methods

Ruling out other causes of fever and giving the corresponding treatment in accordance with the classification of indigestion with food retention. Using treatments like traditional Chinese herbal medicine, preparation, chiropractics, enema and massage therapy with less or no use of antibiotics and antipyretic drugs. Based on the observatory findings of the heat fading conditions and the possible complications, the thesis tries to make further summary, analysis, induction and consolidation.

2.3. Traditional Chinese Medicine (TCM) Zhu San

For two or more symptoms like nausea, vomiting, abdominal distension, distending pain, thick white coating, it belongs to the food retention in the stomach (basic type) and can be treated with Chiropractic Therapy, sanjia, shenling and baikou; For symptoms like vermilion, red tongue, irritability, feverish sensation in the palms and soles, yellow tongue, it belongs to the heat type of children food retention and can be treated with two more reagent like detoxification and calculus bovis; for two or more symptoms like hypodynamia, Emaciation, yellow or white dry coating, and thin sloppy stool, it belongs to the spleen injury type of children food retention and also needs combine with astringent prescription, etc.

2.4. Other Treatments

1) Natrii powder 3 g, pepper 0.5 g, grinded into powder and mixed white vinegar into paste, daily dressing change. Used for heavier infantile indigestion with food retention.

2) Radix et Rhizoma Rhei 30 g, mirabilite 20 g, grinded into powder and then mixed white vinegar into paste, daily dressing change. Applied for symptoms like abdominal distension, abdominal pain and constipation caused by indigestion.

3) Vinasse 100 g, fried hot, put into two bags, alternatively fomenting abdomen. 1 time per day, 2 to 3 hours each time. Used for spleen deficiency syndrome caused by indigestion.

4) Massage Therapy: Push and knead Banmen point 100 times, Qing dachang 100 times, Zhong wan 100 times, Fu yinyang 50 times, and massage abdominal for 2 minutes, Push and knead Zong sanli 100 times, Qi jiegu 100 times, push Spine 10 times and chiropractic 3 - 5 times. For children with inner Ji of milk food, nip Si feng 10 times, Na dujia 3 - 5 times, or combined with needling Si feng. For children with spleen deficiency syndrome caused by indigestion, Push and knead Pitu 100 times, Yun Shui Ru Tu 100 times.

5) Chinese Medicine Enema, Endothelium corneum, medicated leaven, malt, parched hawthorn fruit, radish seed, dried tangerine or orange peel, poria cocos, pinellia, Fried hovenia dulcis, Radix Aucklandiae, etc. for Children with heavy internal heating, mixed with Coptis chinensis, plaster stone, Capejasmine, Forsythia, etc. 2 times a day, and 100 - 200 ml for retention enema.

2.5. Standard for Treatment Effect

Cured: 24 - 48 hours after medication, both temperature and diet return to normal, other symptoms disappear; Significant effective: 24 - 48 hours after medication, temperature returns to normal, diet almost back to normal, most of the main symptoms disappear. Effective: 73 - 96 hours after medication, temperature is significantly lowered, main symptoms are eased. Invalid: either physical signs or symptoms are not changed.

3. Results

For the 566 pediatric cases, 354 cases were cured in 2 or 3 days by taking TCM Zhu san; 123 cases that have difficulty in taking drugs were treated with Chinese medicine enema and were cured in 3 days; the rest 49 cases were cured in 3 to 4 days through not only enema, but also the mixed use of massage therapy and navel administration with Chinese traditional medicine; 20 cases with other symptoms or poor effects were transferred to other treatments. In sum, we have up to 96.3% total effective rate.

4. Discussions

The Word *Shi Ji* (Indigestion with food retention), appeared for the first time in book *Confucians' Duties to Parents* [1]. Shortly after, another book, *Symptom Disease Cause Pulse Manifestation Therapeutic Methods*, specifically spent several chapters discussing the following symptoms which are, Shiji Kesou or Dyspeptic coughs (Cough caused by Indigestion) [2]; Shiji Xiexie or Dyspeptic diarrhea (diarrhea caused by indigestion); Shiji Futong or Dyspeptic abdominalgia (Abdominal pain caused by indigestion) [2] and so on. Then much attention has been paid to symptoms caused by indigestion. Shen Jinao in Qing Dynasty took a further look on the disease: "most pediatric diseases are caused by indigestion of the milk food, or by the six pathogenic factors (wind, cold, summer heat, humidity, dryness and fire) combined with dyspepsia. So Shi Ji is specially listed out and is different from Jipi (literally, Indigestion addiction)" [3]. Shi Ji is resulted from improper feeding. The stagnated food stops in stomach and intestine and leads to spleen dysfunction, which in the end causes spleen-stomach or in other words, digestive system disease. Clinically, it is characterized with no appetite, abdominal distention, eructation with fetid odor, and sour stool or constipation. Shi Ji is also called stagnation, which is similar to indigestion or digestive disorder in Western medicine. The symptom may occur throughout the year and has a higher incidence in summer and autumn due to the summer damp-heat traps the spleen qi. Children of all age groups can be onset but with more frequency in infants, and the disease is often complicated with cold, diarrhea and malnutrition. Infants who have spleen-stomach weakness, innate deficiency or experience artificial feeding are easily attacked by such disease repeatedly. A minority of children who suffer long-time dyspepsia and persistent loss of treatment will have their spleen and stomach function badly damaged, which in turn hinders the absorption of nutrition and the growth of body, and reduces into Gan (malnutrition). That is the reason why our forefathers expressed this way: "Ji is the mother of Gan, if there is no Ji, Gan will be non-existent." *Causes and Manifestations of Children's Miscellaneous Diseases* is the book that originally recorded the disease by using the term *Dyspepsia Syndrome* and *Hyperhagia* [4]. After that *Huo You Xin Shu* applied *Ji syndrome* to name the disease while *Ying Tong Bai Wen* used *Ji Zhi* [5]. Another book *Essentials of the Care of Infants Cold-Heat Syndrome of Shi Ji*) clearly pointed out that Pediatric Shi Ji is resulted from "long-term indigestion of the milk food because of the deficiency cold in spleen and stomach" [6].

As the living standards continue to improve, more and more types of food come onto people's table. In order to supply their children with nutrition, mothers and fathers blindly give their children nutritional supplements. Such high intensity has had serious impact on children's stomach and spleen function. The infantile period is a growing stage for children, during that period many of their body's functions are not in shape, especially the digestive system function is relatively weak, the secretion of digestive fluid is too little and therefore the gastrointestinal absorption ability is very poor. And what's more, children can not control themselves like adults, if parents feed them a bit carelessly; it is likely to cause digestive function disorder. When the milk food comes into the stomach, it can not be properly digested and absorbed, which will damage both stomach and spleen function, and will cause indigestion with food retention. After a period of time this will be transformed into heat, if combined with indigestion, will produce internal heat. If continued, it is bound to lead to fever accompanied by symptoms such as abdominal pain, bloating, belching, sour stool, constipation, and even symptoms like dysphoria, poor sleep, sweating for some children. Based on previous experiences, we can say the fever caused by infantile Shi Ji is not characterized by high temperature but low, and with the feeling of thirst.

Through recent years' observation, we have found it is not uncommon for some of such high fever cases lasting for a long period of time [7] [8]. The treatment of this fever should focus on promoting digestion to eliminate stagnation. Fever will naturally disappear if the stagnation is eliminated. In addition, other treatments like massage, chiropractic therapy could also be used to cure the fever effectively. Western medicine believes that for children, their digestive function is not yet perfect, bacteria planted in their intestinal and antibodies are relatively fewer than normal; indigestion can cause gastrointestinal dysfunction, lower immunity, gastric acid secretion decrease, which in turn causes food indigestion; and besides, enteric pathogenic bacteria breed quickly and are absorbed into the bloodstream through the intestinal mucosa, which may cause fever, multiple organ damage and many complications, even have life-threatening consequence to the children.

According to Chinese medicine, fever caused by Shi Ji, is divided into two categories: exogenous fever and fever of internal injury. The former is initiated by the struggle between vital qi of human body and exogenous pathogenic factors perceived by human body. The latter is related to factors like diet, tiredness or injury of seven emotions namely, joy, anger, worry, fear, love, hate and desire. These factors may result in viscera dysfunction,

Qi-blood imbalance, and excess of either yin or yang, which in turn bring about fever. For children, the circulation of vital energy is not sufficient; the viscera are very delicate, their liver and intestine functions are good, yet the spleen is aesthetically susceptible. And besides, children's feeling of hunger is not quite obvious, they can't tell if it is enough for food and drinks. If given unsuitable or coarse food, they are easily hurt. Pediatric pathogenesis has the following characteristics: they get sick easily; the symptom spreads and changes rapidly; food retention transforms into internal fever easily and can lead to the coexistence of fever and indigestion. Clinically, such cases are more common and the chief complaint is fever. Some doctors often treat the fever with antibiotics, which not only fails to cure the fever, but causes gastrointestinal symptoms, even allergic reactions after the use of antibiotics and antipyretic. In the past, due to the limitation of living condition, there was a shortage of nutrients, even if the function of spleen and stomach is very good, malnutrition still could not be prevented because of the shortage. Now the living standard is obviously improved and the majority of families have only one child, which make the parents overindulge their children. What's more, Media mislead the public to take more nutritional Foods; some parents even force their children to eat, which causes children have strong negative mentality. As time passes it develops into indigestion with food retention, seriously malnutritional stagnation and even all kinds of disease.

Through the discussion of the connection between fever and pediatric indigestion with food retention, the paper tries to explore the theoretical relationship of both Western medicine and Chinese medicine in the area. And furthermore, In order to enhance children's physical quality, reduce the occurrence of disease, and promote the healthy growth of children, the paper tries to give tips on how to feed children scientifically, as well as how to treat the fever by Chinese medicine with less or no use of antibiotics.

References

[1]   Zhang, H.C., *et al*. (1984) Revised Confucians' Duties to Their Parents. Henan Scientific and Technical Publishers.

[2]   Qin, J.M. (1990) Symptom Disease Cause Pulse Manifestation Therapeutic Methods. Shanghai Scientific and Technical Publishers, Shanghai.

[3]   Shen, J.N. (1980) You Ke Shi Mi. Shanghai Scientific and Technical Publishers, Shanghai.

[4]   Chao, Y.F. (2008) Treatise on Causes and Manifestations of Various Diseases. Huaxia Press, Beijing.

[5]   Sun, H.S. (2005) Golden Mirror of Medicine. Youke Xinfayaojue Baihuajie. People's Medical Publishing House, Beijing.

[6]   Chen, F.Z. (2006) You You Ji Cheng. People's Medical Publishing House, Beijing.

[7]   Wang, H.T. (2010) The Self-Made Soup Reach of the Original Cold Solution Heat Treatment 36 Cases of Children with Food Product Efficacy. *Journal of Traditional Chinese Medicine*, **03**, 41-542.

[8]   Liang, J.J. (2004) The Heat-Clearing and Eliminate Stagnation Method Reach of the Original Cold Solution Heat Treatment 30 Cases of Children with Food Product Efficacy. *Journal of Emergency in Traditional Chinese Medicine*, **10**, 640.

15

Establishment of Growth Curves to Full Term Newborns: A Moroccan Study

Mohamed Amine Radouani[1], Salem Ananou[1], Mustapha Mrabet[2], Aicha Kharbach[1], Hassan Aguenaou[3], Amina Barkat[1,4*]

[1]Research Team on Health and Nutrition of Mother and Child, Faculty of Medicine and Pharmacy of Rabat, Mohammed V University of Rabat, Rabat, Morocco
[2]Teaching and Research Unit of Public Health, Research Team on Health and Nutrition of Mother and Child, Faculty of Medicine and Pharmacy of Rabat, Mohammed V University of Rabat, Rabat, Morocco
[3]Joint Research Unit in Nutrition and Food URAC 39 (Ibn Tofaïl University—CNESTEN), Designated Regional Center of Nutrition Partner of AFRA/IAEA, Kenitra, Morocco
[4]Department of Medicine and Neonatal Resuscitation, National Center for Neonatology and Nutrition, Rabat, Morocco
Email: dr.med.radouani@gmail.com, slemananou@gmail.com, aichakh@hotmail.com, mrabetmp@gmail.com, *barakatamina@hotmail.fr

Abstract

Neonatal anthropometric data is an important reflection of the growth and fetal development. Objective: Knowing the anthropometric standards of Moroccan newborns according to sex, gestational age, parity, age and corpulence of women. Materials and Methods: Prospective and cross-sectional study. The information forward newborns alive, healthy, Moroccan parents, from normal pregnancies, born in Rabat Souissi's maternity between January 2008 and December 2013, was gathered. Results: 5000 births were recruited. The ratio was balanced. Anthropometric standards identified according to gestational age and gender were lower than the Frenchs (AUDIPOG) and Tunisians. With our curves, we determined new thresholds for SGA and macrosomia. Factors influencing fetal growth, it was verified, in addition to sex and gestational age of the newborn, age, parity and maternal body mass index (BMI), that have proven determinants of fetal growth in our context. Conclusion: The curves of birth weight, height and head circumference of Moroccan newborns recruited have determined a new thresholds for hypotrophy and macrosomia.

Keywords

Anthropometric Data, Gestational, Age, Parity, Corpulence, Hypotrophy, Macrosomia

---

*Corresponding author.

1. Introduction

The assessment of intrauterine growth based on simple measures of weight, height and head circumference of the newborn, is an important instrument that helps a lot to support adequate and proper care management for newborns. Those measures must be reported on reference curves.

In Morocco, national reference curves don't exist and those Frenchs or North's America used, but that are not necessarily suitable to the standards of our people. However, several factors influence fetal growth [1], like the size and maternal weight [2] [3], ethnicity [4]-[7], socioeconomic's conditions [8] and altitude of the place of residence [9]. The geographical position and socio-economic conditions in Morocco are not like those of European or North America's countries. It is the same for ethnicity and anthropometric measures. So one might ask whether the evaluations carried from these "international" curves are less accurate and less adapted to our context.

This work is a first initiative whose main objective is the evaluation of anthropometric standards of a group of newborns Moroccans aged 37 to 42 completed weeks of gestation. Our results will be compared to:

- AUDIPOG those of the study (Association of Computerized Records Users Perinatology, Obstetrics and Gynecology) recently conducted in France by Mama *et al.* [10]
- For weight curves of the Tunisian experience, conducted by El Mhamdi *et al.* [11] due to the ethnic and geographic similarity we have with Tunisia, but this study is limited to the data weight newborns.
  The secondary objectives are:
- Analysis of the impact of certain factors (especially those related to the mother in addition to the sex of the fetus [12] [13] on fetal growth.

2. Materials and Methods

2.1. Methodology

It was a prospective and cross-sectional study conducted in Maternity Souissi University Hospital of Rabat-Morocco between January 2008 and December 2013. This hospital drains the northern half of Moroccans. Parturients who are admitted Moroccan represent differents ethnicities.

✓ Inclusion criteria: Newborns whose gestational age was between 37 and 42 weeks from Moroccan women, healthy, with no obstetrical pathology, with at least three antenatal consultations, informed and after obtaining their consent. Gestational age, it is calculated by the last menstrual period and/or by the data of early obstetrical ultrasound (before the 12° week of amenorrhea), then checked birth by the score of Dubowitz. They are included newborns whose don't have any clinically detectable malformation.

✓ Exclusion criteria: They are excluded twin pregnancies, those with enamelled complications have disturbed intrauterine growth (hypertension, diabetes, severe anemia, severe malnutrition), those with a dubious term dating and/or discordance with the data clinical examination (a difference of more than a week), parturients having a long-term treatment (anti-bacillary, anti-HIV), newborns parent(s) not Moroccan(s), all malformed and died newborns.

Each newborn was measured in the first hour after birth, weight, height and head circumference.

The weighing was done with a balance accurate to 10 g, the size was taken with six feet and head circumference was measured using a flexible tape measure.

For every woman in labor was established a standardized assessment sheet with the collection of: age, weight, height, Body Mass Index (BMI), the number of pregnancies and the number of parities, if multipare, age at first pregnancy and birth space.

Anthropometric measurements (weight and height) of the women were held during the first consultation and admission to the room of childbirth; we used a Scale-type mechanical balance "Seca viva 750" for weight gain and a fathom of wood to adult for measuring the size.

2.2. Definition of Terms

- Is considered as a newborn "SGA" small for gestational age or "with intrauterine growth restriction" when its weight, based on gestational age, is strictly less than the 10° percentile of the weight curve reference.
- Harmonious hypotrophy: weight, size and head circumference are reduced.
- Dysharmonious hypotrophy: only the weight that is reduced.

- We define "hypertrophy" or "Macrosomia" when the weight exceeds the 90° percentile.
- An Appropriate for gestational age (AGA) if the weight is between the two limits (10° and 90° percentile).

2.3. Statistical Analysis

The data were analyzed by SPSS statistical software (Statistical Package for Social Sciences) version 13.0 for Windows. Quantitative variables were expressed as average and standard deviation), and/or median and quartiles. The qualitative variables were expressed as frequency and percentage. The t-Student test for paired sample was used for comparison of averages. ANOVA has been used for comparison of more than two averages. The test "post hoc" Bonferroni was used for comparison between the subgroups. A value of "p" of less than 0.05 was considered statistically significant.

3. Results

Neonatal Data

During the study period, 5000 births, 2500 boys and 2500 girls were included. The delivery was vaginally in 85% of cases and by caesarean in 15% of cases. Each age group of 37 to 41 WA was composed of 416 male newborns and 416 female newborns. When the group of 42 WA it featured 420 male newborns and 420 female newborns. The birth weight of all infants ranged from 2000 g to 4800 g with an average of 3358.90 g (±493.5) in boys and 3228.82 g (±460.4) in girls with a statistically significant difference ($p < 0.001$).

Table 1 shows the average weights of the newborns according to their genders and ages.

The sizes ranged from 36 cm to 58 cm with an average of 48.90 cm (±3.01) in boys and 48.20 cm (±2.71) in girls with a statistically significant difference ($p < 0.001$). The distribution of average sizes of newborns according to their gender and their AG is presented in **Table 2**.

The values of head circumference (HC) were measured between 28 cm and 40 cm with an average of 33.90 cm (±1.72) in boys and 33.60 cm (±1.65) in girls and the difference was statistically significant ($p < 0.001$). The averages by gender and GA are outlined in **Table 3**.

The 3°, 10°, 25°, 50°, and 75°, 90° and 97° percentile of the various anthropometric parameters of newborns (males) are presented in **Table 4**; and those female newborns in **Table 5**.

Constructed weight curves are shown in **Figure 1** for newborn male and **Figure 2** for newborn female.

The size and head circumference curves produced are shown in **Figure 3** for newborns of male sex and **Figure 4** for newborns of female sex.

4. Discussion

Growth curves are remarkably useful in neonatology units, serving the trophic status of newborns. This status can draw the support scheme and the list of potential risks.

Although the population is not representative of Morocco, these curves we obtained can be considered unique to our center and valid for maternity and neonatal units of the Rabat's region, as they can give an idea about the anthropometric constants of Moroccan neonates. The limitation of this study to full-term newborns is due to the low number of premature births that met our inclusion criteria.

Table 1. Average of weight of term newborns by Sex and the GA.

GA	Boys		Girlsl		p
	Average	SD	Average	SD	
37.00	3174.11	506.10	3045.03	436.07	0.167
38.00	3297.96	625.10	3101.98	386.40	0.095
39.00	3322.82	382.53	3161.10	440.25	**0.007**
40.00	3351.68	502.92	3246.10	468.96	**0.016**
41.00	3524.40	479.50	3355.73	446.61	**0.013**
42.00	3453.41	458.55	3394.29	472.49	0.558
Total	3358.89	493.50	3228.77	460.40	**<0.001**

Table 2. Medium to term newborn by sex and GA.

GA	Boys		Girls		P
	Average	SD	Average	SD	
37.00	47.82	2.465	47.333	3.393	0.356
38.00	48.14	3.011	47.740	2.465	0.445
39.00	48.49	2.777	48.026	2.689	0.223
40.00	49.38	3.184	48.509	2.866	0.001
41.00	49.58	2.494	48.574	2.751	0.010
42.00	48.99	2.593	48.619	2.305	0.466
Total	48.90	3.052	48.312	2.715	0.001

Table 3. HC' averages of full-term infants by sex and GA.

GA	Boys		Girls		p
	Average	SD	Average	SD	
37.00	33.39	1.82	33.25	1.52	0.157
38.00	33.70	1.91	33.50	1.67	0.620
39.00	34.01	1.70	33.38	1.69	**0.042**
40.00	34.11	1.71	33.65	1.70	**0.012**
41.00	34.06	1.34	33.72	1.50	0.087
42.00	33.90	1.72	33.70	1.70	0.613
Total	33.90	1.72	33.60	1.65	**<0.001**

Table 4. Weight distribution, sizes and HC FOR newborn males by gestational age.

	Weight (g)						
37	2175.00	2480.00	2777.50	3140.00	3420.00	3810.00	4020.00
38	2378.50	2564.00	2872.00	3210.00	3573.00	4010.00	4179.00
39	2433.00	2700.00	3010.00	3310.00	3620.00	4020.00	4195.00
40	2500.00	2830.00	3100.00	3355.00	3730.00	4240.00	4578.00
41	2610.00	2960.00	3255.00	3520.00	38,550.00	4275.00	4760.00
42	2470.50	2810.00	3247.50	3440.00	3840.00	4000.00	4398.00
	Size (cm)						
37	40.35	42.00	45.00	48.00	50.00	52.00	52.80
38	40.40	42.90	47.00	48.50	50.00	52.00	53.00
39	40.70	45.00	47.00	49.00	50.00	52.00	53.00
40	41.55	46.20	48.00	50.00	51.00	53.00	54.00
41	43.90	47.00	48.00	50.00	51.00	52.00	55.00
42	42.00	45.00	48.00	49.00	50.00	52.00	54.80
	Head circumference (cm)						
37	29.10	31.000	32.000	34.00	35.00	35.50	36.255
38	30.00	31.00	32.00	34.00	35.00	36.00	36.20
39	30.00	32.00	33.00	34.00	35.00	36.00	36.70
40	30.00	32.00	33.00	34.00	35.00	36.00	37.00
41	31.00	32.00	33.00	34.00	35.00	36.05	37.45
42	30.50	31.20	32.50	34.00	35.00	36.00	37.00

Table 5. Distribution of weights, sizes and HC for newborn females according to GA.

				Weight (g)			
37	2051.00	2515.00	2757.00	3028.00	3301.00	3610.00	3878.00
38	2155.00	2530.00	2750.00	3110.00	3410.00	3635.00	4124.00
39	2303.00	2604.00	2851.00	3152.00	3455.00	3755.00	4140.00
40	2427.00	2695.00	2953.00	3204.00	3555.00	3823.00	4240.00
41	2618.00	2809.00	3054.00	3355.00	3707.00	4163.00	4375.00
42	2604.00	2730.00	3053.00	3305.00	3655.00	3933.00	4369.00
				Size (cm)			
37	40.87	44.10	46.00	48.00	49.70	50.90	51.50
38	41.05	45.00	47.00	48.00	50.00	51.00	52.00
39	41.50	45.00	47.00	48.00	50.00	51.00	52.00
40	41.70	45.00	47.00	49.00	50.00	51.00	53.00
41	43.30	46.30	48.00	49.00	50.00	52.00	54.80
42	42.00	45.20	47.50	48.00	50.00	51.80	54.00
				Head circumference (cm)			
37	29.60	31.00	32.00	33.00	34.000	35.00	35.75
38	30.00	31.00	32.00	33.00	34.85	35.00	36.00
39	30.00	31.00	32.50	34.00	35.00	35.30	36.50
40	30.00	31.00	33.00	34.00	35.00	36.00	37.00
41	31.00	32.00	33.00	34.00	35.00	36.00	37.00
42	30.00	32.00	33.00	34.00	35.00	35.90	36.90

We have analyzed for the first time in Morocco three anthropometric parameters of birth: weight, height and head circumference. The data collected from our sample confirmed elevated anthropometric values (weight, height and head circumference) in newborn boys than girls, according to gestational age, which corroborates the findings of other studies [14]-[18].

By convention, to compare the results of neonatal growth curves, we take as reference point the values obtained at 40 weeks gestation and essentially the average or median age (50 th percentile). Was chosen for the comparison of our curves, those of Mama (France: AUDIPOG study) [10] Dawodu (UAE) [15] and El Mhamdi (Tunisia) [11].

The average weight at birth of our male newborns to 40 weeks gestational age is less than 65 g of UAE [15] and 170 g to that of Tunisian [11]; Similarly, the average weight of our newborn female is less than 52 g of UAE [15] and 148 g that of the Tunisian [11].

The average size and head circumference of boys in our study are lower than those found in the United Arab Emirates [15], 1.70 cm and 0.65 cm in succession; and in our average girls are inferior to those of UAE [14], of 1.80 cm and 0.55 cm successively.

The median (50° percentile) weight in our newborn males 40 weeks gestational age is less than AUDIPOG in the study [10] of 112 g and 148 g compared to Tunisian [11]; and among our newborn females, it is less than 128 g than in France [10] and 195 g than in Tunisia [11]. The median size and head circumference of boys in our study are lower than those of Mama [10], 0.3 cm and 1.1 cm in succession; and with our girls are below the median of 0.6 cm and 0.5 cm in succession. The values of 50° percentile of our weight newborns 38 SA 42 SA are below their corresponding among Tunisians [11] and in AUDIPOG study [10] with the exception of females who are 38 WA weight slightly higher than the French [10], while our values 37 weeks are almost similar to those of Tunisia [11] and slightly larger than that of the French study [10]. Similarly, are the values of 10° percentile except 37 weeks where our results exceed those of Tunisia [11] and French [10]. For values of 90° percentile, they stand between the corresponding values in the Tunisian experience [11] and the study of Udder.

About the values of 10° and 50° percentile of the size and values of 10°, 50° and 90° head circumference

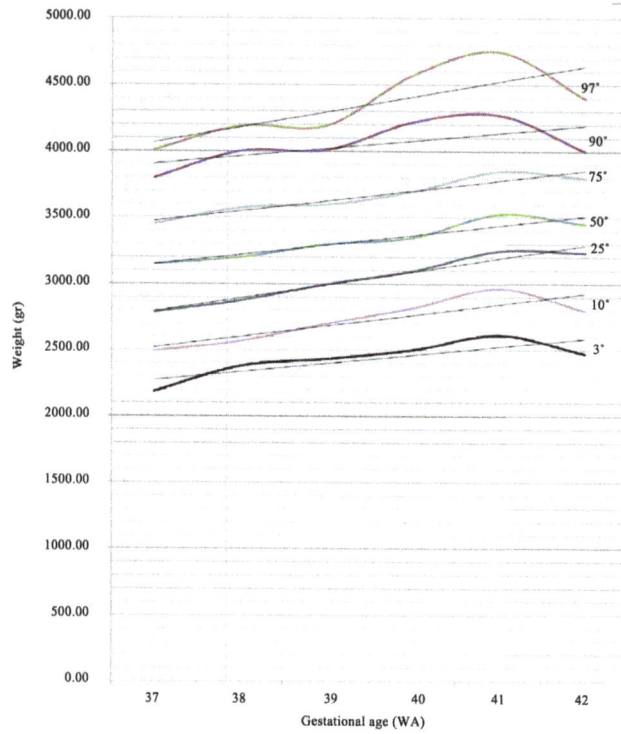

Figure 1. Curves of weight percentiles at birth (boys).

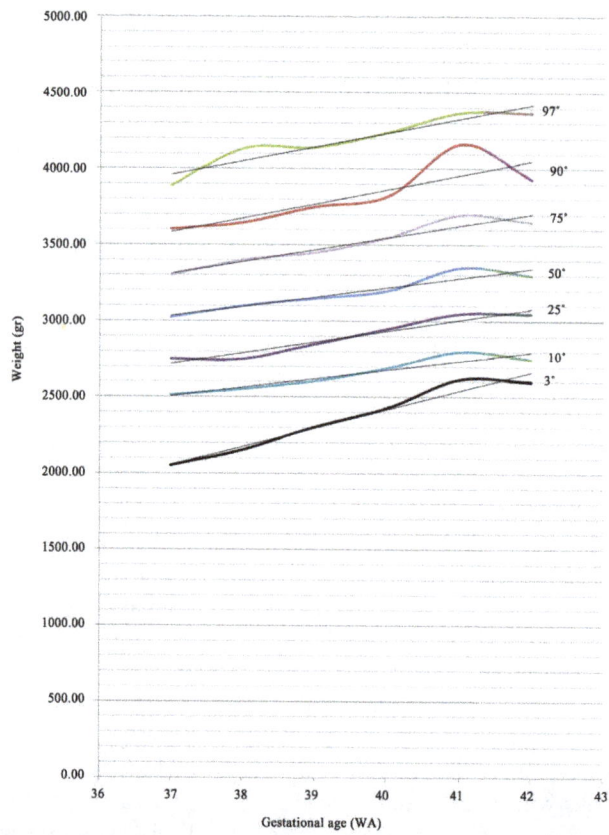

Figure 2. Curves weight percentiles at birth (girls).

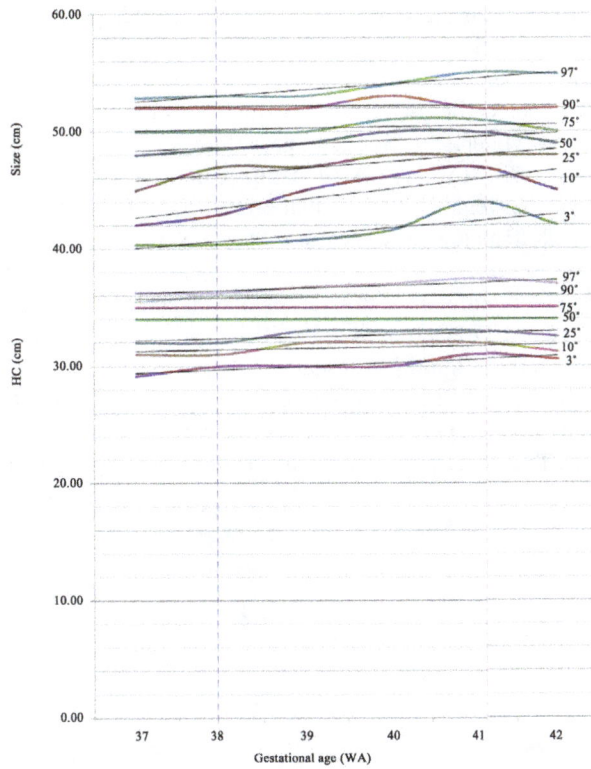

Figure 3. Size and head circumference curves (HC) for boys.

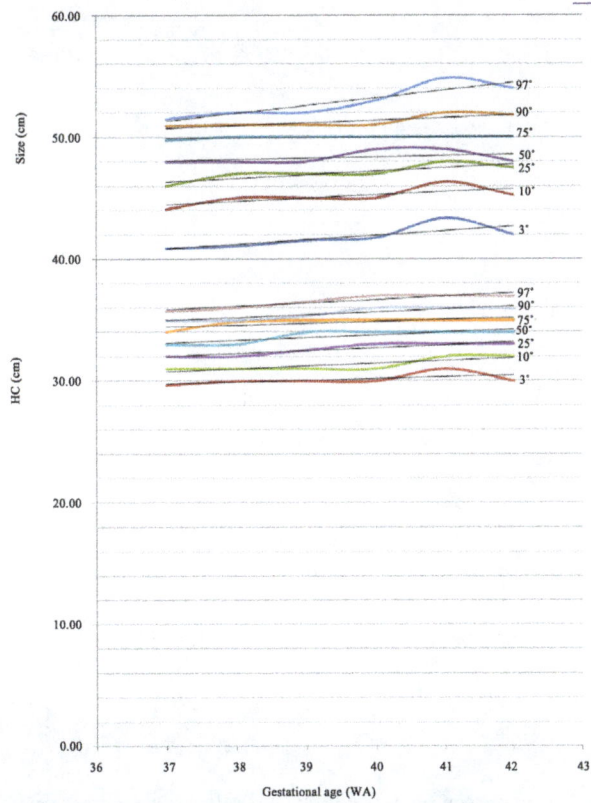

Figure 4. Size and head circumference curves (HC) for girls.

percentiles among our newborns are lower than their corresponding in France [10], while the percentile values of 90° size in our study are higher than Mama [10]. By comparing curves (10° and 90° percentile) with those of the AUDUPOG study [10] and those of the Tunisian study (weight curves) [11]; we find for weight newborn males that our curve 10° percentile (SGA threshold) is below except for 37 weeks, that is to say that the French and Tunisian curves could underestimating fetal growth in our population and 90° percentile curve (macrosomia threshold) is above except 42 SA which means that the comparison curves might consider some of our newborns as macrosomic while have a weight within normal limits according to our new curves (**Figures 5-8**).

On the curves of weight female newborns, our curves are close to those of the AUDIPOG except at 37 and 41 WA (**Figure 5**).

For the size and head circumference, our curves of 90° percentile (threshold macrosomia) are almost superimposed on those of our AUDIPOG and curves 10° percentile (IUGR threshold) are below the French curves (**Figure 6**) for male newborns (**Figure 7**) for females.

In total, we see that there is a difference between our results and those of curves selected for comparison, because of the ethnic and/or geographic factors. Thus one sees that the curves obtained we define new thresholds IUGR and macrosomia. These interesting data must be reinforced by a broader national multicenter study.

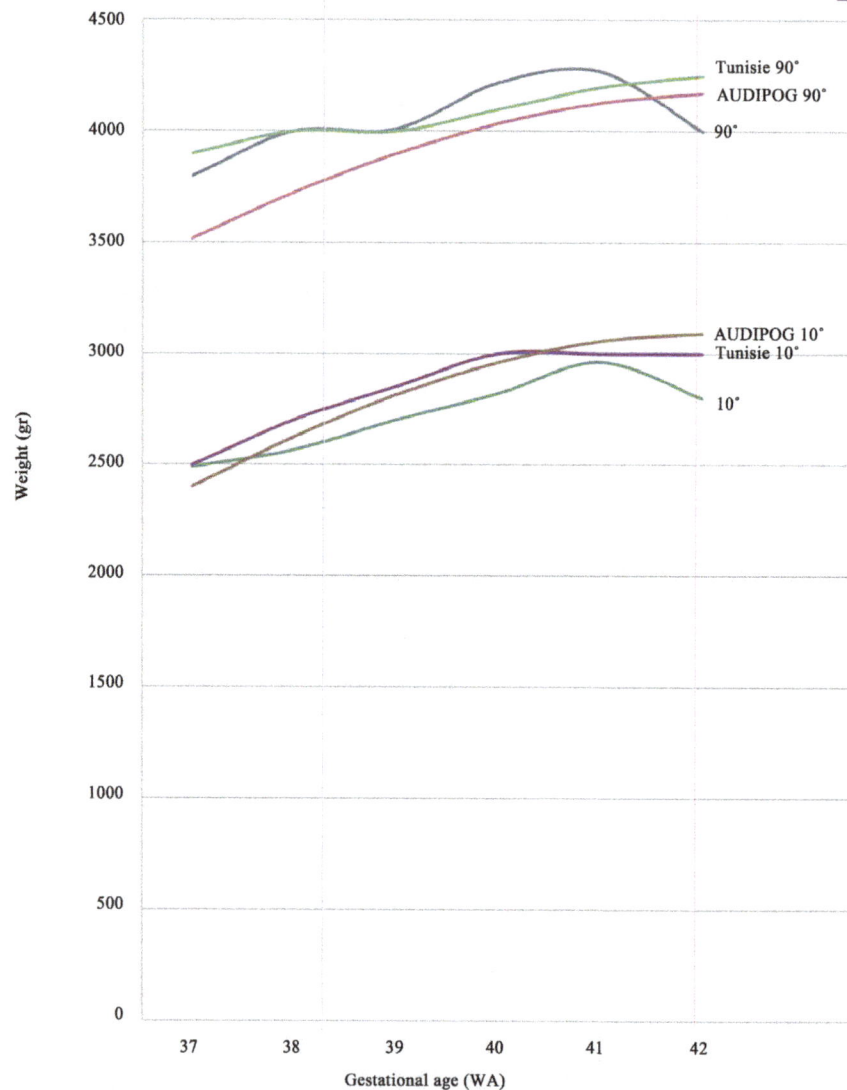

Figure 5. Comparison of 10 and 90th percentiles of weight in newborns of our curves with that of Tunisia and those AUDIPOG (boys).

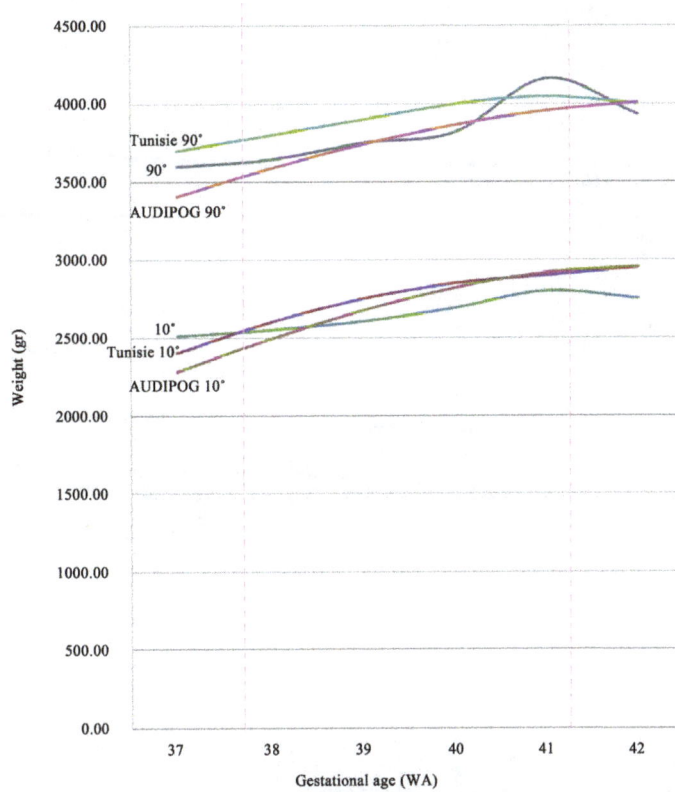

Figure 6. Comparison of 10 and 90th percentiles of weight newborns in our curves with that of AUDIPOG and those Tunisian (girls).

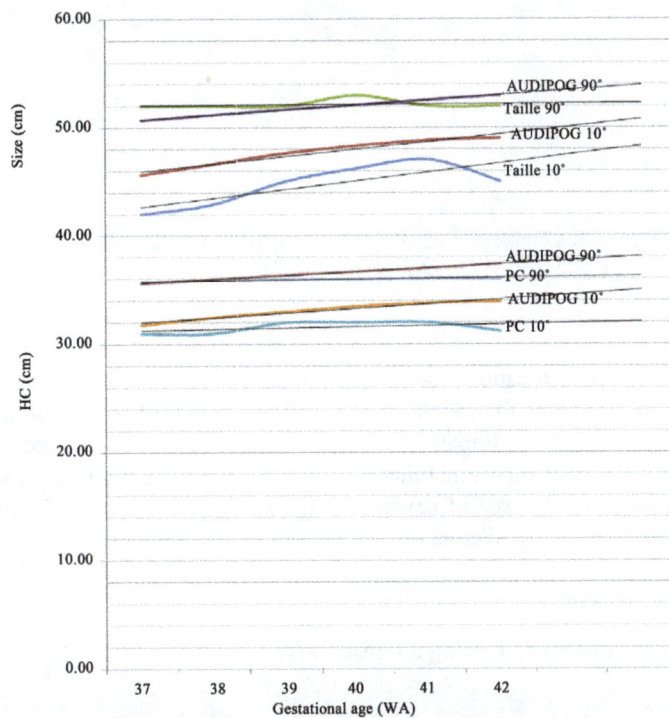

Figure 7. Comparison of 10 and 90th percentiles of sizes and HC newborn male AUDIPOG with our curves.

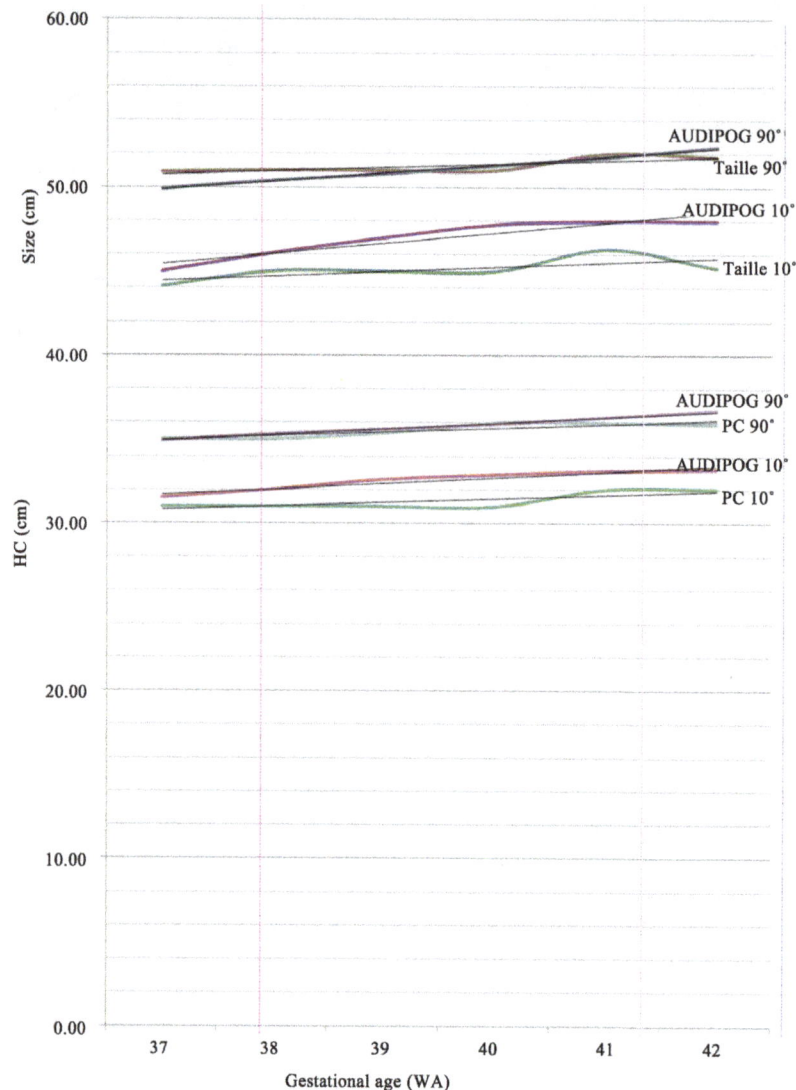

Figure 8. Comparison of 10 and 90th percentile sizes and HC for newborns in our curves with that AUDIPOG (girls).

5. Conclusion

This study, the first of its kind nationwide, is a real contribution to the study of fetal growth in Morocco. On the one hand, it provides us curves for weight, height and head circumference normal births ultimately occurred at the Souissi Maternity Hospital in Rabat. This is a true action research. This model is potentially extrapolated to the Moroccan population and such suitability can be verified by other subsequent studies. Moreover, it became clear through this work that the sex of newborn and gestational age is key factors in its growth. But, maternal body size and parity are major predictors of fetal growth in our population.

Competing Interests

Authors have declared that no competing interests exist.

References

[1] Figueras, F. and Gardosi, J. (2009) Should We Customize Fetal Growth Standards? *Fetal Diagnosis and Therapy*, **25**, 297-303. http://dx.doi.org/10.1159/000235875

[2]   Gardosi, J., Mongelli, M., Wilcox, M. and Chang, A. (1995) An Adjustable Fetal Weight Standard. *Ultrasound in Obstetrics & Gynecology*, **6**, 168-174. http://dx.doi.org/10.1046/j.1469-0705.1995.06030168.x

[3]   Mongelli, M., Figueras, F., Francis, A. and Gardosi, J. (2007) A Customized Birth Weight Centile Calculator Developed for an Australian Population. *Australian and New Zealand Journal of Obstetrics and Gynaecology*, **47**, 128-131. http://dx.doi.org/10.1111/j.1479-828X.2007.00698.x

[4]   Drooger, J.C., *et al.* (2005) Ethnic Differences in Prenatal Growth and the Association with Maternal and Fetal Characteristics. *Ultrasound in Obstetrics & Gynecology*, **26**, 115-122. http://dx.doi.org/10.1002/uog.1962

[5]   Wilcox, M., Gardosi, J., Mongelli, M., Ray, C. and Johnson, I. (1993) Birth Weight from Pregnancies Dated by Ultrasonography in a Multicultural British Population. *BMJ*, **307**, 588-591. http://dx.doi.org/10.1136/bmj.307.6904.588

[6]   Zhang, J. and Bowes, W.A. (1995) Birth-Weight-for-Gestational-Pattern by Race, Sex, and Parity in the United States Population. *Obstetrics & Gynecology*, **86**, 200-208. http://dx.doi.org/10.1016/0029-7844(95)00142-E

[7]   Arntzen, A., Samuelsen, S.O., Bakketeig, L.S. and Stoltenberg, C. (2004) Socioeconomic Status and Risk of Infant Death. A Population-Based Study of Trends in Norway, 1967-1998. *International Journal of Epidemiology*, **33**, 279-288. http://dx.doi.org/10.1093/ije/dyh054

[8]   Yip, R. (1987) Altitude and Birth Weight. *The Journal of Pediatrics*, **111**, 869-876. http://dx.doi.org/10.1016/S0022-3476(87)80209-3

[9]   Bukowski, R., *et al.* (2008) Individualized Norms of Optimal Fetal Growth: Fetal Growth Potential. *Obstetrics & Gynecology*, **111**, 1065-1076. http://dx.doi.org/10.1097/AOG.0b013e3181704e48

[10]   Mamelle, N., Munoz, F. and Grandjean, H. (1996) Fetal Growth from the AUDIPOG Study. Establishment of Reference Curves. *J Gynecol Obstet Biol Reprod* (Paris), **25**, 61-70.

[11]   El Mhamdi, S., Ben Salem, K., Hadded, A., Gaddour, Z. and Soltani, M.S. (2010) Graphic Model of Birth Weight and Gestational Age in Monastir, Tunisia. *Revue d'Épidémiologie et de Santé Publique*, **58**, 121-126. http://dx.doi.org/10.1016/j.respe.2009.12.008

[12]   Mochhoury, L., Razine, R., Kasouati, J., Kabiri, M. and Barkat, A. (2013) Body Mass Index, Gestational Weight Gain, and Obstetric Complications in Moroccan Population. *Journal of Pregnancy*, **2013**, Article ID: 379461.

[13]   Mochhoury, L., Razine, R., Kharbach, A. and Barkat, A. (2013) Prise pondérale maternelle pendant la grossesse et poids des nouveau-nés. Données marocaines. *Revue de Médecine Périnatale*, **5**, 111-119.

[14]   Krasovec, K. and Anderson, M.A., Eds. (1991) Maternal Nutrition and Pregnancy Outcomes. Anthropometric Assessment. Scientific Publication No 529, Pan American Health Organization, Washington DC.

[15]   Dawodu, A., Bener, A., Koutouby, G.A., Varady, E. and Abdulrazzaq, Y. (2008) Size at Birth in a Rapidly Developing Economy: Intrauterine Growth Pattern of UAE Infants. *Annals of Human Biology*, **35**, 615-623. http://dx.doi.org/10.1080/03014460802385439

[16]   Brenner, W.E., Edelman, D.A. and Hendricks, C.H. (1976) A Standard of Fetal Growth for the United States of America. *American Journal of Obstetrics & Gynecology*, **26**, 555-564.

[17]   Thomson, A.M., Billewicz, W.Z. and Hytten, F.E. (1968) The Assessment of Fetal Growth. *BJOG: An International Journal of Obstetrics and Gynaecology*, **75**, 903-916. http://dx.doi.org/10.1111/j.1471-0528.1968.tb01615.x

[18]   Amini, S.B., Catalano, P.M., Hirsch, V. and Mann, L.I. (1994) An Analysis of Birth Weight by Gestational Age Using a Computerized Perinatal Data Base, 1975-92. *Obstetrics & Gynecology*, **83**, 342-352.

Abbreviations

UAE: United Arabic Emirates;
IUGR: Intrauterine Growth Restriction;
GA: Gestational Age;
WA: Weeks of Amenorrhea;
HC: Head Circumference;
BMI: Body Maternal Index;
SGA: Small for Gestational Age;
AGA: Appropriate for Gestational Age.

16

Resolution of Late Steroid-Responsive Nephrotic Syndrome in a Patient with Alport Syndrome Treated with Atorvastatin

Jia-Feng Chang[1,2], Wei-Ning Lin[1], Chien-Chen Tsai[3]*

[1]Graduate Institute of Basic Medicine, Fu Jen Catholic University, Taipei, Taiwan
[2]Division of Nephrology, Department of Internal Medicine, Far Eastern Memorial Hospital, New Taipei City, Taiwan
[3]Department of Anatomic Pathology, Far Eastern Memorial Hospital, New Taipei City, Taiwan
Email: *cjf6699@yahoo.com.tw

Academic Editor: Ashraf Mohamed Abdel-Basset Bakr, Mansoura University Children's Hospital, Egypt

Abstract

Experimental and clinical studies have pointed out the lipid-induced renal damage, and statins may have pleiotropic effects on renoprotection. We reported a girl with X-linked Alport syndrome whose late steroid-responsive nephrotic syndrome (NS) was resolved by atorvastatin. She had been in a nephrotic condition despite of prednisone therapy 60 mg/day for 8 weeks. Renal biopsy dispicted extreme foamy appearance of tubular epithelial cells with detachment led to luminal obliteration. Atorvastatin was started on the ninth week of prednisone therapy due to severe hypercholesterolemia. Partial remission of NS was dramatically achieved with unchanged dosage of prednisone at the end of the twelfth week. Our case provides a pathology-based evidence to support the use of statins in profoundly hyperlipidemic patients with NS. In patients with NS and profound hyperlipidemia, early initiation of statin therapy is required in combination with immunosuppressive therapy.

Keywords

Nephrotic Syndrome, Statin

1. Introduction

Experimental and clinical studies have pointed out the lipid-induced renal damage [1], and statins may have

---
*Corresponding author.

pleiotropic effects on renoprotection [2]. Lowering serum concentrations of cholesterol and triglycerides by lipid-apheresis or statin therapy improves the response to steroids in pediatric nephrotic syndrome (NS) [3]-[6]. We reported the case of a girl with X-linked Alport syndrome whose late steroid-responsive nephrotic syndrome (NS) was resolved by atorvastatin. To our best knowledge, there was no study showing pathology-based evidence to support the use of statins in profoundly hyperlipidemic patients with NS.

2. Case Report

A 12-year-old girl presented with puffy face, bilateral lower-leg edema and frothy urine in recent two months. Biochemical studies showed nephrotic range proteinuria, hematuria > 30 erythrocytes per high-power field, lipiduria, serum cholesterol 10.1 mmol/l, albumin 16 g/l, and creatinine 30.5 mmol/l. Her blood pressure was 108/70 mmHg, and renin-angiotensin system blockers were not used. A kidney biopsy was performed for her nephrotic-nephritic syndrome with unclear etiology. Light microscopic examination with hematoxylin and eosin stain revealed rigidity and moderate thickening of the glomerular basement membrane (GBM), and segmental glomerular sclerosis. Accumulating an excessive amount of neutral fats in renal tubular cells led to extremely foamy appearance and luminal obliteration (**Figure 1**). Such fatty change is followed by necrosis of injured cells and detachement from the basement membranes compounding luminal obliteration. Electron microscopy depicted irregular distribution of GBM with basket-weave appearance (thinning, thickening, splitting and lamination of lamina densa) and diffuse effacement of podocyte foot processes (**Figure 2**). Myriad intracellular lipid droplets were noted within tubulointerstitial lipid-laden foamy macrophages (**Figure 3**).

The pathological finding pointed out the burden of lipid-induced renal damage. Compatible with her renal pathology, she had been in a nephrotic condition despite of prednisone therapy 60 mg/day for 8 weeks. Atorvastatin was started at a dose of 10 mg/day on the ninth week of prednisone therapy due to her progressive hypercholesterolemia (16.0 mmol/l). Partial remission of NS (proteinuria < 3 g/24 h) was dramatically achieved at the end of the twelfth week. The dosage of prednisone (60 mg/day) had not been changed since the inclusion of atorvastatin. Therefore, atorvastatin may resolve proteinuria by improving hyperlipidemia and lipid-induced renal damage.

3. Discussion

Studies have reported statins have pleiotropic effects on improving glomerular damage, preventing glomerulosclerosis and tubulointerstitial fibrosis [2]. Lowering serum concentrations of cholesterol and triglycerides by lipid-apheresis or statin therapy improves the response to steroids in pediatric NS [3]-[6]. In obese animal models,

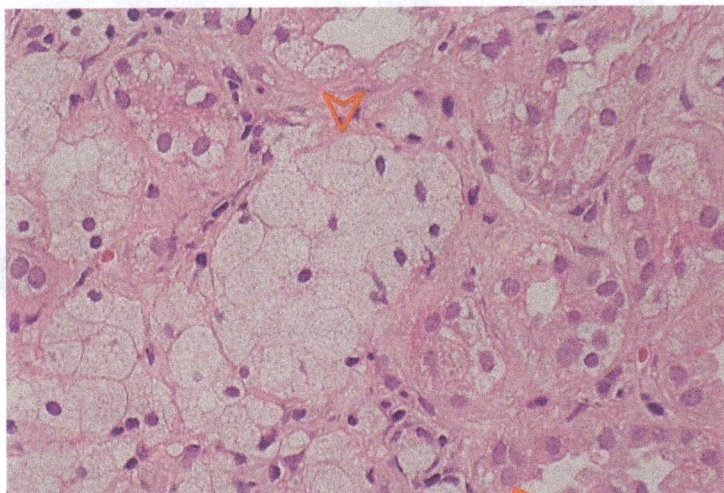

Figure 1. Light microscopy depicted accumulating excessive lipids in renal tubular cells led to extremely foamy appearance and luminal obliteration (arrow). Such fatty change is followed by necrosis of injured cells and detachement from the basement membranes (arrow) compounding luminal obliteration.

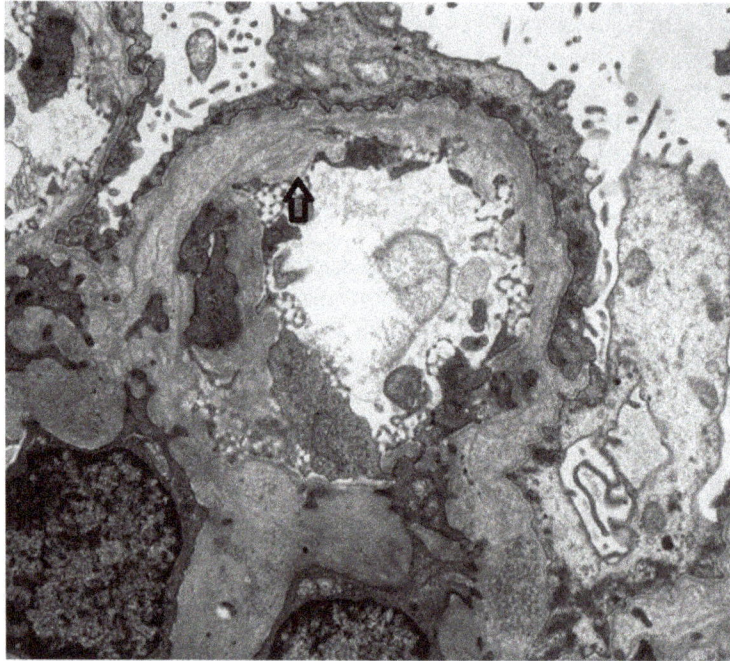

Figure 2. Electron microscopy demonstrated irregular distribution of glomerular basement membrane with basket-weave appearance (thinning, thickening, splitting and lamination of lamina densa; arrow), and effacement of podocyte foot processes.

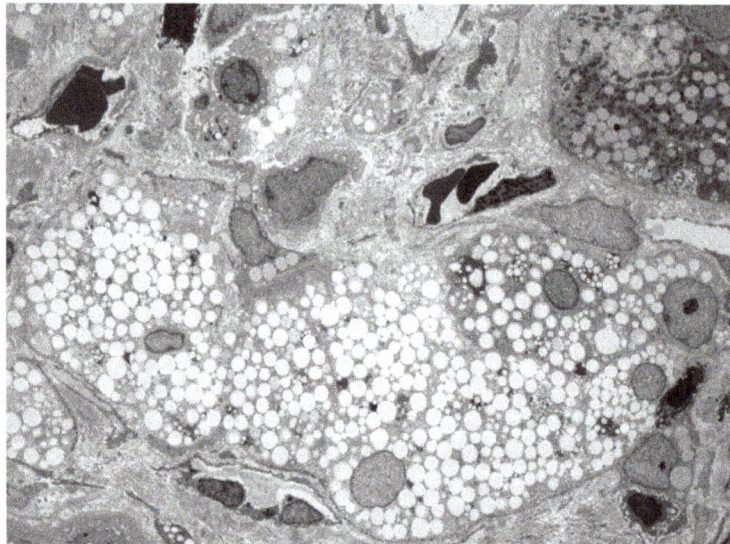

Figure 3. Myriad intracellular lipid droplets were noted within tubulointerstitial lipid-laden foamy macrophages.

lipid accumulation in kidneys accentuated glomerulosclerosis and proteinuria [7]. Compared with non-treated obese animals, statins attenuated lipid accumulation in the proximal tubules and reduced glomerular hypertrophy [8]. In experimental anti-glomerular basement membrane glomerulonephritis, the anti-proteinuric effect of ator-vastatin is mediated through anti-inflammatory responses [9] [10].

To our best knowledge, this is the first case of a hyperlipidemic patient whose late steroid-responsive NS was resolved by atorvastatin with a pathology-based evidence of lipid-induced kidney injury. The renal pathology revealed extremely foamy tubular cells and detachment of injured cells from the basement membranes. Such re-sults led to obliterate renal tubular lumens, increased intratubular pressure, tubulointerstitial edema and decreased glomerular filtration rate. Thus we initiated atorvastatin in this patient to treat her progressive hypercholesterolemia and lipid-induced kidney injury. Her nephritic range proteinuria and severe hypercholesterolemia were significantly ameliorated with atorvastatin, accompanied with elevated serum albumin level and edema resolution. The baseline therapeutic doses of prednisone and diuretic regimen were not changed. The reasons why the combination therapy of prednisone and atorvastatin became more effective for NS included but not limited to the following. On one hand, statins have direct anti-proteinuric effects on both podocytes and renal tubular epithelial cells by preventing oxidized low-density lipoprotein-induced damage [11] [12]. On the other hand, pleiotropic effects of statins include modification of endothelial function, immunomodulation and anti-inflammation [13]. Based on the pathological evidence, atorvastatin may have an effect on ameliorating the extremely foamy change of renal tubular cells with subsequent apoptosis, and thereby relieving renal tubular obstruction. The appropriateness of statins in pediatric patients is the major concern [14]. Adverse effects of statins, such as muscle injury and liver toxicity, were not found in our patient. Study reported short-term use of statins is safe and efficient in the hyperlipidemic pediatric patients, but long-term safety is unknown [15]. Implementing statin therapy in children with nephrotic syndrome should be carefully followed up [16].

4. Conclusion

Our case provided a pathology-based evidence to support the use of statins in profoundly hyperlipidemic patients with NS. It suggests statins have anti-proteinuric effects by lowering lipid-induced renal damage and improve the response to steroid treatment. In profoundly hyperlipidemic patients with NS, early initiation of statin therapy is required in combination with immunosuppressive therapy.

References

[1]   Kiss, E., Kränzlin, B., Wagenblaβ, K., Bonrouhi, M., Thiery, J., Gröne E., Nordström, V., Teupser, D., Gretz, N., Malle, E. and Gröne, H.J. (2013) Lipid Droplet Accumulation Is Associated with an Increase in Hyperglycemia-Induced Renal Damage: Prevention by Liver X Receptors. *The American Journal of Pathology*, **182**, 727-741. http://dx.doi.org/10.1016/j.ajpath.2012.11.033

[2]   Trevisan, R., Dodesini, A.R. and Lepore, G. (2003) Lipids and Renal Disease. *Journal of the American Society of Nephrology*, **17**, S145-S147. http://dx.doi.org/10.1681/ASN.2005121320

[3]   Hattori, M., Chikamoto, H., Akioka, Y., Nakakura, H., Ogino, D., Matsunaga, A., Fukazawa, A., Miyakawa, S., Khono, M., Kawaguchi, H. and Ito, K. (2003) A Combined Low-Density Lipoprotein Apheresis and Prednisone Therapy for Steroid-Resistant Primary Focal Segmental Glomerulosclerosis in Children. *American Journal of Kidney Diseases*, **42**, 1121-1130. http://dx.doi.org/10.1053/j.ajkd.2003.08.012

[4]   Ito, S., Machida, H., Inaba, A., Harada, T., Okuyama, K., Nakamura, T., Aihara, Y. and Yokota, S. (2007) Amelioration of Steroids and Cyclosporine-Resistant Nephrotic Syndrome by Pravastatin. *Pediatric Nephrology*, **22**, 603-606. http://dx.doi.org/10.1007/s00467-006-0371-4

[5]   Prescott Jr., W.A., Streetman, D.A. and Streetman, D.S. (2004) The Potential Role of HMG-CoA Reductase Inhibitors in Pediatric Nephrotic Syndrome. *Annals of Pharmacotherapy*, **38**, 2105-2114. http://dx.doi.org/10.1345/aph.1D587

[6]   Sanjad, S.A., Al-Abbad, A. and Al-Shorafa S. (1997) Management of Hyperlipidemia in Children with Refractory Nephrotic Syndrome: The Effect of Statin Therapy. *The Journal of Pediatrics*, **130**, 470-474. http://dx.doi.org/10.1016/S0022-3476(97)70213-0

[7]   Jiang, T., Wang, Z., Proctor, G., Moskowitz, S., Liebman, S.E., Rogers, T., Lucia, M.S., Li J. and Levi, M. (2005) Diet-Induced Obesity in C57BL/6J Mice Causes Increased Renal Lipid Accumulation and Glomerulosclerosis via a Sterol Regulatory Element-Binding Protein-1c-Dependent Pathway. *The Journal of Biological Chemistry*, **280**, 32317-32325. http://dx.doi.org/10.1074/jbc.M500801200

[8]   Gotoh, K., Masaki, T., Chiba, S., Ando, H., Fujiwara, K., Shimasaki, T., Tawara, Y., Toyooka, I., Shiraishi, K., Mitsutomi, K., Anai, M., Itateyama, E., Hiraoka, J., Aoki, K., Fukunaga, N., Nawata, T. and Kakuma, T. (2013) Effects of Hydrophilic Statins on Renal Tubular Lipid Accumulation in Diet-Induced Obese Mice. *Obesity Research & Clinical Practice*, **7**, e342-e352. http://dx.doi.org/10.1016/j.orcp.2013.04.001

[9]   Eller, P., Eller, K., Wolf, A.M., Reinstadler, S.J., Tagwerker, A., Patsch, J.R., Mayer, G. and Rosenkranz, A.R. (2010) Atorvastatin Attenuates Murine Anti-Glomerular Basement Membrane Glomerulonephritis. *Kidney International*, **77**, 428-435. http://dx.doi.org/10.1038/ki.2009.478

[10] Fujita, E., Shimizu, A., Masuda, Y., Kuwahara, N., Arai, T., Nagasaka, S., Aki, K., Mii, A., Natori, Y., Iino, Y., Katayama, Y. and Fukuda, Y. (2010) Statin Attenuates Experimental Anti-Glomerular Basement Membrane Glomerulonephritis Together with the Augmentation of Alternatively Activated Macrophages. *The American Journal of Patholo-*

gy, **177**, 1143-1154. http://dx.doi.org/10.2353/ajpath.2010.090608

[11] Bussolati, B., Deregibus, M.C., Fonsato, V., Doublier, S., Spatola, T., Procida, S., Di Carlo, F. and Camussi, G. (2005) Statins Prevent Oxidized LDL-Induced Injury of Glomerular Podocytes by Activating the Phosphatidylinositol 3-Kinase/AKT-Signaling Pathway. *Journal of the American Society of Nephrology*, **16**, 1936-1947. http://dx.doi.org/10.1681/ASN.2004080629

[12] Chu, G., Jia, R. and Yang, D. (2006) Fluvastatin Prevents Oxidized Low-Density Lipoprotein-Induced Injury of Renal Tubular Epithelial Cells by Inhibiting the Phosphatidylinositol 3-Kinase/Akt-Signaling Pathway. *Journal of Nephrology*, **19**, 286-295.

[13] Steffens, S. and Mach, F. (2006) Drug Insight: Immunomodulatory Effects of Statins—Potential Benefits for Renal Patients? *Nature Clinical Practice Nephrology*, **2**, 378-387. http://dx.doi.org/10.1038/ncpneph0217

[14] Stein, E.A. (2007) Statins and Children: Whom Do We Treat and When? *Circulation*, **116**, 594-595. http://dx.doi.org/10.1161/CIRCULATIONAHA.107.717777

[15] Vuorio, A., Kuoppala, J., Kovanen, P.T., Humphries, S.E., Strandberg, T., Tonstad, S. and Gylling, H. (2010) Statins for Children with Familial Hypercholesterolemia. *Cochrane Database of Systematic Reviews*, **7**, CD006401.

[16] Prescott Jr., W.A., Streetman, D.A. and Streetman, D.S. (2004) The Potential Role of HMG-CoA Reductase Inhibitors in Pediatric Nephrotic Syndrome. *Annals of Pharmacotherapy*, **38**, 2105-2114. http://dx.doi.org/10.1345/aph.1D587

17

NPHS2 Gene Mutation and Polymorphisms in Indonesian Children with Steroid-Resistant Nephrotic Syndrome

Dedi Rachmadi[1*], Ani Melani[2], Leo Monnens[3]

[1]Department of Child Health, Faculty of Medicine, Universitas Padjadjaran Bandung, Bandung, Indonesia
[2]Medical Faculty, Health Research Unit, Universitas Padjadjaran Bandung, Bandung, Indonesia
[3]Department of Pediatrics, Radboud University Medical Centre Nijmegen, Nijmegen, The Netherlands
Email: [*]dedirachmadi@yahoo.com

Academic Editor: Carl E. Hunt, George Washington University School of Medicine and Health Sciences, USA

Abstract

Objective: Although several NPHS2 gene mutations and polymorphisms were described and associated with clinical manifestation of steroid-resistant nephrotic syndrome (SRNS), the occurrence of these genetic abnormalities or variants appeared to be influenced by race and ethnic group. We have investigated probable mutations and variants in NPHS2 gene involved in SRNS and their association with clinical manifestations. Methods: We examined 28 children with primary SRNS who visited the pediatric nephrology division of 10 teaching hospitals in Indonesia. Molecular genetic studies of the NPHS2 gene were conducted through screenings for the exon 1, exon 2, and exon 8. The mutational analysis of NPHS2 was performed by DNA sequencing. Fisher's Exact Test was used to determine the correlation between NPHS2 polymorphisms and clinical manifestations. Results: Seven females (25%) and 21 males (75%) participated in the study. The mean age of the subjects with 95% CI is: 7.6 (6.1 - 9.0) years while the mean age at onset of disease with 95% CI is: 5.4 (3.9 - 7.0) years. Sixteen patients (57.14%) were younger than 6 years at the onset of disease. Seventeen (60.7%) subjects had normal eGFR, while 11 (39.3%) had chronic renal insufficiency. The mean eGFR of the subjects with 95% CI is: 111.4 (87.7 - 135.1) ml/min/1.73 m^2. The mean systolic blood pressure with 95% CI is: 117.0 (108.9 - 125.1) mmHg and the mean diastolic blood pressure with 95% CI is: 77.0 (70.3 - 83.7) mmHg. We identified 6 NPHS2 polymorphisms, i.e. g.-52G>T, c.101A>G, g.-117C>T, c.288C>T, c.954C>T, and c.1038A>G and no mutation was found. There was no correlation between NPHS2 polymorphisms and clinical manifestations (p > 0.05). Conclusion: The results demonstrate no mutation of NPHS2 gene, and the 6 NPHS2 gene polymorphisms that were identified

---

[*]Corresponding author.

have no correlation with the clinical manifestation in Indonesian children with SRNS.

Keywords

Steroid-Resistant Nephrotic Syndrome, NPHS2 Gene, Polymorphism

---

1. Introduction

Steroid-resistant nephrotic syndrome (SRNS) is defined as a condition where nephrotic syndrome patients do not achieve remission after a full dose of single drug prednison therapy during the first four weeks [1] [2]. Other authors suggested a period of after 4 - 6 weeks [3] and 8 weeks of standard steroid treatment with no remission [4]. Steroid-resistant nephrotic syndrome accounts about 10% - 15% of nephrotic syndrome in children and tends to progress to end stage-renal disease within 10 years [5]. Molecular genetic studies have demonstrated that mutations in NPHS2 gene are responsible for structurally defective podocytes or deficient basement membrane, resulting in severe proteinuria [6]-[9].

About 50 NPHS2 gene mutations and variants and/or nonsilent polymorphisms have been reported and recognized as potentially involved in proteinuria [6]. Information about NPHS2 variants for different racial and ethnic groups are lacking in terms of the variant population frequency and their association with clinical manifestations. The available data as described in HuGe review suggest that large epidemiological studies to examine the association between NPHS2 variants and nephrotic syndrome are warranted [10]. In Indonesia, knowledge on NPHS2 mutations and variants in children with SRNS is lacking. We decided to evaluate the presence of probable mutations and variants in NPHS2 gene which are involved in SRNS and their association with clinical manifestations.

2. Materials and Methods

Subjects were patients with steroid resistant nephrotic syndrome (SRNS) who visited the pediatric nephrology division of several educational hospitals in Indonesia. The inclusion criteria were Indonesian, aged between 1 - 14 years old, with primary SRNS. This study was approved by the ethical committee of the Faculty of Medicine, Universitas Padjadjaran/Dr. Hasan Sadikin General Hospital, Bandung. The definitions for nephrotic syndrome (NS) and steroid resistant nephrotic syndrome (SRNS) used were definitions as defined by the International Study of Kidney Disease in Children (ISKDC) criteria, *i.e.* edema, severe proteinuria, and hypoalbuminemia (<2.5 g/dL) for NS [11] while SRNS was defined as NS patients who do not achieve remission after the full-dose single drug prednisone therapy during the first four weeks [1]. NS and SRNS were diagnosed by pediatric nephrologists or pediatricians supervised by pediatric nephrologists. Renal insufficiency was defined as an estimated glomerulo filtration rates (eGFR) of <90 mL/min per 1.73 m^2. Data analysis was performed using SPSS^{TM} version 20.0. Fisher's Exact Test was used to determine the correlation between NPHS2 polymorphisms and clinical manifestations, *i.e.* eGFR, hematuria, and hypertension.

1) Mutation analysis

DNA was extracted and purified from peripheral blood which was collected after informed consent from the subjects was obtained in accordance with the standard protocol. These procedures were conducted at the Health Research Unit of the Faculty of Medicine, Universitas Padjadjaran, Bandung. The mutation analysis was then performed at the Laboratory of Pediatrics and Neurology of the Radboud University Medical Centre Nijmegen. The exons of the NPHS2 gene were PCR-amplified using specific primers. Three sets of primers were designed to cover the sequences of introns adjacent to each NPHS2 exon. The sequences of the forward and reverse primers, PCR conditions, and the sizes of PCR products are given in **Table 1**.

2) Sequence reaction protocol

We sequence a PCR product (single bright band on agarose gel), by adding to each primer: 2.5 uL diluted PCR product (10 × diluted with MilliQ), 0.5 uL RR-sequence mix (keep on ice containing 2.5 × sequence buffer), 1.75 uL 5 × sequence buffer, 0.25 uL 10M primer, and 5.0 uL MilliQ-water. We spin the content and then put the tube(s) in a PCR machine and run the sequence program with the following instructions: 0.96°C for 60 sec; 1. 96°C for 60 sec; 2. Ramp 1°C/sec to 50°C; 3. 50°C for 5 sec; 4. Ramp 1°C/sec to 60°C; 5. 60°C for 2 min

NPHS2 Gene Mutation and Polymorphisms in Indonesian Children with Steroid-Resistant...

109

Table 1. Primers and PCR conditions used in the study, NPHS2 Genbank References: NM_014625, AJ279254, NP_055440.

Exon	Primer sequences 5' → 3'	T anneal (°C)	Fragment (bp)
1	F: GCA GCG ACT CCA CAG GGA CT	56	420
	R: TCC ACC TTA TCT GAC GCC CC		
2	F: AGG CAG TGA ATA CAG TGA AG	58	203
	R: GGC CTC AGG AAA TTA CCT A		
8	F: GGT GAA GCC TTC AGG GAA TG	58	380
	R: TTC TAT GGC AGG CCC CTT TA		

0 sec; 6. Go to 1.27 times; 7.15°C forever; 8. End.

We add 1 uL 125 mM EDTA and 1 uL 3 M NaAc and mix the content and add 30 uL abs. EtOH.

We leave the samples at room temperature for 15 minutes and centrifuge for 30 minutes at 3000 g −4°C, then remove the supernatant by short-spinning the opened tubes upside down on a tissue and then wash the samples by adding 35 uL 70% EtOH and centrifuge for 15 minutes at 1650 g −40°C. We store the pellets at −20°C until electrophoresis. Just before electrophoresis, we dissolve the pellet in 10uL HiDi, denature 1 minute at 92°C, cool on ice and run the samples in the automatic DNA sequencer.

3. Results

The study population consisted of 59 Indonesian pediatric patients with primary steroid resistant nephrotic syndrome. Subjects were recruited from patients who visited the pediatric nephrology division of 10 education hospitals in several cities in Indonesia, *i.e.* Bandung, Jakarta, Yogyakarta, Semarang, Surabaya, Denpasar, Medan, Palembang, Makassar, and Manado. The molecular genetic studies of the NPHS2 gene were performed for all subjects but only 28 subjects were successfully screened for exon 1, exon 2, and exon 8. The other subjects and the other exons were failed to performed. The 28 subjects consisted of 7 females (25%) and 21 males (75%). The mean age of the subjects with 95% CI: 7.6 (6.1 - 9.0) years while the mean age at onset of disease with 95% CI: 5.4 (3.9 - 7.0) years. Seventeen (60.7%) subjects had normal eGFR, while 11 (39.3%) had chronic renal insufficiency (eGFR < 90 mL/min/1.73 m^2). The mean eGFR of the subjects with 95% CI: 111.4 (87.7 - 135.1) ml/min/1.73 m^2. The mean systolic blood pressure with 95% CI: 117.0 (108.9 - 125.1) mmHg and the mean diastolic blood pressure with 95% CI: 77.0 (70.3 - 83.7) mmHg. The clinical characteristics of the patients with NPHS2 gene polymorphisms are presented in **Table 2**.

The nomenclature for describing the sequence variations of NPHS2 used here was based on the reference sequence NM_014625, AJ279254, NP_055440 (Gen Bank Database). DNA sequence analysis of exon 1, exon 2, and exon 8 of the subjects did not find any mutation, but six polymorphisms were detected. In exon 1, 3 kinds of polimorfisms were revealed, *i.e.* g.-52G>T (heterozygous) in 4 of 28 patients (14%), c.101A>G (homozygous) in 12 of 28 patients (43%), and g.-117C>T (heterozygous 8 and 1 homozygous) in 9 patients (32%). Polymorphism c.288C>T (heterozygous) in exon 2 was found in 4 of 28 patients (14%), whereas in exon 8 polymorphism c.954C>T were detected in 24 patients (85.7%), which consisted of 15 heterozygous and 9 homozygous. heterozygous c.1038A>G polymorphism was also found in exon 8 of 5 of 28 patients (17.8%). The polymorphisms are presented in **Table 3**.

The results of the univariate analysis with Fisher's Exact Test on the correlation between NPHS2 polymorphisms and clinical manifestations, *i.e.* eGFR < 90 (ml/min/1.73 m^2), hematuria, and hypertension, were not significant (**Table 4**).

4. Discussion

Almost 50 NPHS2 gene mutations and variants and/or non-silent polymorphisms have been reported as potentially involved in structurally defective podocytes or deficient basement membrane that lacks perm-selectivity, causing proteinuria [6]. Previous studies have shown that NPHS2 gene mutations and variants were associated with different clinical features, such as early childhood onset proteinuria, rapid progression to ESRD, late onset nephrotic syndrome, and renal histology of FSGS [5] [12] [13]. In sporadic SRNS, these mutations are responsible for 10% - 30% of diseases [13]-[17]. Most published studies on SRNS cases associated

Table 2. Characteristics of the subject (n = 28).

No	Characteristics	n (%)
1	Sex	
	Male	21 (75)
	Female	7 (25)
2	Hematuria	
	(+)	8 (28.6)
	(-)	20 (71.4)
3	Hypertension	
	(+)	12 (42.9)
	(-)	16 (57.1)
4.	Age (years)	
	Mean (SD): 7.6 (3.8)	
	Median: 7.0	
	Range: 2.5 - 13.9	
5.	Age onset (years)	
	Mean (SD): 5.4 (4.1)	
	Median: 4.1	
	Range: 1.0 - 13.0	
6	Creatinine (mg/dL)	
	Mean (SD): 0.91 (1.07)	
	Median: 0.6	
	Range: 0.2 - 6.0	
7	eGFR (ml/min/1.73 m^2)	
	Mean (SD): 111.4 (61.2)	
	Median: 96.5	
	Range: 12 - 295	

Table 3. NPHS2 polymorphisms in 28 patients with steroid-resistant nephrotic syndrome.

Exon	Polymorphism	Effect	Heterozygous/ Homozygous	Patients (n = 28)
1	g.-52G>T	p.Arg6Arg	Heterozygous	4 (14.2%)
1	c.101A>G	p.Arg34Arg	Homozygous	12 (42.8%)
1	g.-117C>T	p.Phe39Phe	Heterozygous	8 (28.5%)
			Homozygous	1 (3.5 %)
2	c.288C>T	p.Ser96Ser	Heterozygous	4 (14.2%)
8	c.954C>T	p.Ala318Ala	Heterozygous	15 (53.5%)
			Homozygous	9 (32.1%)
8	c.1038A>G	p.Leu346Leu	Heterozygous	5 (17.8%)

with biopsy-proven focal segmental glomerulosclerosis (FSGS) [5] [10] [15]. In addition, NPHS2 gene mutation studies in different populations and countries have shown that ethnicity plays an important role in disease genes [5] [18] [19]. NPHS2 412C→T and 419delG gene mutations are the risk factors for SRNS in Indonesian children [20].

The result of this study shows a ratio of male and female of 3:1, which is similar to those from previous SNRS studies. The ISKDC has reported a male and female ratio of 2:1 [11]. However, Caridi *et al.* observed a male to female ratio of patients with an NPHS2 gene mutation of 7:2 [14]. A study about NPHS2 412C→T and

Table 4. Correlation between NPHS2 polymorphisms and clinical manifestations in 28 patients with steroid-resistant nephrotic syndrome.

Polymorphisms	eGFR < 90 (ml/min/1.73 m²)		p^*	Hematuria		p^*	Hypertension		p^*
	+	−		+	−		+	−	
g.-52G>T			1.000			1.000			0.113
+	2	2		1	3		0	4	
−	9	15		7	17		12	12	
c.101A>G			0.705			0.691			0.136
+	4	8		4	8		3	9	
−	7	9		4	12		9	7	
g.-117C>T			1.000			0.091			0.434
+	4	5		5	5		3	7	
−	7	12		3	15		9	9	
c.288C>T			1.000			0.555			1.000
+	2	2		2	2		2	2	
−	9	15		6	18		10	14	
c.954C>T			0.355			0.311			1.000
+	10	12		5	17		9	13	
−	1	5		3	3		3	3	
c.1038A>G			0.353			0.123			1.000
+	3	2		3	2		2	3	
−	8	15		5	18		10	13	

*Fisher's Exact Test.

419delG gene mutations in Indonesian children with SRNS concluded that male gender was risk factor for SRNS [20]. The age at onset of disease in this study is 1 to 13 years with 57% of the patients who were younger than 6years at the disease onset. Weber *et al.*, found that NPHS2 gene mutation R138Q in SRNS patients is associated with early onset (12 ± 3 months) [13]. Polymorphism of NPHS2 gene R229Q is associated with late-onset nephrotic syndrome [21] as well as increased risk of microalbuminuria in the general population [22]. This R229Q variant presents in approximately 4% of Western population, encoding a protein with lower affinity for binding to nephrin [23]. About 36% patients with SRNS exhibited progression to ESRD 5 - 6 years after onset. Aucella *et al.*, studied 33 patients adult onset FSGS which showed that glomerular filtration rate (GFR) was in the normal range in 19 subjects and 14 patients had a variable degree of renal failure [24]. In our study, 17 (60.7%) of the subjects had normal eGFR, while 11 (39.3%) had chronic renal insufficiency (eGFR < 90 mL/min/1.73 m²). Our previous study about NPHS2 412C→T and 419delG gene mutations shows that no differencein clinical manifestations is found between SRNS with mutation and SRNS without mutation, except for serum creatinin in 412C→T mutation [25].

This study reports the identification of 6 NPHS2 polymorphisms, *i.e.* g.-52G>T, c.101A>G, g.-117C>T, c.288C>T, c.954C>T, and c.1038A>G, in patients with clinical diagnosis of SRNS. Homozygous NPHS2 c.101A>G polymorphism was found in 12 subjects, leading to p.Arg34Arg. Homozygous NPHS2 g.-117C>T was found only in 1 subject and Homozygous NPHS2 c.954C>T was found in 9 subjects, leading to p.Ala318Ala. The other NPHS2 polymorphisms were heterozygous. The NPHS2 homozygous and heterozygous polymorphisms have not been implicated in clinical manifestation of SRNS, such as decrease of GFR, hypertension and hematuria, in this study (**Table 4**).

In our study, we could not find any mutation of NPHS2 gene as causative SNRS, suggesting that NPHS2 gene mutations are not major cause of SNRS in Indonesian children. In addition, we also suggests that there is an inter-ethnic difference in the occurrence of NPHS2 gene mutations or their variants, so the 6 NPHS2 gene polymorphisms that were identified have no correlation with the clinical manifestation. The strength of our study lies in the collection of sample from multicenter of various teaching hospitals in Indonesia, while the weakness of this study is only 28 of 59 samples were successfully screened, due to limitation of time and research finance.

5. Conclusion

In conslusion, no mutation was found in this study; however, due to our limitations, more studies are needed. Other exons of podocin or other podocyte proteins in Indonesian children may play a role in the pathogenesis of SRNS.

Acknowledgements

We thank to Prof Bert vanden Heuvel for supervising our research with mutation analysis of NPHS2 gen that performed at The Laboratory of Pediatrics and Neurology of the Radboud University Medical Centre Nijmegen.

References

[1]   Clark, A.G. and Barrat, T.M. (1999) Steroid Responsive Neprotic Syndrome. In: Barrat, T.M., Avner, E.D. and Harmon, W.E., Eds., *Pediatric Nephrology*, 4th Edition, Lippincott Willams & Wilkins, Baltimore, 731-747.

[2]   Fydryk, J. and Querfeld, U. (2002) The Nephrotic Syndrome-Idiopathic Steroid Resistant Nephrotic Syndrome. In: Cochat, P., Ed., *European Society for Paediatric Nephrology Handbook*, ESPN, Switzerland, 259-262.

[3]   Roth, K.S., Amaker, B.H. and Chan, J.C.M. (2002) Nephrotic Syndrome: Pathogenesis and Management. *Pediatrics in Review*, **23**, 237-247. http://dx.doi.org/10.1542/pir.23-7-237

[4]   Hogg, R.J., Portman, R.J., Milliner, D., Lemley, K.D., Eddy, A. and Ingelfinger, J. (2000) Evaluation and Management of Proteinuria and Nephrotic Syndrome in Children: Recommendations from a Pediatric Nephrology Panel Established at the National Kidney Foundation Conference on Proteinuria, Albuminuria, Risk, Assessment, Detection, and Elimination (PARADE). *Pediatrics*, **105**, 1242-1249. http://dx.doi.org/10.1542/peds.105.6.1242

[5]   Kitamura, A., Tsukaguchi, H., Iijima, K., Araki, J., Hattori, M., Ikeda, M., *et al.* (2006) Genetics and Clinical Features of 15 Asian Families with Steroid-Resistant Nephrotic Syndrome. *HealthNephrology Dialysis Transplantation*, **21**, 3133-3138. http://dx.doi.org/10.1093/ndt/gfl347

[6]   Caridi, G., Perfumo, F. and Ghiggeri, G.M. (2005) NPHS2 (Podocin) Mutations in Nephrotic Syndrome. Clinical Spectrum and Fine Mechanisms. *Pediatric Research*, **57**, 54R-61R. http://dx.doi.org/10.1203/01.PDR.0000160446.01907.B1

[7]   Niaudet, P. (2004) Genetic Form of Nephrotic Syndrome. *Pediatric Nephrology*, **19**, 1313-1318. http://dx.doi.org/10.1007/s00467-004-1676-9

[8]   Bagga, A. and Mantan, M. (2005) Nephrotic Syndrome in Children. *Indian Journal of Medical Research*, **122**, 13-28.

[9]   Antignac, C. (2002) Genetic Models: Clues for Understanding the Pathogenesis of Idiopathic Nephrotic Syndrome. *Journal of Clinical Investigation*, **109**, 447-449. http://dx.doi.org/10.1172/JCI0215094

[10]   Franceschini, N., Karl, N., Jeffrey, K., Louise, M. and Cheryl, W. (2006) NPHS2 Gene, Nephrotic Syndrome and Focal Segmental Glomerulosclerosis: A HuGE Review. *Genetics in Medicine*, **8**, 63-75. http://dx.doi.org/10.1097/01.gim.0000200947.09626.1c

[11]   International Study of Kidney Disease in Children (ISKDC) (1981) The Primary Nephrotic Syndrome in Children. Identification of Patients with Minimal Change Nephrotic Syndrome from Initial Response to Prednison. *The Journal of Pediatrics*, **98**, 561-564. http://dx.doi.org/10.1016/S0022-3476(81)80760-3

[12]   Hinkes, B., Vlangos, C., Heeringa, S., Mucha, B., Gbadegesin, R., Liu, J., *et al.* (2008) Specific Podocin Mutations Correlate with Age of Onset in Steroid-Resistant Nephrotic Syndrome. *Journal of the American Society of Nephrology*, **19**, 365-371. http://dx.doi.org/10.1681/ASN.2007040452

[13]   Weber, S., Gribouval, O., Esquivel, E.L., Moriniere, V., Tête, M.J., Legendre, C., *et al.* (2004) *NPHS2* Mutation Analysis Show Genetic Heterogeneity of Steroid-Resistant Nephrotic Syndrom and Lowpost-Transplant Recurrence. *Kidney International*, **66**, 571-579. http://dx.doi.org/10.1111/j.1523-1755.2004.00776.x

[14]   Caridi, C., Berteli, R., Carrea, A., Di Duca, M., Catarsi, P., Artero, M., *et al.* (2001) Prevalence, Genetics, and Clinical

Features of Patients Carrying Podocin Mutations in Steroid-Resistant Nonfamilial Focal Segmental Glomerulosclerosis. *Journal of the American Society of Nephrology*, **12**, 2742-2746.

[15] Karle, S., Uetz, B., Ronner, V., Glaeser, L., Hildebrandt, F. and Fuchshuber, A., Members of the APN Study Group (2002) Novel Mutations in *NPHS2* Are Detected in Familial as Well as Sporadic Steroid Resistant Nephritic Syndrome. *Journal of the American Society of Nephrology*, **13**, 388-393.

[16] Caridi, G., Bertelli, R., Di Duca, M., Dagnino, M., Emma, F. and Muda, A.O. (2003) Broadening the Spectrum of Diseases Related to Podocin Mutations. *Journal of the American Society of Nephrology*, **14**, 1278-1286. http://dx.doi.org/10.1097/01.ASN.0000060578.79050.E0

[17] Ruf, R.G., Lichtenberger, A., Karle, S.M., Haas, J.P., Anacleto, F.E., Schultheiss, M., *et al.*, The APN Study Group (2004) Patients with Mutations in *NPHS2* (Podocin) Do Not Respond to Standard Steroid Treatment of Nephrotic Syndrome. *Journal of the American Society of Nephrology*, **15**, 722-732. http://dx.doi.org/10.1097/01.ASN.0000113552.59155.72

[18] Yu, Z.H., Ding, J., Huang, J.P., Yao, Y., Xiao, H.J., Zhang, J.J., *et al.* (2005) Mutations in *NPHS2* in Sporadic Steroid-Resistant Nephrotic Syndrome in Chinese Children. *Nephrology Dialysis Transplantation*, **20**, 902-908. http://dx.doi.org/10.1093/ndt/gfh769

[19] Otukesh, H., Ghazanfari, B., Fereshtehnejad, S.M., Bakhshayesh, M., Hashemi, M., Hoseini, R., *et al.* (2009) *NPHS2* Mutations in Children with Steroid-Resistant Nephritic Syndrome. *Iranian Journal of Kidney Diseases*, **3**, 99-102.

[20] Rachmadi, D., Hilmanto, D., Idjradinata, P. and Sukadi, A. (2011) *NPHS2* Gene Mutation, Atopy and Gender as Risk Factors for Steroid-Resistant Nephrotic Syndrome in Indonesian. *Paediatrica Indonesiana*, **51**, 272-276.

[21] Tsukaguchi, H., Sudhakar, A., Le, T.C., Nguyen, T., Yao, J., Schwimmer, J.A., Schachter, A.D., *et al.* (2002) *NPHS2* Mutations in Late-Onset Focal Segmental Glomerulosclerosis: R229Q Is a Common Disease-Associated Allele. *Journal of Clinical Investigation*, **110**, 1659-1666. http://dx.doi.org/10.1172/JCI0216242

[22] Pereira, A.C., Pereira, A.B., Mota, G.F., Cunha, R.S., Herkenhoff, F.L., Pollack, M.R., *et al.* (2004) *NPHS2* R229Q Functional Variant Is Associated with Microalbuminuria in the General Population. *Kidney International*, **65**, 1026-1030. http://dx.doi.org/10.1111/j.1523-1755.2004.00479.x

[23] Obeidova, H., Merta, M., Reiterova, J., Maixnerova, D., Stekrova, J., Rysava, R., *et al.* (2006) Genetic Basis of Nephrotic Syndrome—Review. *Prague Medical Report*, **107**, 5-16.

[24] Aucella, F., De Bonis, P., Gatta, G., Muscarella, L.A., Vigilante, M., Di Giorgio, G., *et al.* (2004) Molecular Analysis of *NPHS2* and *ACTN4* Genes in a Series of 33 Italian Patients Affected by Adult-Onset Nonfamilial Focal Segmental Glomerulosclerosis. *Nephron Clinical Practice*, **99**, 31-36. http://dx.doi.org/10.1159/000082864

[25] Rachmadi, D., Hilmanto, D., Idjradinata, P. and Sukadi, A. (2011) *NPHS2* (412 C→T and 419delG) Gene Mutation and Their Clinical Manifestation in Indonesian Steroid-Resistant Nephrotic Syndrome. *Majalah Kedokteran Bandung*, **43**, 193-198. http://dx.doi.org/10.15395/mkb.v43n4.69

18

Management of Specific Complications after Congenital Heart Surgery (I)

A. Sánchez Andrés[1], C. González Miño[2], E. Valdés Diéguez[3], L. Boni[3], J. I. Carrasco Moreno[1]

[1]Pediatric Cardiology Unit, Hospital Universitario y Politécnico La Fe, Valencia, Spain
[2]Pediatric Intensive Care Unit, Hospital General de Castellón, Castellon, Spain
[3]Pediatric Surgery Unit, Hospital Universitario y Politécnico La Fe, Valencia, Spain
Email: tonisanchan@hotmail.com

Abstract

In addition to the general consequences of surgery and cardiopulmonary by-pass, lesion-specific complications can occur after surgery for congenital heart disease. It is important for the pediatric intensive care specialist to fully understand the preoperative anatomy and the intraoperative details of these patients. This allows a timely and appropriate treatment of general and lesion-specific complications. In this article we provide a list of commonly-performed surgical procedures and possible associated problems to be anticipated in the early postoperative period. Then it follows a discussion about the diagnosis and management of these complications, based on their pathophysiological features.

Keywords

Congenital Heart Diseases, Pediatric Heart Surgery, Postoperative

1. Introduction

1) Congenital heart disease is the most common birth defect. Recent prevalence estimates range from 6 to 10 per 1000 live births. Many of these infants require surgery to correct or palliate their heart defect; several of them require surgery in the newborn period [1].

2) Optimal management of the postoperative pediatric cardiac surgical patient requires a thorough understanding of patient anatomy, physiology, surgical procedure and clinical condition [2].

3) Cardiopulmonary bypass, specific surgical procedure, anesthesia and other medications have the potential to produce multisystemic effects [2]. Postoperative care focuses on anticipating potentially deleterious effects and a timely intervention to restore cardiopulmonary homeostasis and prevent end organ damage [3].

4) Multidisciplinary approach: as these patients are currently managed in intensive care units, a multiduscip-

linar collaborative effort is required to achieve a better outcome. An accurate and timely determination of cardiac output, systemic O_2 delivery, and tissue oxygenation is essential to optimizing outcomes [4].

5) Severity of illness scores have been developed to predict postoperatory outcomes, based on bed side collected data, such us lactate levels or drugs employed for haemodynamic support (VIS score); recently, Kyle G. Miletic *et al.* [3] have reported a novel vasoactive-ventilation-renal score (VVR) incorporating postoperative markers of cardiovascular, pulmonary and renal dysfunction, the three most commonly affected organ systems in children after surgery for congenital heart disease (CHD).

6) Relative to the amount of information avaliable about CPB and general complications after pediatric cardiac surgery, updated literature about lesión specific complications is lagging [5].

The main objective of this article is to provide a list of commonly-performed surgical procedures and possible associated problems to be anticipated in the early postoperative period. The diagnosis and management of these complications, based on their pathophysiological features are also discussed.

2. Complications after Cardiac Procedures

The following tables show the most common problems to be anticipated in the early postoperative period according to the general pathophysiological mechanism underlying the congenital heart disease, as well as the specific procedure performed.

1) Repair of left to right shunts (**Table 1**).

2) Repair of right-sided obstructions (**Table 2**).

3) Repair of left-sided obstructions (**Table 3**).

4) Palliative procedures (**Table 4**).

5) Miscellaneous: including procedures for anatomic and physiologic correction of D-transposition of the great arteries and repair of anomalous origin of coronary artery from pulmonary artery and surgery on the mitral valve (**Table 5**).

3. Diagnosis and Management of Specific Complications

3.1. Residual Left to Right Shunts (Table 1)

It is the case of an incorrect septal defect closure or a residual shunt at other levels (e.g.: systemic-pulmonary collateral arteries or apical muscular VSDs), either preoperatively unrecognized or recognized but intentionally left untreated. The pathophysiology of these shunts include the development of pulmonary edema secondary to increased pulmonary blood flow, pulmonary hypertension, ventricular volume overload, and in some circumstances systemic cardiac output limitation. The most common signs and symptoms include a pulmonary (or VSD type) ejection murmur, high left atrial filling pressures, cardiomegaly with signs of increased pulmonary blood flow on chest radiograph, and variable degrees of low cardiac output [6].

Residual shunts at atrial level are rarely a problem, unless other factors increase the shunt volume. The development of congestive heart failure should guide the clinician to rule out mitral stenosis or regurgitation, small size and/or dysfunction of the systemic ventricle, and systemic ventricular outflow tract obstruction [7].

Residual shunts at ventricular or arterial level are clinically more relevant because of the systemic ventricle volume overload and the pressure and volume overload of the pulmonary circulation. In general, shunts with a Qp:Qs smaller than 1.5 - 2.1 without pulmonary hypertension are well tolerated. Larger shunts are almost always associated with congestive heart failure. Patients with large preoperative left to right shunt usually tolerate residual shunts better than patients who were cyanotic before surgery. For example, a patient with a residual ventricular septal defect after repair of tetralogy of Fallot, moves from a situation in which the left ventricle is normally loaded preoperatively to a new situation in which it is overloaded with volume. At pulmonary level, from a situation of reduced pulmonary flow we pass to the opposite scenario of pulmonary overload. These factors make the residual defect poorly tolerated [8].

Once the diagnosis of residual shunt is made, the right treatment must be chosen, balancing the risks and benefits of a surgical or a percutaneous intervention. Some injuries are not repairable and these patients need to be managed with conservative measures. Maneuvers that reduce pulmonary vascular resistances must be avoided because they increase the shunt magnitude. Examples of these are the use of high oxygen concentrations or

Table 1. Repair of left to right shunts.

General Complications

-Residual defects: leading to various degrees of left to right shunt.

-Pulmonary hypertension: this is the most predictable complication in older patients who had time to develop pulmonary vascular disease, in neonates and in patients with pulmonary venous obstruction.

-Arrhythmias: any arrhythmia can occur after any cardiac surgical procedure, but the patients with ventricular or atrioventricular septal defects have a greater risk of complete heart block (CHB) and junctional ectopic tachycardia (JET).

Specific Complications

▪ *Repair of atrial septal defects*

  -Sinus-Node dysfunction.

  -Acute left-ventricular failure (in older children and adults).

▪ *Repair of ventricular septal defects*

  -Pulmonary Hypertension.

  -Arrhythmias: JET and CHB.

  -Insufficiency or stenosis of the right atrioventricular valve.

▪ *Ligation of patent ductus arteriosus*

  -Recurrent laryngeal nerve injury.

  -Damage or ligation of the left pulmonary artery or aorta.

▪ *Repair of truncus arteriosus*

  -Pulmonary hypertension.

  -Truncal valve stenosis or regurgitation.

  -Right ventricular dysfunction.

▪ *Repair of aorto-pulmonary window*

  -Pulmonary hypertension.

▪ *Repair of anomalous pulmonary venous return*

  -Pulmonary hypertension.

  -Arrhythmias.

  -Residual stenosis of the pulmonary veins or anastomosis.

  -High left ventricular filling pressures due to the small size of the left chambers.

hyperventilation. Inotropic support, mechanical ventilation, afterload reducers, and the use of diuretics are usually needed. As soon as the heart recovers from the deleterious effects of surgery, the residual shunt will become better tolerated, allowing a decrease of the medical treatment [9].

3.2. Residual Obstruction of the Ventricular Outflow Tracts

Residual obstructions should be sought after any surgery on the ventricular outflow tracts (**Tables 2-3**), such as repair of subaortic stenosis, aortic or pulmonary valve commisurotomy, Fallot repair. Furthermore, systemic ventricle obstruction may occur after repair of atrio-ventricular septal defects or after interventions that reduce the ventricular volume preload when the underlying anatomy includes subvalvular hypertrophy (often septal). Ventricular hypertrophy can cause obstruction of the foramen narrowing subvalvular ventricular bulb.

Signs and symptoms of systemic ventricle obstruction include an ejection systolic murmur, left atrial hypertension,

Table 2. Repair of right-sided obstructions.

General Complications
• *Residual stenosis or regurgitation.*
• *Right ventricular dysfunction*: both systolic and diastolic. The latter is more common due to the right ventricle hypertrophy and its poor compliance, particularly if a right ventriculotomy is performed.

Specific Complications
• *Repair of Fallot's tetralogy and its variants*
-Right ventricular dysfunction.
-Arrhythmias: JET, CHB.
-Pulmonary regurgitation.
-Residual pulmonary stenosis.
-Residual ventricular septal defect.
• *Repair of absent pulmonary valve syndrome*
-Tracheobronchomalacia.
• *Repair of pulmonary atresia with intact ventricular septum*
-Right ventricular dysfunction.
-Myocardial ischemia (in case of right ventricular dependent coronary circulation).
-Circular shunt: if it is used both systemic to pulmonary fistula type modified Blalock-Taussig shunt and a patch on the right ventricular outflow tract.
-Hypoxia (particularly in the first postoperative hours)

pulmonary edema and a low cardiac output state (according to the degree of the residual defect) [10].

In the interpretation of the diagnostic tests (including echocardiography and cardiac catheterization), special emphasis must be placed in the anatomical details of the obstruction, especially in presence of ventricular dysfunction, when a severe stenosis may not produce an accordingly severe gradient. Unlike adult patients with systemic ventricle obstruction, the use of beta-adrenergic agonists is not usually associated with myocardial ischemia, provided that cardiac output and myocardial oxygen delivery are assured.

Special attention must be paid when the obstruction is dynamic, since an increase in myocardial contractility may worsen the lesion. Therefore in this setting inotropes are contraindicated. The presence of systemic ventricular obstruction is also a relative contraindication to the use of vasodilation agents. In fact systemic vasodilation in presence of ventricular outflow obstruction may cause severe hypotension, due to the inability of the heart to increase cardiac output [11] [12].

Patients who had a significant relief of systemic outflow tract obstruction easily develop systemic arterial hypertension, due to a maintained hyperdynamic state of the heart and vessels. Treatment of hypertension is particularly important in the first 24 hours after surgery, to protect the surgical repair (sutures) and to minimize the risk of bleeding. The most effective drugs include vasodilators, beta-blockers and inhibitors of angiotensin converting enzyme (ACEi).

3.3. Dysfunction of the Mitral or Tricuspid Valve

Residual atrio-ventricular (AV) valve regurgitation or stenosis may occur after any reparative surgery of the valve itself or when closing a septal defect unmasks valvular stenosis in one side of the heart.

AV valve insufficiency results in elevated atrial pressures on the affected side. If atrial pressure is being monitored directly, it can get drawn with very prominent V waves and a regurgitant murmur may be listened. Because of the associated ventricular volume overload, signs of ventricular failure may develop.

AV valve stenosis is also associated with high pressure in the atria, but not with ventricular volume overload. Systemic or pulmonary edema is very common in AV valve stenosis as a consequence of systemic or pulmonary

Table 3. Repair of left-sided obstructions.

General Complications
• *Residual stenosis.*
• *Systemic arterial hypertension.*
• *Left ventricular diastolic dysfunction.*

Specific Complications
• *Repair of aortic stenosis*
-Valvotomy: residual stenosis/aortic regurgitation.
-Ross operation: myocardial ischemia.
-Konno operation: myocardial Ischemia, right ventricular outflow tract obstruction and arrhythmias.
• *Repair of subaortic stenosis*
-Residual stenosis.
-Iatrogenic mitral valve regurgitation.
-Arrhythmias.
• *Repair of supravalvar aortic stenosis*
-Residual aortic stenosis.
-Aortic regurgitation due to valve injury.
-Myocardial ischemia.
• *Repair of aortic coarctation*
-Residual stenosis.
-Paraplegia.
-Postcoarctectomy syndrome.
-Aortic stenosis unmasked.
-Recurrent laryngeal nerve injury.
• *Repair of interrupted aortic arch*
-Residual stenosis (normally at anastomosis site).
-Left bronchial compression (by the advanced aorta).
-Hypocalcemia (if DiGeorge Syndrome associated).
• *Repair of mitral stenosis*
-Pulmonary hypertension.
-Residual stenosis or regurgitation.
-Left ventricular dysfunction.

venous hypertension respectively. Cardiac output may be limited in case of severe A-V valve stenosis or insufficiency, especially in acute onset [6].

In case of a hemodinamically significative lesion—and if the valve is amenable of surgical repair—the patient should be brought back to the OR without delay. If the alternative is a prosthetic valve implantation, palliative medical treatment should be considered, given the poor outcome of prosthetic valves in young patients. The medical management of AV valve regurgitation focuses on afterload reduction with inotropic support when necessary. Systemic vasodilators are useful in mitral regurgitation, while diuretics may be useful in both AV valve

Table 4. Palliative procedures.

Systemic to pulmonary shunts (Modified Blalock-Taussig, Central shunts)
▪ *Excessive pulmonary blood flow.*
▪ *Arterial hypotension.*
▪ *Shunt thrombosis (acute hypoxemia).*
Pulmonary Artery Banding
▪ Cyanosis.
▪ Excessive pulmonary blood flow.

Table 5. Miscellaneous.

Arterial switch operation for D-transposition of great arteries
▪ *Myocardial ischemia and left ventricular dysfunction.*
▪ *Aortic regurgitation.*
▪ *Supravalvar pulmonary stenosis.*
Atrial switch operation (Mustard or Senning)
▪ Tunnel stenosis (pulmonary and/or systemic venous obstruction).
▪ Arrhythmias.
Repair of anomalous left or right coronary artery from pulmonary artery
▪ Myocardial failure with or w/o mitral regurgitation (secondary to ischemia).
Mitral valve surgery
▪ Residual stenosis or regurgitation.
▪ Pulmonary hypertension.

regurgitation and stenosis. Even though medical treatment of an AV valve stenosis is usually poorly effective, associated conditions (such as pulmonary hypertension) require aggressive treatment [13] [14].

3.4. Left or Right Ventricular Diastolic Dysfunction

Ventricular diastolic dysfunction should be expected after any cardiac surgery on a hypertrophied heart, such as after repair of obstructive lesions of either ventricular outflow tract. When a right ventriculotomy is needed (especially in a hypertrophied ventricle) both diastolic and systolic dysfunction may develop. Furthermore, due to its anatomical location, the right ventricle is particularly exposed to the operating room temperature, so that myocardial preservation by means of systemic cooling may be less effective.

Diastolic dysfunction is characterized by high pressures at atrial level and has similar characteristics to those seen in AV valve dysfunction. The presence of a residual shunt at atrial level exacerbates the symptoms of cardiac failure in case of left (systemic) ventricular dysfunction, while it may be useful in maintaining the cardiac output in case of right (pulmonary) ventricular dysfunction (e.g., TOF repair). In this case, a certain degree of cyanosis must be expected, but it is normally well tolerated.

The need to maintain high filling pressures of a ventricular chamber (see treatment here below) results in increased upstream hydrostatic pressures which, in turn, favors the extravasation of fluids and leads to pulmonary or generalized (systemic) edema, depending on the side affected [15] [16].

The first-line treatment of diastolic dysfunction is the administration of IV fluids to maintain an adequate ventricular preload, although this will come at the expense of an increase in systemic and pulmonary venous pressures. Thus, fluids administration may be limited by the consequences of pulmonary or systemic venous hypertension, such as hypoxia or severe peripheral edema and effusions respectively [17]. The use of inodilators, such as milrinone, is also very useful. Especially the right ventricle responds very well to the initial administration of fluids, but—as seen—high hydrostatic pressures easily lead to the appearance of pleural effusions and/or ascites. Without adequate drainage of these effusions the intra-thoracic and intra-abdominal pressures will increase. This will lead, in the first case, to higher airway pressures which will be transmitted to the pulmonary vasculature. This situation of increased pulmonary vascular resistance will negatively affect the already depressed right ventricle, thus maintaining a vicious circle, apart from altering the gas exchange. Increased intra-abdominal pressure may result in decreased renal perfusion and eventually kidney failure, complicating the fluids and electrolytes management. All this triggers a downward spiral in which, finally, cardiac output is affected and it is difficult to restore. Effective treatment includes timely drainage of pleural effusions and ascites, together with an appropriate hidroelectrolyte management. In cases of refractory right ventricular dysfunction, mechanical assistance with ECMO may be needed. In general, right ventricular diastolic function improves within days, as far as the right ventricle recovers from surgery and becomes more distensible (and assuming that the intervention restored normal or near-normal RV systolic pressures). Diastolic dysfunction can be managed in a similar way, but more likely to be associated with prolonged cardiac arrest and/or cardiac transplantation.

3.5. Pulmonary Hypertension

Early repair of cardiac defects characterized by increased pulmonary blood flow has reduced the incidence of postoperative pulmonary hypertension. However the use of cardiopulmonary bypass during most pediatric cardiac interventions can produce pulmonary hypertension in patients with underlying risk factors. Neonates, patients with obstruction of pulmonary veins or mitral valve dysfunction, and those with high preoperative pulmonary vascular resistance, are at higher risk. Pain, agitation, tracheal aspirations or hypoventilation may trigger a pulmonary hypertensive crisis. Signs and symptoms of pulmonary hypertension depend on the acuity of changes in lung (pulmonary vascular resistance) resistance and the underlying anatomy. Chronic pulmonary hypertension that doesn´t worsen acutely with cardiopulmonary bypass may be well tolerated during the postoperative period while the acute crisis can produce severe life-threatening symptoms.

A patent foramen ovale, ASD, VSD or systemic-pulmonary shunts are responsible of the major clinical manifestation of an acute elevation in pulmonary pressure, which is the cyanosis (due to a right to left shunt). Pulmonary hypertension in absence of septal defects can cause acute right ventricular failure and low cardiac output, without significant changes in saturation. A sudden drop in blood pressure or saturation in a patient with known pulmonary vascular disease or significant risk factors for pulmonary hypertension should immediately make the clinician consider this diagnosis and consequently establish the adequate treatment. The presence of a pulmonary artery pressure catheter can help in the establishment of a diagnosis. Most commonly there will be a drop in systemic arterial pressure while pulmonary pressure will not change. The increase of pulmonary to systemic pressure ratio is diagnostic of increased pulmonary resistance.

The increase in pulmonary arterial pressure is transmitted to the right ventricle and as a consequence the interventricular septum will be shifted leftward, compromising the function of the left ventricle. Tachycardia is a common sign that shows how the heart struggles to maintain systemic output at low-volume filling. Other clinical manifestations include the sudden drop in lung compliance or the development of bronchospasm.

The most effective measure to manage patients at high risk of pulmonary hypertension in the postoperative period is prevention. The establishment and maintenance of proper analgesia and sedation, especially during painful stimuli (such as OT tube suctioning), is very important. The induction of respiratory alkalosis may be helpful in a pulmonary hypertensive crisis, but maintaining a pH above 7.5 for long periods of time can have deleterious effects on cerebral perfusion. Therefore, a practical approach would be to prevent and timely treat common problems that lead to hypoxia and respiratory acidosis, such as pneumothorax, selective right bronchus intubation or the presence of bronchial secretions, and try to maintain pH between 7.4 and 7.5. Then one would try to normalize the pH and reduce the sedation day by day with caution, paying attention to the appearance of any symptoms of pulmonary artery hypertension. When pulmonary hypertension persists for more than 4 - 7 days, it is suggestive of the existence of residual lesions or chronic injury of the pulmonary vasculature.

If prophylactic measures fail, aggressive treatments such as nitric oxide, sildenafil, bosentan, or even mechanical circulatory support are indicated. Numerous studies have shown that low doses of nitric oxide (2 - 20 parts per million-ppm) are as effective as high doses (40 - 80 ppm) and are associated with fewer side effects, such as methemoglobinemia or secondary hypotension. Sildenafil and bosentan can be used as a transition from inhaled nitric oxide to chronic oral therapy, given that the use of exogenous NO inhibits the production of endogenous NO. Other intravenous vasodilators, including calcium channel blockers, nitrates and prostaglandins, have been used, but they have the limitations of systemic hypotension due to the lack of pulmonary selectivity. Prostacyclin has proved to be an effective drug that can reverse the changes in the pulmonary vasculature before they become permanent [18].

All these strategies are based on an attempt to dilate the pulmonary vascular bed to increase pulmonary blood flow. If this is not possible, the next option is to try to alter the balance between pulmonary and systemic vascular resistances, by increasing systemic ones:

- First of all an adequate preload should be guaranteed, for which colloid or crystalloid administration at 30 - 40 mL/kg is useful.
- Arterial pH should be maintained around 7.45 to 7.50, and blood $PaCO_2$ between 30 and 35 mmHg. Serum bicarbonate should be kept at the higher limit of its range. High frequency ventilation may be used to achieve these goals and sodium bicarbonate boluses or infusion may be administered if necessary.
- Simultaneously we can introduce inhaled nitric oxide (iNO) at 10 - 20 ppm.
- If oxygen saturations are still low, the next step is to increase mean systemic arterial pressure to 60 - 70 mmHg (depending on the patient's age), which can be achieved with an infusion of norepinephrine (being this drug much more selective on the peripheral vascular bed than on the pulmonary one) or high-dose dopamine.
- We can try the administration of intravenous magnesium (due to its smooth muscle relaxant effect, being a calcium antagonist, and also being effective as skeletal muscle relaxant, sedative and antiarrhythmic drug) in bolus or continuous infusion to maintain serum magnesium concentrations between 3 to 5.5 mmol/L.
- Finally we can use intravenous adenosine starting with a bolus of 50 microgrs/kg and then infused at 25 - 50 microgrs/kg/minute.

With this therapeutic strategy we can successfully manage patients with such low oxygenation rates that would usually be treated with an ECMO device, without significant differences in mortality [19].

3.6. Acute Low Cardiac Output

Many congenital heart defects produce pressure and volume ventricular overload, which if maintained for long time lead to myocyte damage and death. This will lead to ventricular dysfunction and eventually low cardiac output syndrome. To avoid these deleterious effects, early primary repair of cardiac defects is nowadays the preferred strategy in many centers.

Another cause of cellular damage is the relative myocardial ischemia during the aortic cross clamp phase of most cardiac operations. Coronary artery blood flow is interrupted and a cardioplegic solution (rich in potassium) is infused into them to stop the heart in diastole and to protect the myocytes. Many advances are needed to create the ideal cardioplegic solution to keep the heart viable in absence of coronary perfusion, and to prevent ventricular failure. Another factor during surgery that predispose to ventricular failure is the need to perform a ventriculotomy. This creates a scar without contractile capacity, which may lead to acute (or chronic) postoperative ventricular failure [20]. Other factors accounting for postoperative low cardiac output are: 1) residual cardiac lesion; 2) inflammatory response triggered by CPB; 3) changes in systemic vascular resistances and pulmonary vascular resistances; 4) arrhythmias and 5) cardiac tamponade [2].

The aims of the management of the patient in low cardiac output state are to reverse the cause of ventricular dysfunction, to optimize its preload, to increase the contractility with medications that do not increase oxygen consumption, and to decrease the ventricular afterload. Actually the most important aspect is to reduce the afterload, as this improves contractility and reduces myocardial oxygen consumption, although in patients with left ventricular outflow tract obstruction this measure should be applied with caution [21].

When high inotropic doses are needed and especially if the patient does not improve (with progressive increase in serum lactate and persistence of low mixed venous saturation) a circulatory mechanical support device should be implanted, to prevent the deleterious consequences of maintained low cardiac output state and multiple organ dysfunction.

In the pharmacological treatment, we will make a special mention of Levosimendan, a drug with promising results in postoperative adult patients and whose effects are currently being studied in the pediatric population, with promising results in several published clinical trials. This drug sensitizes the myocardium to the action of calcium, stabilizing the troponin molecule in the cardiac muscle and prolonging the effect of calcium on the contractile proteins. It has vasodilatory properties and has also been shown to increase cardiac output and to decrease wedge pressure and pulmonary resistance in patients with heart failure [22] [23].

A published study in pediatric patients [24] has shown the effectiveness of Levosimendan administration in 26 patients (21 postoperative and 5 with dilated cardiomyopathy and severe ventricular dysfunction). The doses used in continuous intravenous infusion were 0.1 mcgrs/kg/min which increased after two hours to 0.2 mcgrs/kg/min, and this was maintained for 24 hours. All patients were monitored and the administration of intravenous vasodilators (nitroprusside) was suspended during the infusion of Levosimendan. A side effect considered mild (which necessitated dose reduction) was hypotension requiring increase in ordinary inotropic infusion and increase in volume needs. Serious side effects (requiring drug suspension) were the onset of dangerous ventricular arrhythmias.

The drug's safety was demonstrated, since only one case of treatment discontinuation due to serious ventricular arrhythmia was reported. This patient was treated with additional antiarrhythmic therapy and the problem was resolved in three days. Mild adverse effects can be minimized by adjusting the arterial pressure, the central venous pressure and the serum ions prior to the drug administration and monitoring vital signs during the treatment.

The most immediate beneficial effect was the reduction of serum lactates and central venous pressure. The hemodynamic improvement in most patients allowed removing hemofiltration in those patients who were being treated with it, as well as weaning patients who were on mechanical ventricular assistance. It also showed improvement of patients as a bridge to heart transplantation. Levosimendan doses may be repeated weekly (according to its metabolite half-life).

Thus, the authors of this study conclude that patients who would mostly take advantage of Levosimendan are those with moderate-severe heart failure on waiting list for cardiac transplantation, because the drug would allow them to maintain their clinical situation and avoid worsening. On the other hand, patients with postoperative acute-moderate heart failure also benefit from the use of Levosimendan, in order to achieve myocardial recovery as fast as possible with the lowest dose of intravenous inotropes.

4. Discussion

Compared to adults, children need a much closer monitorization in the postoperative period, due to the onset of minute by minute changes related to conditions such as age, maturation, growth, development, preoperative condition and type of surgery performed. This observation currently requires a highly specialized staff who is familiar with the management of these patients. Postoperative course is different weather the patient is a newborn, a child or an infant. Especially the newborn due to conditions of immaturity, mainly cardiovascular, respiratory, neurological and renal levels can develop a greater number of complications increasing morbidity and mortality.

Preoperative patient condition is very important since children with complex heart anomalies and varying degrees of heart failure, shock or respiratory failure, are patients at risk of a storm and difficult to handle postoperative. Not surprisingly, these patients need more complex surgeries and therefore their mortality rate is higher. Currently, most of the centers worldwide report an mortality about 6%, while the overall mortality for adults is around 3%.

Pediatric cardiac surgery has improved considerably during the last several years. Yet, general and lesion specific complications are to be expected during the early postoperative period. The knowledge and understanding of these complications and their physiology is crucial for an optimal management of these patients. Optimal management of the postoperative pediatric cardiac surgical patient requires a thorough understanding of patient anatomy, physiology, surgical repair or palliation, and clinical condition. Postoperative care focuses on anticipating potentially deleterious events and instituting a proactive approach in managing patients. Intervention strategies are directed at preventing low cardiac output and avoiding adverse sequelae in major organ systems. Acute low cardiac output, diastolic disfunction or pulmonary hypertension are some of the most important general complications, whereas residual shunts, residual obstruction of ventricular outflow tracts, or valve disfunction should be expected after some specific heart diseases and surgical procedures. A residual lesion is a lesion that is present at the time of the completion of an operation or intervention. Residual lesions may be secondary to three etiologies: 1) Attempted therapy to treat the lesion may have failed; 2) The lesion may have been intentionally not treated and purposefully left present, and 3) Knowledge of the lesion may not have existed until completion of the operation or intervention.

Postoperative management of pediatric patients undergoing cardiac surgery requires an understanding of basic principles of tissue oxygenation, cardiovascular physiology and anatomy and pathophysiology of congenital heart disease. Signs and symptoms of low cardiac output syndrome should be treated timely and aggressively and the diagnoses and treatment strategies should take into account both the general problems of any post-operative cardiac patient as well as the specific heart disease and type of surgery performed.

References

[1] Krishnamurthy, G., Ratner, V. and Bacha, E. (2013) Neonatal Cardiac Care, a Perspective. *Seminars in Thoracic and Cardiovascular Surgery: Pediatric Cardiac Surgery Annual*, **16**, 21-31. http://dx.doi.org/10.1053/j.pcsu.2013.01.007

[2] Beke, D.M., Braudis, N.J. and Lincoln, P. (2005)Management of the Pediatric Postoperative Cardiac Surgery Patient. *Critical Care Nursing Clinics of North America*, **17**, 405-416. http://dx.doi.org/10.1016/j.ccell.2005.08.006

[3] Miletic, K.G., Spiering, T.J., Delius, R.E., *et al.* (2014) Use of a Novel Vasoactive-Ventilation-Renal Score to Predict Outcomes after Paediatric Cardiac Surgery. *Interactive CardioVascular and Thoracic Surgery*, **20**, 289-295.

[4] Bronicki, R.A. and Chang, A.C. (2011) Management of the Postoperative Pediatric Cardiac Surgical Patient. *Critical Care Medicine*, **39**, 1974-1984. http://dx.doi.org/10.1097/CCM.0b013e31821b82a6

[5] Pouard, P. and Bojan, M. (2013) Neonatal Cardiopulmonary Bypass. *Seminars in Thoracic and Cardiovascular Surgery: Pediatric Cardiac Surgery Annual*, **15**, 59-61. http://dx.doi.org/10.1053/j.pcsu.2013.01.010

[6] Ungerleider, R.M. (2005) Optimizing Response of the Neonate and Infant to Cardiopulmonary Bypass. *Cardiology in the Young*, **15**, 142-148. http://dx.doi.org/10.1017/S1047951105001186

[7] Wessel, D.L. (1992) Postoperative Management of the Open Heart Surgery Patient. In: Gioia, F.R., Stidham, G.L. and Yeh, T.S., Eds., *Pediatric Clinical Care Medicine*, 135-152.

[8] Cyran, S.E., Hannon, D.W., Daniels, S.R., Gelfand, M.J., Bailey, W.W., Wilson, J.M. and Kaplan, S. (1987) Predictors of Postoperative Ventricular Dysfunction in Infants Who Have Undergone Primary Repair of a Ventricular Septal Defect. *American Heart Journal*, **113**, 1144-1148. http://dx.doi.org/10.1016/0002-8703(87)90926-4

[9] Kavey, R.E. (2006) Optimal Management Strategies for Patients with Complex Congenital Heart Disease. *Circulation*, **113**, 2569-2571. http://dx.doi.org/10.1161/CIRCULATIONAHA.106.629154

[10] Cullen, S., Shore, D. and Redington, A. (1995) Characterization of Right Ventricular Diastolic Performance after Complete Repair of Tretralogy of Fallot: Restrictive Physiology Predicts Slow Postoperative Recovery. *Circulation*, **91**, 1782-1789. http://dx.doi.org/10.1161/01.CIR.91.6.1782

[11] Jonas, R. (2004) Left Ventricular Outflow Tract Obstruction: Aortic Valve Stenosis, Suaortic Stenosis, Supravalvar Aortic Stenosis. In: Jonas, R., Nardo, D. and James, A., *et al.*, Eds., *Comprehensive Surgical Management of Congenital Heart Disease*, Atnold, London, 320-340.

[12] Uva, M.S., Galetti, L., Gayet, F.L., Piot, D., Serraf, A., Bruniaux, J., Comas, J., Roussin, R., Touchot, A., Binet, J.P., *et al.* (1995) Surgery for Congenital Mitral Valve Disease in the First Year of Life. *The Journal of Thoracic and Cardiovascular Surgery*, **109**, 164-174. http://dx.doi.org/10.1016/S0022-5223(95)70432-9

[13] Yoshimura, N., Yamaguchi, M., Oshima, Y., Oka, S., Ootaki, Y., Murakami, H., Tei, T. and Ogawa, K. (1999) Surgery for Mitral Valve Disease in the Pediatric Age Group. *The Journal of Thoracic and Cardiovascular Surgery*, **118**, 99-106. http://dx.doi.org/10.1016/S0022-5223(99)70148-0

[14] Vargas, F.J., Mengo, G., Granja, M.A., Gentile, J.A., Rannzini, M.E. and Vazquez, J.C. (1998) Tricuspid Annuloplasty and Ventricular Placation for Ebstein's Malformation. *The Annals of Thoracic Surgery*, **65**, 1755-1757. http://dx.doi.org/10.1016/S0003-4975(98)00290-2

[15] Lipshultz, S.E. (2000) Ventricular Dysfunction Clinical Research in Infants, Children and Adolescents. *Progress in Pediatric Cardiology*, **12**, 1-28. http://dx.doi.org/10.1016/S1058-9813(00)00076-X

[16] Tede, N. and Child, J. (2000) Diastolic Dysfunction in Patients with Congenital Heart Disease. *Cardiology Clinics*, **18**, 491-499. http://dx.doi.org/10.1016/S0733-8651(05)70157-0

[17] Yano, M., Kohno, M., Ohkusa, T., Mochizuki, M., Yamada, J., Kohno, M., *et al.* (2000) Effect of Milrinone on Left Ventricular Relaxation and Calcium Uptake Function of Cardiac Sarcoplasmic Reticulum. *American Journal of Physiology—Heart and Circulatory Physiology*, **279**, H1898-H1905.

[18] Wessel, D.L., Adatia, I., Giglia, T.M., Thompson, J.E. and Kulik, T.J. (1993) Used of Inhaled Nitric Oxide and Acetylcholine in the Evaluation of Pulmonary Hypertension and Endothelial Function after Cardiopulmonary By-Pass. *Circulation*, **88**, 2128-2138. http://dx.doi.org/10.1161/01.CIR.88.5.2128

[19] Petros, A.J. and Pierce, C.M. (2006) The Management of Pulmonary Hypertension. *Pediatric Anesthesia*, **16**, 816-821.

[20] Balaguru, D., Artman, M. and Auslender, M. (2000) Management of Heart Failure in Children. *Current Problems in Pediatrics*, **30**, 1-35. http://dx.doi.org/10.1016/S0045-9380(00)80035-3

[21] Kay, J.D., Colan, S.D. and Graham Jr., T.P. (2001) Congestive Heart Failure in Pediatric Patients. *American Heart*

Journal, **142**, 923-928. http://dx.doi.org/10.1067/mhj.2001.119423

[22] Egan, J.R., Clarke, A.J., Williams, S., Cole, A.D., Ayer, J., Jaceobe, S., *et al.* (2006) Levosimendan for Low Cardiac Output: A Pediatric Experience. *Journal of Intensive Care Medicine*, **21**, 183-187. http://dx.doi.org/10.1177/0885066606287039

[23] Namachivayam, P., Crossland, D.S., Butt, W.W. and Shekerdemian, L.S. (2006) Early Experience with Levosimendan in Children with Ventricular Dysfunction. *Pediatric Critical Care Medicine*, **7**, 445-448. http://dx.doi.org/10.1097/01.PCC.0000235251.14491.75

[24] Camino, M., Riaño, B., Martínez, C. and Zunzunegui, J.L. (2008) Levosimendan Experience in Paediatric Population. *Med Clin Monogr (Barc)*, **9**, 18-21.

19

Seroprevalence of Dengue Virus IgG among Children 1 - 15 Years, Selected from an Urban Population in Karachi, Pakistan: Population Based Study

Shakeel Ahmed[1,2]*, Syed Rehan Ali[1], Farhana Tabassum[1]

[1]Department of Paediatrics and Child Health, Aga Khan University Hospital, Karachi, Pakistan
[2]Department of Paediatrics, Bahria University Medical and Dental College, Karachi, Pakistan
Email: *shakeel.ahmed@aku.edu

Abstract

Objectives: This was to estimate the proportion of Dengue virus specific IgG ELISA among asymptomatic children between the ages of 1 year to 15 years, residing in an urban population of Karachi. Design: Cross-sectional study. Settings: Subjects were selected from Garden, Karachi; an urban area located adjacent to the Central district of Karachi. Participants: Children of ages 1 year to 15 years, of either sex, residing in the urban area of Garden, Karachi for more than 1 year were selected for the study. Those with a history of yellow fever or using corticosteroids within 1 month of recruitment were excluded. Outcome measures: Data were collected on socioeconomic status of households, medical history, including previous dengue infection, general examination findings and anthropometric indices. Blood samples were collected and sent to Research Laboratories, AKU for determining complete blood counts and serum IgG antibodies for Dengue. All collected information was then analyzed for ascertaining the predicting factors for positive IgG among children less than 15 years. Results: From a total of 900 subjects, 46% were found to have positive IgG in their bloods. Our results revealed that a male child of age more than 10 years was more likely to be IgG positive. Other risk factors identified with the seropositivity included lower household income and absence of anemia, thrombocytopenia and lack of hand washing. Conclusions: The study indicated a significant proportion of children under 15-year-old infected with Dengue virus, with a potential risk of severe complications, if re-infected with dengue. Stringent measures are still needed by both public and private authorities to contain dengue outbreaks, and reducing the proportion of associated mortality, as seen in the previous years. Trial registration: Seed Money Grant (ID# SM090101) was awarded to the corresponding author by Research Committee, Faculty of Health Sciences, Aga Khan University, Pakistan.

---

*Corresponding author.

Keywords

Dengue Virus, IgG, Cross-Sectional, Thrombocytopenia, Hand-Washing, Anemia

1. Introduction

With an estimated 50 million infections per year across many countries, Dengue is now recognized as one of the major public health problems worldwide [1]. It is a mosquito-borne illness belonging to the genus *flavivirus* and consisting of 4 distinct serotypes, namely DENV-1, DENV-2, DENV-3 and DENV-4 [2]. In majority of the cases, the illness is self-limiting with mild symptoms such as fever, rash and joint pain (Dengue Fever). However, this may predispose to a severe form (dengue hemorrhagic fever) with infection with a different serotype [3] [4].

Today, dengue is endemic in more than 100 countries across Asia, Africa, America, Eastern Mediterranean, and West Pacific. Central to this is the enlarging habitat of its vectors, *Aedes aegypti* and *Aedes albopictus*. *Aedes aegypti* in particular, is highly adaptive in crowded areas; hence epidemics have been seen in cities with un-planned urbanization and overcrowding [5] [6].

Pakistan also had its share of dengue outbreaks in the recent years owing to the factors mentioned above. Epidemics have been reported especially in urban areas of Karachi and Lahore; situation worsening especially after monsoonal rains and floods. In October 2010, a total of 1809 cases were suspected out which 881 cases were confirmed of Dengue infection [7]. In 2011, worst outbreak occurred in the country when more than 14,000 people were affected with dengue with over 300 deaths [8].

Considering the current situation of Dengue virus and unavailability of data in Pakistan urgent attention and oversight is required to ensure effective preventive and curative program development. The objective of this study was to estimate the proportion of Dengue virus specific IgG ELISA among asymptomatic children between the ages of 1 year to 15 years, residing in an urban population of Karachi. When re-infected this population would potentially be at a higher risk of developing severe forms of dengue hemorrhagic fever.

2. Methodology

2.1. Study Design/Selection Criteria

A cross sectional survey was conducted from September 2011 to February 2012 to estimate the prevalence of dengue virus. The study cohort consisted of children between one to 15 years of age. The study participants were stratified by geographical zone and age group. There were four zones (East, West, North and South) in the Garden area. The participants were divided into three age groups of 1 - 5 years, 6 - 10 years and 11 - 15 years. Seventy five children were included from each age group in each zone to ensure that the sample was representative not only 1 zone that why each zone was divided equally. Thus a total of 900 children were enrolled in the study and for the selection of respondents systematic random sampling technique was used.

2.2. Selection of Households

After the distribution of zones and ages the second stage was selection of the household's. To select the 1st household Right Hand Rule was followed. Selection of households was done through Systematic Random technique within the starting point of zone. Interview was conducted from every 10th house hold where having at least one child under the age of 1 - 15 years and where the child's family gave informed written consent, before consent full explanation of the study was provided.

2.3. Selection of Respondents

As mentioned earlier, every 10th household was selected for the interview .If there were two or more family with having eligible targeted children in one selected HH only 1 child was selected.

House hold selection was made by using the Health Facility Utilization Survey 2010 conducted by Department of Paediatrics & Child Health, Aga Khan University Karachi.

2.4. Data Collection

After taking written consent from the parents/guardians, data was collected by research medical officers using a questionnaire, specially prepared for this survey. Information was collected on household socioeconomic status, medical history of febrile episodes including previous dengue infection followed by general clinical examination. Anthropometry height (in cms) and weight (in kilograms) was also performed. Blood samples were collected from the subjects and sent to Research Laboratory, Aga Khan University, Pakistan for determining complete blood counts and serum IgG antibodies for Dengue. Complete blood counts were tested using automated hematology analyzer (Beckman).Dengue IgG antibodies was determined by Enzyme Linked ImmunoSorbent Assay (ELISA), using Pan Bio Kits (Dia. Pro Diagnostic BioprobesSrl—Via Columella, 31 Milan—Italy).

2.5. Sample Size

The sample size was calculated using point estimation. We assumed that if 5% of the population has been infected with dengue virus, the minimum estimated number to recruit was 852 subjects, at 5% level of significance and precision of 0.02.

2.6. Statistical Analysis

Data was analyzed using IBM SPSS (Statistical Package for Social Sciences) for Windows version 19 (IBM® SPSS® Statistics, IBM Corporation, Somers, NY, USA). Frequencies were expressed in Means (±standard deviations) calculated for quantitative variables, while proportions were assessed for categorical variables. Factors predicting likelihood to positive IgG among subjects was assessed by multiple logistic regressions. p-value if less than 0.05 was considered significant.

2.7. Ethical Approval

The study was approved by the Ethics Review Committee of the Aga Khan University, Pakistan.

3. Results

Table 1 shows the different characteristics of the population by IgG positivity. A total of 900 subjects, comprising of 461 males and 439 females, were surveyed, from which 419 (46%) had IgG antibodies in their blood. The mean age for IgG positive subjects was relatively higher to the IgG negative subjects (9.5 ± 3.7 years vs. 6.7 ± 4.2 years; p-value < 0.001). About 61% children, with positive IgG were of the age of more than 10 years (**Figure 1**).

   Household characteristics revealed that likelihood for previous dengue infection is more when hand washing is not practiced and no water purifying measures are taken. Likelihood for previous dengue infection is more if the average monthly income is less than Rupees 8000 (**Table 1**).

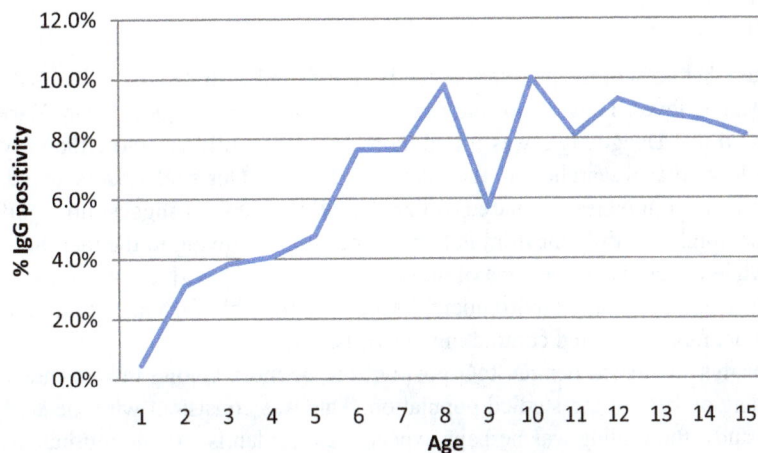

Figure 1. Trends of IgG positivity across age groups of subjects.

Table 1. Characteristics of the population with respect to positive IgG (n = 900).

Characteristics		Total	IgG + ve[1]	Wald X^2	df	p-value	OR (95% CI)
Age groups	1 - 5 years	391	122 (31)				1
	6 - 10 years	258	143 (55)	1.84	1	<0.001	2.74 (1.98 - 3.80)
	More than 11 years	251	154 (61)	54.7	1	<0.001	3.50 (2.51 - 4.88)
Sex	Female	439	192 (44)				1
	Male	46	227 (49)	2.74	1	0.09	1.25 (0.96 - 1.62)
Water purification	Yes	235	91 (39)				1
	No	665	328 (49)	7.79	1	0.01	1.54 (1.14 - 2.09)
Hand washing	Yes	497	212 (43)				1
	No	403	207 (51)	6.77	1	0.01	1.42 (1.09 - 1.85)
Average monthly income	More than Rs 15,000	168	65 (39)				1
	Rs 10,001 - 15,000	179	86 (48)	3.08	1	0.08	1.46 (0.96 - 2.25)
	Rs 8000 - 10,000	315	136 (43)	0.91	1	0.34	1.20 (0.82 - 1.76)
	Less than Rs 8000	238	132 (55)	10.97	1	0.001	1.97 (1.32 - 2.95)
Anemia	Present	142	36 (25)				1
	Absent	758	383 (50)	28.7	1	<0.001	3.02 (2.01 - 4.52)
Thrombocytopenia	Present	18	3 (17)				1
	Absent	882	416 (47)	5.6	1	0.02	4.50 (1.29 - 15.66)
Hepatosplenomegaly	Absent	770	354 (46)				1
	Present	130	65 (50)	0.72	1	0.4	1.20 (0.80 - 1.70)

[1]Expressed as n (%).

Table 2 summarizes the adjusted logistic regression model signifying preponderance patterns for IgG positive subjects. Male children of increasing age were more likely to be IgG positive. The data also shows that children with anemia or thrombocytopenia were less likely to have had a previous dengue infection. The adjusted model revealed that households with lower average income and no water purifying method employed resulted in greater preponderance of previous dengue infection among the target population.

4. Discussion

Our study indicated that 46% of the population had been infected with dengue virus, making them susceptible to severe forms of dengue fever. To date, no study of this sort had been conducted from Karachi, Pakistan.

Our study showed that Dengue IgG was found more in elderly children (more than 5 years). This finding has also been reported by other researchers in their settings [9]-[11]. Our study also showed greater preponderance of dengue IgG antibodies in males compared to females. Where reports suggest no significant differences associated with sex that might be different from Pakistan's perspective owing to the fact that majority of the females remain indoors while males spend their maximum time outside [11]-[13]. As mentioned previously, the dengue vectors are highly adaptable to any environment, hence it is probable for male children of such ages to become exposed to its habitat more often and contracting the virus.

In our study, analysis revealed dengue IgG positivity to be more among lowest categories of socioeconomic position, comprising of 19% of the studied population. This was consistent with the study reported from Brazil [13] [14]. In our study, the finding was perhaps expected as Garden is a modern urban area with high rise buildings and inhabited by affluent communities.

Table 2. Adjusted odds ratios (with 95% CI) computed using multiple logistic regression.

Characteristics		Wald X^2	df	p-value	OR (95% CI)
Age groups	1 - 5 years				1
	6 - 10 years	24.9	1	<0.001	2.40 (1.70 - 3.38)
	More than 10 years	44.4	1	<0.001	3.34 (2.34 - 4.76)
Sex	Female				1
	Male	4.34	1	0.04	1.35 (1.02 - 1.80)
Water purification	Yes				1
	No	4.5	1	0.03	1.43 (1.02 - 2.00)
Average monthly income	More than Rs 15,000				1
	Rs 10,001-15,000	4.54	1	0.03	1.65 (1.04 - 2.61)
	Rs 8000-10,000	1.35	1	0.25	1.28 (0.85 - 1.93)
	Less than Rs 8000	13.1	1	<0.001	2.26 (1.45 - 3.51)
Anemia	Present				1
	Absent	14.7	1	<0.001	2.32 (1.51 - 3.57)
Thrombocytopenia	Present				1
	Absent	4.54	1	0.03	4.07 (1.12 - 14.8)

Employing strategies for water purification was also found to be important in the study, indicating a more likelihood to prior dengue infection in absence of water purification. In our analyses, 39% reported to purify water for consumption, using methods such boiling (15%), filtering (0.02%) and chlorination (0.001%). It can be conceived that untreated water would be the possible niche for the *Aedes* mosquitoes to breed and multiply.

Unique in this study is the positive association of stunting with IgG positivity ($X^2 = 4.12$, df = 1, p-value = 0.042). Our analysis also revealed a lesser likelihood of IgG positivity in presence of anemia and thrombocytopenia. These 3 conditions are pretty prevalent in this part of the world, each clinical correlate limiting us to offer any interpretation to its significance with IgG positivity.

Some limitations are to note in this study. For instance we opted to collect information from a relatively affluent community of Karachi. Though previous studies on Dengue from around the world have indicated Dengue to be a threat for the urban areas, including squatter settlements would have provided a comparative picture showing proportional associations of positive IgG with overcrowding, sanitation and presence of domestic animals [6] [7]. The important and interesting aspect is to assess the serotype of the most prevalent dengue virus in these settings, as limited literature suggests DENV-2 and DENV-3 to be most prevailing in Pakistan [7].

5. Conclusion

The study indicates a significant part of the population of children less than 15 years in Garden, Karachi is infected with Dengue virus. Though severe dengue infections occur in a comparatively smaller population, but the children identified in this study are definitely at risk of severe complications in case of re-infection [6]. New cases are reported with the advent of monsoons and monsoonal rains. Pakistan has received its share of monsoon rains and potentially at risk for another dengue outbreak. Despite public and private measures for containing the infection, we are far away from reducing the rates of dengue in our population. Serious measures are needed to control the mosquito vector populations and reduce the associated morbidity and mortality, as seen in the previous years.

Acknowledgements

The study was carried out using the Aga Khan University Seed Money Grant awarded to SA.

Competing Interests

The authors declare no competing interests.

Authors' Contributions

SA, SRA and FT were involved in data collection, entry, analysis, revision and manuscript writing.

SA was involved in study conception, manuscript writing, data collection, entry, analysis editing and overall supervision.

All authors have read and approved the final manuscript.

Data Sharing Statement

There is no additional data available.

References

[1] World Health Organization (2009) Dengue: Guidelines for Treatment, Prevention, and Control. World Health Organization, Geneva.

[2] Sharma, Y., *et al.* (2012) Seroprevalence and Trend of Dengue Cases Admitted to a Government Hospital, Delhi—5-Year Study (2006-2010): A Look into the Age Shift. *International Journal of Preventive Medicine*, **3**, 537-543.

[3] World Health Organization (1997) General Considerations. Dengue Hemorrhagic Fever: Diagnosis, Treatment, Prevention and Control. World Health Organization.

[4] Idrees, S. and Ashfaq, U.A. (2012) A Brief Review on Dengue Molecular Virology, Diagnosis, Treatment and Prevalence in Pakistan. *Genetic Vaccines and Therapy*, **10**, 6. http://dx.doi.org/10.1186/1479-0556-10-6

[5] Black, W.C.T., *et al.* (2002) Flavivirus Susceptibility in *Aedes aegypti. Archives of Medical Research*, **33**, 379-388. http://dx.doi.org/10.1016/S0188-4409(02)00373-9

[6] Simmons, C.P., *et al.* (2012) Dengue. *New England Journal of Medicine*, **366**, 1423-1432. http://dx.doi.org/10.1056/NEJMra1110265

[7] Jahan, F. (2011) Dengue Fever (DF) in Pakistan. *Asia Pacific Family Medicine*, **10**, 1. http://dx.doi.org/10.1186/1447-056X-10-1

[8] Rai, M.A. (2011) Epidemic: Control of Dengue Fever in Pakistan. Nature, **479**, 41. http://dx.doi.org/10.1038/479041d

[9] Gupta, P., *et al.* Assessment of World Health Organization Definition of Dengue Hemorrhagic Fever in North India. *Journal of Infection in Developing Countries*, **4**, 150-155. http://dx.doi.org/10.3855/jidc.708

[10] Thai, K.T., *et al.* (2005) Seroprevalence of Dengue Antibodies, Annual Incidence and Risk Factors among Children in Southern Vietnam. *Tropical Medicine International Health*, **10**, 379-386. http://dx.doi.org/10.1111/j.1365-3156.2005.01388.x

[11] Yamashiro, T., *et al.* (2004) Seroprevalence of IgG Specific for Dengue Virus among Adults and Children in Santo Domingo, Dominican Republic. *American Journal of Tropical Medicine and Hygiene*, **71**, 138-143.

[12] World Health Organization (2011) Taking Sex and Gender into Account in Emerging Infectious Disease Programmes: An Analytical Framework. World Health Organization, Geneva.

[13] Siqueira, J.B., *et al.* (2004) Household Survey of Dengue Infection in Central Brazil: Spatial Point Pattern Analysis and Risk Factors Assessment. *American Journal of Tropical Medicine and Hygiene*, **71**, 646-651.

[14] Teixeira, M.G., *et al.* (2012) Risk Factors for the Incidence of Dengue Virus Infection in Preschool Children. *Tropical Medicine & International Health*, **17**, 1391-1395. http://dx.doi.org/10.1111/j.1365-3156.2012.03086.x

20

Herpes Zoster in Childhood

Alexander K. C. Leung[1,2]*, Benjamin Barankin[3]

[1]University of Calgary, Calgary, Canada
[2]Alberta Children's Hospital, Calgary, Canada
[3]Toronto Dermatology Centre, Toronto, Canada
Email: *aleung@ucalgary.ca

Abstract

Herpes zoster is caused by reactivation of latent varicella-zoster virus that resides in a dorsal root ganglion. Herpes zoster can develop at any time after a primary infection or varicella vaccination. The incidence among children is approximately 110 per 100,000 person-years. Clinically, herpes zoster is characterized by a painful, unilateral vesicular eruption in a restricted dermatomal distribution. In young children, herpes zoster has a predilection for areas supplied by the cervical and sacral dermatomes. Herpes zoster tends to be milder in children than that in adults. Also, vaccine-associated herpes zoster is milder than herpes zoster after wild-type varicella. The diagnosis of herpes zoster is mainly made clinically, based on a distinct clinical appearance. The most common complications are secondary bacterial infection, depigmentation, and scarring. Chickenpox may develop in susceptible individuals exposed to herpes zoster. Oral acyclovir should be considered for uncomplicated herpes zoster in immunocompetent children. Intravenous acyclovir is the treatment of choice for immunocompromised children who are at risk for disseminated disease. The medication should be administered ideally within 72 hours of rash onset.

Keywords

Varicella-Zoster Virus, Reactivation, Vesicular Eruption, Dermatome, Acyclovir

1. Introduction

Herpes zoster, also known as shingles, is caused by reactivation of endogenous latent varicella-zoster virus that resides in a sensory dorsal root ganglion usually after primary infection with varicella-zoster virus (*i.e.*, varicella

---
*Corresponding author.

or chickenpox) [1]. Herpes zoster can develop at any time after a primary infection or varicella vaccination [1]. The activated virus travels back down the corresponding cutaneous nerve to the adjacent skin, causing a painful, unilateral vesicular eruption in a restricted dermatomal distribution.

2. Epidemiology

Herpes zoster occurs more commonly after varicella infection than after varicella vaccination [2]. Herpes zoster usually occurs in persons with relative cell-mediated immunologic compromise such as elderly individuals or patients with an immunosuppressive illness or receiving immunosuppressive therapy [3]. The cumulative lifetime incidence among the general population is approximately 10% to 30%, with the risk increasing sharply after 50 years of age [4]-[6]. In the study by Insigna et al, the overall age- and sex-adjusted incidence of herpes zoster was 320 per 100,000 person-years in the United States from 2000 to 2001 [7]. The rate was higher among females (390 per 100,000 person-years) than among males (260 per 100,000 person-years).The incidence among children aged 0 to 14 years was 110 per 100,000 person-years [7]. Kawai et al performed a systematic review of 63 studies from 22 countries on the incidence of herpes zoster [4]. The authors found the incidence rate of herpes zoster ranged between 300 to 500 per 100,000 person-years in the general population in North America, Europe, and Asia-Pacific, based on studies using prospective surveillance, electronic medical record data or administrative data with medical record review. The incidence is twice in whites when compared to blacks [8]. Immunocompromised individuals have a 20 to 100 times greater risk than immunocompetent individuals of the same age [9] [10].

In general, herpes zoster is uncommon in individuals younger than 10 years of age and rare in infants [3] [5]. The younger a child is when he/she has varicella, the greater the likelihood that herpes zoster will develop in childhood or early adulthood [6]. In this regard, infantile herpes zoster is more commonly associated with intrauterine varicella-zoster virus infection than postnatal infection. In approximately 2% of children exposed to varicella-zoster virus in utero, subclinical varicella develops, and therefore they are at risk for herpes zoster after birth [3]. Enders et al prospectively followed 1373 women who had varicella during the first 36 weeks of gestation [11]. Herpes zoster in infancy or early childhood was reported in 10 children who were asymptomatic at birth. The observed risk of herpes zoster after maternal varicella between 13 and 24 weeks and between 25 and 36 weeks was 4/477 (0.8%) and 6/345 (1.7%), respectively. Eight of these children had herpes zoster during the first year of life.

At times, herpes zoster may result from varicella vaccination as the vaccine strain of varicella-zoster virus may become latent and later reactivate to cause herpes zoster [3] [12] [13]. In one study, the incidence of herpes zoster among varicella vaccine recipients is about 14 cases per 100,000 person-years, compared with 20 to 63 cases per 100,000 person-years after natural varicella infection [14]. In another study, the incidence of laboratory-confirmed herpes zoster was 48 cases per 100,000 person-years in vaccinated children (wild type and vaccine-strain) and 230 cases per 100,000 person-years in unvaccinated children (wild type only) [15]. Several studies have shown that the incidence of herpes zoster in both healthy and immunocompromised children who received varicella vaccine is less than that experienced by healthy and immunocompromised children who experienced natural varicella infection, respectively [12] [15]-[17]. The lower incidence may be related to a lower rate of reactivation of the attenuated vaccine strain of varicella-zoster virus and the lower rate of rash following vaccination compared with wild-type varicella [12].

3. Pathogenesis

A primary infection with either wild-type or vaccine-type varicella-zoster virus is a prerequisite for herpes zoster [3]. Activation of latent varicella-zoster virus in a partially immune host results in herpes zoster. Defects in immunity, especially cell-mediated immunity, resulting from an immunosuppressive illness or immunosuppressive therapy are important factors in the pathogenesis. Predisposing factors include increasing age, fatigue, and emotional stress. In children, asthma is a risk factor for herpes zoster [18].

The vaccine-type virus strain is known to establish a latent infection in the dorsal root ganglia [14]. The virus reaches the sensory ganglia through sensory nerves at the injection site. The relative risk of herpes zoster developing in a vaccine recipient is higher in individuals who had a vaccine-associated rash or breakthrough infection [14]. In the majority of cases, the zoster lesions occur on the same side as the vaccine injection site [3]. Varicella vaccine is composed of a mixture of varicella zoster virus strains. Viruses sampled from herpes zoster vesicles are single clones, suggesting that a single strain is selected between the time of inoculation and development of the rash [19].

4. Clinical Manifestations

The onset of disease may be heralded by pain within the dermatome and precedes the lesions by 48 to 72 hours [1] [12]. The pain is due to acute neuritis and is related to viral replication, inflammation, and cytokine production leading to neuronal destruction and increased sensitivity of pain receptors [20]. At times, there may be paresthesia, burning, or itching in the affected area [12]. An area of erythema might follow and precede the development of a group of vesicles in the distribution of the dermatome that corresponds to the infected dorsal root ganglion (**Figure 1**) [12]. Usually 1 or, less commonly, 2 or 3 adjacent dermatomes are affected [5] [20]. In young children, herpes zoster has a predilection for areas supplied by the cervical and sacral dermatomes [21]. In adults, the lesions are more common in the lower thoracic and upper lumbar dermatomes and may involve the trigeminal nerve [12]. In both children and adults, the lesions usually do not cross the midline [12]. Vesicles may coalesce to form bullous lesions [1]. The vesicular and bullous lesions may become pustular or occasionally hemorrhagic and ultimately crust in 7 to 10 days [20]. There may be regional lymphadenopathy [12].

Herpes zoster may involve the eyelids when the ophthalmic branch of the trigeminal nerve is affected. Appearance of skin lesions at the side of the nose represents involvement of the nasociliary branch of ophthalmic nerve (Hutchinson's sign) and predicts a higher likelihood of ocular involvement [11] [22].

Herpes zoster tends to be milder in children than in adults [2] [3] [4]. Also, vaccine-associated herpes zoster is milder than herpes zoster after wild-type varicella [2] [3].

In individuals with immunodeficiency, the lesions may involve multiple contiguous, non-contiguous, bilateral,

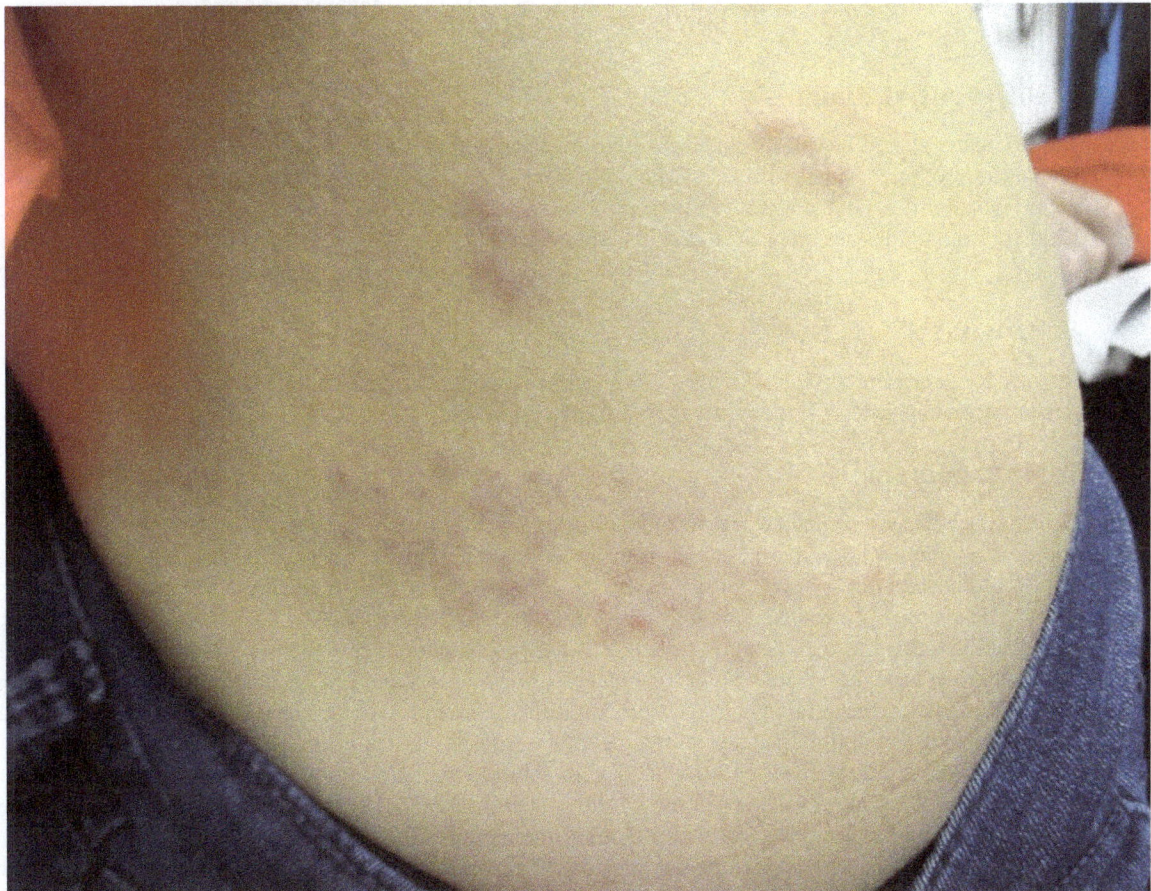

Figure 1. Multiple grouped papules and vesicles on an erythematous base, present unilaterally on the right flank in a dermatomal distribution.

or unusual dermatomes [4] [12]. The lesions may disseminate to other organs such as the liver, kidneys, lungs, and central nervous system. Also, the illness is more severe and prolonged.

5. Complications

The most common complications are secondary bacterial infection, post-inflammatory depigmentation, and scarring [12]. Necrotizing fasciitis is a potential complication if there is secondary bacterial infection [12]. Herpes zoster ophthalmicus may lead to severe eye pain, conjunctivitis, lid ulceration, retinal necrosis, ophthalmoparesis/plegia, sclerokeratitis, anterior uveitis, and optic neuritis [23]. Postherpetic neuralgia, which represents a continuum of pain that does not resolve following the acute episode of herpes zoster, is uncommon in children [1] [2] [5]. Other rare complications include Ramsay Hunt syndrome, Guillain-Barré syndrome, pneumonia, aseptic meningitis, encephalitis, meningoencephalitis, ventriculitis, transverse myelitis, granulomatous cerebral angiitis, cranial nerve paresis/palsies, and peripheral nerve paresis/palsies [17] [20] [24] [25]. Inflammatory skin lesions following herpes zoster may occur within the same dermatome (Wolf's isotopic phenomenon) [12].

Complications are uncommon in vaccine-induced herpes zoster in healthy children. In contrast, in immunocompromised patients, complications are more common and severe.

6. Diagnosis

The diagnosis of herpes zoster is mainly made clinically, based on the distinctive clinical appearance and symptomatology. Laboratory tests usually are not necessary. A Tzanck smear, performed by scraping the base of the lesion, can demonstrate giant cells [1]. The diagnosis can be confirmed if necessary by the demonstration of specific viral antigens in skin scrapings or vesicles using direct fluorescent (FDA) assay. Viral DNA analysis of the lesion by polymerase chain reaction (PCR) can be used to distinguish between wild-type and vaccine-type viruses (genotyping) [14].

7. Differential Diagnosis

Herpes zoster should be differentiated from zosteriform herpes simplex. In zosteriform herpes simplex, there is no painful prodrome, small vesicles of almost uniform size, less number of grouped vesicles, and more likely to recur. Other differential diagnoses include zosteriform lichen planus, drug eruption, insect bites, folliculitis, hand-foot-mouth disease, contact dermatitis, atopic dermatitis, phytophotodermatitis, and dermatitis herpetiformis.

8. Prognosis

Recurrence is uncommon in the immunocompetent individual. Approximately 5% of immunocompetent patients have a second episode of herpes zoster [5]. Three or more episodes are rare [5] [20].

9. Management

Affected patients are contagious because the virus can be transmitted by direct contact with herpes zoster lesions and, less commonly, by airborne spread from aerosolization of virus from skin lesions [11] [14]. Affected children should be kept out of school or day care until crusting appears and contact with pregnant women in particular is to be avoided [1]. Chickenpox may develop in susceptible individuals exposed to herpes zoster [1]. General preventive measures include good personal hygiene, with particular emphasis on hand washing, proper clothing, and covering exposed lesions with bandages. Fingernails should be trimmed to reduce injury from scratching. If secondary bacterial infection occurs, topical or systemic antibiotic therapy is indicated.

The goals of antiviral therapy are to reduce viral shedding, hasten healing of cutaneous lesions, prevent new lesion formation, reduce the pain associated with acute neuritis and possibly decrease complications from the disease [11] [20]. Oral acyclovir (20 mg/kg/dose, maximum 800 mg/dose) five times per day for 5 to 7 days should be considered for uncomplicated herpes zoster in immunocompetent children [5]. Intravenous acyclovir (10 mg/kg or 500 mg/m^2 every 8 hours) for 7 to 10 days is the treatment of choice for immunocompromised children who are at risk for disseminated disease [1] [5]. The medication should be administered ideally within 72 hours of rash onset [20]. Relapse of herpes zoster can be treated with a second course of acyclovir with similar dosing and duration as for a primary episode.

10. Prevention

It is known that vaccine-associated herpes zoster is milder than herpes zoster after wild type-varicella [26]. As such, there is a need for prevention of varicella-zoster virus infection though universal childhood immunization [26] [27]. The Advisory Committee for Immunization Practices of the Centers for Disease Control and Prevention and the American Academy of Pediatrics recommend a routine two-dose varicella vaccination program for children, with the first dose administered at 12 to 18 months and the second dose at 4 to 6 years of age [2]. The Advisory Committee on Immunization Practices further recommends two doses of varicella vaccine, 4 to 8 weeks apart, for all susceptible adolescents and adults and a catch-up second dose for everyone who receives one dose of varicella vaccine previously [28].

References

[1]   Leung, A.K., Robson, W.L. and Leong, A.G. (2006) Herpes Zoster in Childhood. *Journal of Pediatric Health Care*, **20**, 300-303. http://dx.doi.org/10.1016/j.pedhc.2006.01.004

[2]   American Academy of Pediatrics (2012) Varicella Zoster Infections. In: Pickering, L.K., Baker, C.J., Kimberlin, D.W. and Long S.S., Eds., *Red Book*: 2012 *Report of the Committee on Infectious Diseases*, 29th Edition, American Academy of Pediatrics, Elk Grove Village, 774-789.

[3]   Leung, A.K. (2011) Herpes Zoster. In: Leung, A.K., Ed., *Common Problems in Ambulatory Pediatrics: Specific Clinical Problems*, Vol. 1, Nova Science Publishers, Inc., New York, 285-289.

[4]   Kawai, K., Gebremeskel, B.G. and Acosta, C. (2014) Systematic Review of Incidence and Complications of Herpes Zoster: Towards a Global Perspective. *BMJ Open*, **4**, e004833. http://dx.doi.org/10.1136/bmjopen-2014-004833

[5]   LaRussa, P.S. and Marin, M. (2011) Varicella-Zoster Virus Infection. In: Kliegman, R.M., Stanton, B.F., St Geme, J.W., Schor, N.F., Behrman, R.E., *Nelson Textbook of Pediatrics*, 19th Edition, Elsevier, Philadelphia, 1104-1110. http://dx.doi.org/10.1016/B978-1-4377-0755-7.00245-1

[6]   Stein, M., Cohen, R., Bromberg, M., *et al.* (2012) Herpes Zoster in a Partially Vaccinated Pediatric Population in Central Isreal. *Pediatric Infectious Disease Journal*, **31**, 906-909. http://dx.doi.org/10.1097/INF.0b013e31825d33f9

[7]   Insinga, R.P., Itzler, R.F., Pellissier, J.M., *et al.* (2005) The Incidence of Herpes Zoster in a United States Administrative Database. *Journal of General Internal Medicine*, **20**, 748-753. http://dx.doi.org/10.1111/j.1525-1497.2005.0150.x

[8]   Schmader, K., George, L.K., Burchett, B.M., *et al.* (1995) Racial Differences in the Occurrence of Herpes Zoster. *Journal of Infectious Diseases*, **171**, 701-704. http://dx.doi.org/10.1093/infdis/171.3.701

[9]   O'Connor, K.M. and Paauw, D.S. (2013) Herpes Zoster. *Medical Clinics of North America*, **97**, 503-522. http://dx.doi.org/10.1016/j.mcna.2013.02.002

[10] Staikov, I., Neykov, N., Marinovic, B., *et al.* (2014) Herpes Zoster as a Systemic Disease. *Clinics in Dermatology*, **32**, 424-429. http://dx.doi.org/10.1016/j.clindermatol.2013.11.010

[11] Enders, G., Bolley, I., Miller, E., Cradock-Watson, J. and Ridehalgh, M. (1994) Consequences of Varicella and Herpes Zoster in Pregnancy: Prospective Study of 1739 Cases. *The Lancet*, **343**, 1548-1551. http://dx.doi.org/10.1016/S0140-6736(94)92943-2

[12] Chun, C., Weinman, S., Riedlinger, K., Mullooly, J.P., Houston, H., Schmid, D.S. and Seward, J.F. (2011) Laboratory Characteristics of Suspected Herpes Zoster in Vaccinated Children. *The Pediatric Infectious Disease Journal*, **30**, 719-721. http://dx.doi.org/10.1097/INF.0b013e3182137e35

[13] Tseng, H.F., Smith, N., Marcy, S.M., Sy, L.S. and Jacobsen, S.J. (2009) Incidence of Herpes Zoster among Children Vaccinated with Varicella Vaccine in a Prepaid Health Care Plan in the United States, 2002-2008. *The Pediatric Infectious Disease Journal*, **28**, 1069-1072. http://dx.doi.org/10.1097/INF.0b013e3181acf84f

[14] Uebe, B., Sauerbrei, A., Burdach, S. and Horneff, G. (2002) Herpes Zoster by Reactivated Vaccine Varicella Zoster Virus in a Healthy Child. *European Journal of Pediatrics*, **161**, 442-444. http://dx.doi.org/10.1007/s00431-002-0981-1

[15] Weinmann, S., Chun, C., Schmid, D.S., Roberts, M., Vandermeer, M., Riedlinger, K., *et al.* (2013) Incidence and Clinical Characteristics of Herpes Zoster among Children in the Varicella Vaccine Era, 2005-2009. *Journal of Infectious Diseases*, **208**, 1859-1868. http://dx.doi.org/10.1093/infdis/jit405

[16] Civen, R., Chaves, S.S., Jumaan, A., Wu, H., Mascola, L., Gargiullo, P. and Seward, J.F. (2009) The Incidence and Clinical Characteristics of Herpes Zoster among Children and Adolescents after Implementation of Varicella Vaccination. *The Pediatric Infectious Disease Journal*, **28**, 954-959. http://dx.doi.org/10.1097/INF.0b013e3181a90b16

[17] Rentier, B. and Gershon, A.A., The Members of the European Working Group on Varicella (Euro Var) (2004) Consensus: Varicella Vaccination of Healthy Children: A Challenge for Europe. *The Pediatric Infectious Disease Journal*, **23**, 379-389. http://dx.doi.org/10.1097/01.inf.0000122606.88429.8f

[18] Kim, B.S., Mehra, S., Yawn, B., Grose, C., Tarrell, R., Lahr, B. and Juhn, Y.J. (2013) Increased Risk of Herpes Zoster in Children with Asthma: A Population-Based Case-Control Study. *Journal of Pediatrics*, **163**, 816-821.

[19] Quinlivan, M.L., Gershon, A.A., Steinberg, S.P. and Breuer, J. (2004) Rashes Occurring after Immunization with a Mixture of Viruses in the Oka Vaccine Are Derived from Single Clones of Virus. *The Journal of Infectious Diseases*, **190**, 793-796. http://dx.doi.org/10.1086/423210

[20] Albrecht, M.A. (2014) Clinical Manifestations of Varicella-Zoster Virus Infection: Herpes Zoster. In: Post, T.W., Ed., *UpToDate*, UpToDate, Inc., Waltham, MA.

[21] Leung, A.K. and Rafaat, M. (2003) Herpes Zoster. *American Family Physician*, **67**, 1045-1046.

[22] Zaal, M.J., Volker-Dieben, H.J. and D'Amaro, J. (2003) Prognostic Value of Hutchinson's Sign in Acute Herpes Zoster Opthalmicus. *Graefe's Archive for Clinical and Experimental Ophthalmology*, **241**, 187-191. http://dx.doi.org/10.1007/s00417-002-0609-1

[23] De Freitas, D., Martins, E.N., Adan, C., Alvarenga, L.S. and Pavan-Langston, D. (2006) Herpes Zoster Ophthalmicus in Otherwise Healthy Children. *American Journal of Ophthalmology*, **142**, 393-399. http://dx.doi.org/10.1016/j.ajo.2006.03.059

[24] Ong, O.L., Churchyard, A.C. and New, P.W. (2010) The Importance of Early Diagnosis of Herpes Zoster Myelitis. *Medical Journal of Australia*, **193**, 546-547.

[25] Ruppert, L.M., Freeland, M.L. and Stubblefield, M.D. (2010) Segmental Zoster Paresis of the Left Upper Limb in a Pediatric Patient. *American Journal of Physical Medicine Rehabilitation*, **89**, 1024-1029. http://dx.doi.org/10.1097/PHM.0b013e3181e7204b

[26] Leung, A.K. and Barankin, B. (2015) Bilateral Symmetrical Herpes Zoster in an Immunocompetent 15-Year-Old Boy. *Case Reports in Pediatrics*, **2015**, Article ID: 121549.

[27] Leung, A.K., Kellner, J.D. and Davies, H.D. (2009) Chickenpox: An Update. *The Pediatric Infectious Disease Journal*, **4**, 343-350.

[28] Marin, M., Güris, D., Chaves, S.S., Schmid, S. and Seward, J.F., Advisory Committee on Immunization Practices, Centers for Disease Control and Prevention (CDC) (2007) Prevention of Varicella: Recommendations of the Advisory Committee on Immunization Practices (ACIP). *The MMWR Recommendations and Reports*, **56**, 1-40.

21

The Differences of Urinary Neutrophil Gelatinase-Associated Lipocalin (NGAL) Levels between Asphyxiated and Non-Asphyxiated Neonates

Nur Dian Firmani*, Tetty Yuniati, Dedi Rachmadi

Department of Child Health, Faculty of Medicine, Universitas Padjadjaran, Bandung, Indonesia
Email: *nurdian.firmani@gmail.com

Abstract

Objective: To evaluate the differences of urinary NGAL levels between asphyxiated and non-asphyxiated neonates. Methods: This was a cross-sectional observational analytic study, including 34 newborns in Dr. Hasan Sadikin Hospital, Bandung, Indonesia. Sample collection was conducted from December 2014 to March 2015. Urine NGAL levels were evaluated using enzyme-linked immunosorbent assays (ELISA) technique. To determine the differences of urinary NGAL levels between asphyxiated and non-asphyxiated group we used Mann-Whitney U test, and to determine the differences of gestational age and birth weight between these two groups we used Fisher's exact test. Results: Twenty males (60%) and 14 females (40%) neonates participated in the study. From 34 subjects, 17 neonates were diagnosed with asphyxia and 17 neonates without asphyxia. The results showed that urine NGAL levels had significantly increased in asphyxiated neonates. The median urine NGAL level in asphyxiated group is 95% CI: 506.7 (60.0 - 651.7) ng/mL, while the median urine NGAL level in non-asphyxiated group is 95% CI: 6.7 (0.1 - 53.0) ng/mL. Statistically, there were significant urine NGAL levels differences between asphyxiated and non-asphyxiated neonates ($p < 0.001$). There were no differences in gestational age and birth weight between asphyxiated and non-asphyxiated neonates ($p > 0.05$). Conclusions: Urinary NGAL levels in asphyxiated neonates were significantly higher than those in non-asphyxiated neonates. There were significant differences of urine NGAL levels between the groups.

Keywords

Neutrophil Gelatinase-Associated Lipocalin, Asphyxia, Neonates

---

*Corresponding author.

1. Introduction

Neonatal asphyxia is still the leading cause of high morbidity and mortality in developed countries, as well as in developing countries including Indonesia. Global estimates for asphyxia-related neonatal deaths vary from 0.7 to 1.2 million, and about 99% of neonatal deaths are due to asphyxia occurred in low- and middle-income countries [1]. Incidence of neonatal asphyxia in Indonesia is about 3% - 5% of all live births [2].

Asphyxia could reduce renal blood flow and might cause organ dysfunction and tubular renal damage [3]-[6]. Damaged tubular cells will produce and secrete biological substances that related to innate immune response and inflammation process including protein [7]-[9]. Neutrophil gelatinase-associated lipocalin (NGAL) is a protein that is secreted by immune cells, hepatocytes, and renal tubular cells. Neutrophil gelatinase-associated lipocalin could be overly expressed after renal ischemic and it could be detected with higher concentration in urine [10]-[13].

Neutrophil gelatinase-associated lipocalin has been used as a biomarker for acute kidney injury (AKI) in critically ill neonates and children. From previous studies, Askenazi *et al.* [14] described urine NGAL levels in very low birth weight newborns which were diagnosed with AKI, and showed elevated urine NGAL levels. Krawczeski *et al.* [15] compared serum and urine NGAL levels in neonates and children after cardiopulmonary bypass (CPB), and showed elevated serum and urine NGAL levels 2 hours after CPB and it can be used for biomarker of AKI. Sarafidis *et al.* [16] compared serum and urine cystatin-c levels, serum and urine NGAL levels, and urine kidney injury molecule-1 (KIM-1) levels with serum creatinin levels in term asphyxiated and non-asphyxiated newborn, and showed a significant elevated serum cystatin-c levels, also elevated serum and urine NGAL levels in asphyxiated newborn. Serum and urine NGAL levels elevated in asphyxiated newborn with AKI inspite of non-AKI asphyxiated newborn [14]-[16].

The aim of this study is to evaluate the differences between urinary NGAL levels in asphyxiated neonates and non-asphyxiated neonates.

2. Materials and Methods

This cross-sectional study was performed in Neonatology Division of Dr. Hasan Sadikin Hospital Bandung, Indonesia from December 2014 to March 2015. Subjects of this study were calculated by unpaired data analysis for two independent groups, and minimum sample size estimation was 17 each group. Seventeen neonates were diagnosed as asphyxia based on 2 from the following American Academy of Pediatrics' criteria [17]: 1) umbilical cord arterial pH less than 7; 2) Apgar score of 0 to 3 for longer than 5 minutes; 3) neurologic manifestations (eg, seizures, coma, hypotonia); and 4) multisystemic organ dysfunction, and 17 neonates were born without asphyxia. The exclusion criteria were baby born with multiple congenital anomaly and mother with infection risks. This study was approved by the ethical committee of the Faculty of Medicine, Universitas Padjadjaran/Dr. Hasan Sadikin General Hospital Bandung, Indonesia.

Urine samples were collected after informed consent from their parents. Urine NGAL examination was performed with ELISA technique. Data were presented as mean, standard deviation, and median with range. Statistical parameters were calculated using SPSS^{TM} version 20.0. Due to unnormally distributed data, the nonparametric Mann-Whitney U test was used to determine the differences of urinary NGAL levels between the groups. The Fisher's exact test was used to determine the differences of gestational age and birth weight in both groups. p values < 0.05 were considered as significant.

3. Results

Thirty four babies, who were born in Neonatology Division of Dr. Hasan Sadikin General Hospital in Bandung, Indonesia, consisted of 20 males and 14 females were divided into 17 asphyxiated neonates group and 17 non-asphyxiated neonates group. The clinical characteristics of the subjects are presented in **Table 1**, while factors which associated with urine NGAL levels are presented in **Table 2**.

The results from data analysis with Fisher exact test on the differences of gestational age and birth weight between asphyxiated and non-asphyxiated neonates were not significant (**Table 2**). The differences of urine NGAL levels between asphyxiated and non-asphyxiated neonates were analyzed using Mann-Whitney U test, and they are presented in **Table 3**.

The median urine NGAL levels in both groups were statistically significant different (p < 0.001).

Table 1. Characteristics of the subjects (n = 34).

Characteristics	Asphyxiated neonates (n = 17)	Non-asphyxiated neonates (n = 17)
Gestational age, n		
≤36 weeks	9	5
>36 weeks	8	12
Birth weight (gram), mean (SD)	2190 (756)	2727 (760)
Gender, n		
Male	10	10
Female	7	7
Type of delivery, n		
Vaginal delivery	8	6
Caesarian section	8	10
Vacuum extraction	1	1
Seizure, n		
Yes	3	0
No	14	17

SD: standard deviation.

Table 2. Factors associated with urine NGAL levels.

Variables	Asphyxiated neonates (n = 17)	Non-asphyxiated neonates (n = 17)	p Value
Gestational age, n			0.163[*]
≤6 weeks	9	5	
>36 weeks	8	12	
Birth weight, n			1.0[*]
≤1500 gram	2	1	
>1500 gram	15	16	

[*]Fisher's exact test.

Table 3. Urinary NGAL levels.

Urine NGAL levels (ng/mL)	Asphyxiated neonates (n = 17)	Non-asphyxiated neonates (n = 17)	p Value
Median	506.7	6.7	<0.001[†]
Range	60.0 - 651.7	0.1 - 53.0	

[†]Mann-Whitney U test.

4. Discussion

Asphyxiated group had gestational age ≤ 36 weeks more than >36 weeks while the mean gestational age was 34 (26 - 40) weeks, and the mean birth weight was 2190 (800 - 3400) gram. Non-asphyxiated group had gestational age >36 weeks more than ≤36 weeks while the mean gestational age was 37 (32 - 42) weeks, and the mean birth weight was 2727 (1500 - 3920) gram. This study is different from previous studies. Sarafidis *et al.* [16] and El-Salam *et al.* [18] included term neonates and excluded preterm and very low birth weight neonates.

This study also determined the differences of gestational age and birth weight as factors which were associated with urine NGAL levels between asphyxiated and non-asphyxiated neonates. There were no significant differences in gestational age and birth weight between the groups (p = 0.163; p = 1.0).

The results of this study showed the median urinary NGAL levels in asphyxiated group was 506.7 (60.0 - 651.7) ng/mL, elevated significantly from normal value. The median urinary NGAL levels in non-asphyxiated group was 6.7 (0.1 - 53.0) ng/mL. Statistically, there were significant differences of urinary NGAL levels between asphyxiated and non-asphyxiated group (p < 0.001).

Neonatal asphyxia is a leading cause of renal hypoxia and ischemia. Reduced renal blood flow is a major cause of overly NGAL express in tubular renal [12]. Normally, circulating NGAL is filtered in the glomerulus and reabsorbed by the proximal tubule. Consequently, low levels of NGAL are detected in plasma and urine [12]-[14]. In renal tubular damage, circulating NGAL were not well reabsorbed by proximal tubule and induced synthesis NGAL de novo in distal tubule [11] [19]. Neutrophil gelatinase-associated lipocalin could elevate and could be detected in the higher concentration of urine before progressive renal damage and death cells [12] [20].

Previous studies with different subject had been conducted beforehand. Sarafidis *et al.* [16] compared urine NGAL levels between asphyxiated and non-asphyxiated term neonates, and showed that there were significant differences of urinary NGAL levels in both groups (p = 0.006), and urinary NGAL levels showed elevated in asphyxiated neonates with AKI inspite of non-AKI asphyxiated neonates. El-Salam *et al.* [18] reported urinary NGAL levels in term asphyxiated neonates had a significant elevation in 48 hours after birth and before the rising of creatinin serum levels than in control group (p = 0.01).

Limitation of this study is asphyxia based on AAP's criteria not to evaluate all of the criteria, but only from the Apgar score and pH in arterial blood gas because we required more time to observe other criteria. We also did not exclude multiple congenital anomaly condition from objective examination, but only from physical examination. NGAL examination was only to evaluate differences in asphyxiated and non-asphyxiated neonates, not including creatinin serum examination and not to observe occurrence of AKI. However, due to our limitations, more studies are required.

5. Conclusion

Urinary NGAL levels in asphyxiated neonates were significantly higher than those in non-asphyxiated neonates. There were significant differences of urine NGAL levels between the groups.

Acknowledgements

Our study was conducted with private funding. We thanked Professor Abdurachman Sukadi and Professor Herry Garna for initial manuscript preparation counseling. NDF, TY, and DR contributed to conception and design of the study, acquisition of data, interpretation and analysis of data, revising the article and final approval of the version submitted. We also thank to the parents for their children's participation in the present study.

References

[1]   Lawn, J., Shibuya, K. and Stein, C. (2005) No Cry at Birth: Global Estimates of Intrapartum Stillbirths and Intra-partum-Related Neonatal Deaths. World Health Organization, Geneva, 83, 409-417.

[2]   Alisjahbana, A., Hidayat, S., Mintardaningsih, Primadi, A., Harliany, E., Sofiatin, Y., *et al.* (1999) Management of Birth Asphyxia at Home and Health Center. *Paediatrica Indonesiana*, 39, 88-101.

[3]   Askenazi, D.J., Ambalavanan, N. and Goldstein, S.L. (2009) Acute Kidney Injury in Critically Ill Newborns: What Do We Know? What Do We Need to Learn? *Pediatric Nephrology*, 24, 265-274. http://dx.doi.org/10.1007/s00467-008-1060-2

[4]   Aggarwal, A., Kumar, P., Chowdary, G., Majumdar, S. and Narang, A. (2005) Evaluation of Renal Function in Asphyxiated Newborns. *Journal of Tropical Pediatrics*, 51, 295-299. http://dx.doi.org/10.1093/tropej/fmi017

[5]   Andreoli, S.P. (2004) Acute Renal Failure in the Newborn. *Seminars in Perinatology*, 8, 112-123. http://dx.doi.org/10.1053/j.semperi.2003.11.003

[6]   Agras, P.I., Tarcan, A., Baskin, E., Cengiz, N., Gurakan, B. and Saatci, U. (2004) Acute Renal Failure in the Neonatal Period. *Renal Failure Journal*, 26, 305-309. http://dx.doi.org/10.1081/JDI-200026749

[7]   Theocharis, P.G.V., Tsampoura, Z., Basioti, M. and Andronikou, S. (2011) Renal Glomerular and Tubular Function in Neonates with Perinatal Problems. *The Journal of Maternal-Fetal & Neonatal Medicine*, 24, 142-147. http://dx.doi.org/10.3109/14767058.2010.482602

[8]   Durkan, A.M. and Alexander, R.T. (2011) Acute Kidney Injury Post Neonatal Asphyxia. *The Journal of Pediatrics*, 158, e29-e33. http://dx.doi.org/10.1016/j.jpeds.2010.11.010

[9]   Jetton, J.G. and Askenazi, D.J. (2012) Update on Acute Kidney Injury in Neonate. *Current Opinion in Pediatrics*, 24, 1-6. http://dx.doi.org/10.1097/MOP.0b013e32834f62d5

[10] Liborio, A.B., Branco, K.M. and Bezerra, C.T. (2014) Acute Kidney Injury in Neonates: From Urine Output to New Biomarkers. *BioMed Research International*, **2014**, 1-8. http://dx.doi.org/10.1155/2014/601568

[11] Schmidt-Ott, K.M., Mori, K., Li, J.Y. and Kalandadze, A. (2007) Dual Action of Neutrophil Gelatinase-Associated Lipocalin. *Journal of the American Society of Nephrology*, **18**, 407-413. http://dx.doi.org/10.1681/asn.2006080882

[12] Clerico, A., Galli, C., Fortunato, A. and Ronco, C. (2012) Neutrophil Gelatinase-Associated Lipocalin (NGAL) as Biomarker of Acute Kidney Injury: A Review of the Laboratory Characteristics and Clinical Evidences. *Clinical Chemistry and Laboratory Medicine*, **50**, 1505-1517. http://dx.doi.org/10.1515/cclm-2011-0814

[13] Schmidt-Ott, K.M., Mori, K., Kalandadze, A., Liand, J.Y., Paragas, N., Nicholas, T., *et al.* (2006) Neutrophil Gelatinase-Associated Lipocalin-Mediated Iron Traffic in Kidney Epithelia. *Current Opinion in Nephrology and Hypertension*, **15**, 442-449. http://dx.doi.org/10.1097/01.mnh.0000232886.81142.58

[14] Askenazi, D.J., Montesanti, A., Hunley, H., Koralkar, R., Pawar, P., Shuaib, F., *et al.* (2011) Urine Biomarkers Predict Acute Kidney Injury and Mortality in Very Low Birth Weight Infants. *The Journal of Pediatrics*, **159**, 907-912. http://dx.doi.org/10.1016/j.jpeds.2011.05.045

[15] Krawczeski, C.D., Woo, J.G., Wang, Y., Bennett, M.R., Ma, Q. and Devarajan, P. (2011) Neutrophil Gelatinase-Associated Lipocalin Concentrations Predict Development of Acute Kidney Injury in Neonates and Children after Cardiopulmonary Bypass. *The Journal of Pediatrics*, **158**, 1009-1015. http://dx.doi.org/10.1016/j.jpeds.2010.12.057

[16] Sarafidis, K., Tsepkentzi, E., Agakidou, E., Diamanti, E., Taparkou, A., Soubasi, V., *et al.* (2012) Serum and Urine Acute Kidney Injury Biomarkers in Asphyxiated Neonates. *Pediatric Nephrology*, **27**, 1575-1582. http://dx.doi.org/10.1007/s00467-012-2162-4

[17] American Academy of Pediatrics and American College of Obstetricians and Gynecologists (2002) Care of the Neonate. In: Gilstrap, L.C. and Oh, W., Eds., *Guidelines for Perinatal Care*, 5th Edition, American Academy of Pediatrics, Elk Grove Village, 196-197.

[18] El-Salam, M.A., Zaher, M.M., Mohamed, R.A.E., Al Shall, L.Y., Saleh, R.A.M. and Hegazy, A.A. (2014) Comparison of Some Urinary Biomarkers of Acute Kidney Injury in Term Newborn with and without Asphyxia. *Clinical Medicine and Diagnostics*, **4**, 23-28.

[19] Hooman, N., Nakhali, S. and Sharif, M.R. (2014) Update on Acute Kidney Injury in Pediatrics. *Journal of Pediatric Nephrology*, **2**, 56-62.

[20] Myjak, B.L. (2010) Serum and Urinary Biomarkers of Acute Kidney Injury. *Blood Purification*, **29**, 357-365. http://dx.doi.org/10.1159/000309421

Hepatitis B, Hepatitis C and HIV among Children 6 to 59 Months in the Community in the Democratic Republic of Congo

Jeff Maotela Kabinda[1,2,3], Tony Shindano Akilimali[2], Ahuka Serge Miyanga[1], Philippe Donnen[4,5,6], Dramaix-Wilmet Michèle[3,4,5]

[1]Provincial Blood Transfusion Centre of Bukavu, Bukavu, Congo
[2]Catholic University of Bukavu, Bukavu, Congo
[3]Research Centre in Biostatistics and Epidemiology, Brussels, Belgium
[4]Free University of Brussels, Brussels, Belgium
[5]School of Public Health, Brussels, Belgium
[6]Centre for Policy and Health Systems/International Health, Brussels, Belgium
Email: kabindaalu@yahoo.fr

Abstract

Objectives: To determine the prevalence of HBV, HCV and HIV among children 6 to 59 months and determine the risk factors. Materials and Methods: Descriptive and analytical study on children aged 6 to 59 months of community Maniema (DRC) conducted between 24 June and 24 July 2013. We enrolled 781 children aged 6 to 59 months. For association between the presence of viral markers and potential risk factors the chi-square test of Pearson was applied, the odds ratios (OR) and their 95% confidence intervals (95% CIs) were calculated. The Fisher exact test was used when the conditions for application of the chi-square test of Pearson were not met. Results: The median age of the children was 34 months, 51% of female children. Ten percent of children had a history of blood transfusion; 6.6% and 64% had fever and anemia. The prevalence of HBsAg was 3.6%, the prevalence of antibodies against hepatitis C was 2.8% and HIV was 3.7%. The risk factors were HBsAg, male gender (5.5% male vs 2.0 % female; OR = 2.8(1.3 - 6.9) p = 0.001) and urban areas (5.0% rural vs 0.5% urban, OR = 0.1 (0.01 - 0.72), p = 0.01). For HCV and HIV, these factors were the history of blood transfusion in the child and the mother. For HCV 7.6% of children with blood transfusion history; OR = 3.2 (1.1 - 8.5); p = 0.05 and 11.1% history's mother blood transfusion, OR = 5.6 (2.1 - 14.1). For HIV 11.4% of children with blood transfusion history, OR = 3.8, p = 0.005 and 9.8% history's mother blood transfusion, OR = 2.9, p = 0.04. Conclusion: Vaccination against hepatitis B in children must be widespread, educational messages to the population must target the risk factors for these viruses. A screening of hepatitis in pregnant women must be

coupled with rigorous selection policy for blood donors before each donation and qualification of any unit of blood.

Keywords

HBV, HCV, HIV, Child

1. Introduction

Chronic infection with the virus of hepatitis B virus (HBV) or C virus (HCV) affects more than 170 million people worldwide. It is considered a public health problem comparable to a silent epidemic [1] because of its risk of progression to cirrhosis and liver cancer. According to data from 2005 published in 2013, Central Africa, the prevalence of hepatitis C was between 1.5% and 3.5% [2] and in the age group of less than 5 years, the prevalence was 2.6%. For hepatitis B, the prevalence in Central Africa varied between 5% and 7% in children 5 to 9 years [3]. HIV is the leading cause of child mortality in Africa, where 1700 children are newly infected every day [4] [5]. These three viruses share the same procedure for sending in children. HIV transmission in children is mainly through blood products and from mother to child. But the use of short course antiretroviral regimes in the third trimester allows for transmission rates <5% [4]. For hepatitis B virus, outside the transmission by blood products [6] [7], the mother-to-child transmission remains the main infection diffusion modality in highly endemic countries, as is the case in sub-Saharan Africa [8]. This hepatitis B transmission rates from mother to child is estimated at between 40% and 45% [7]. For hepatitis C transmission in children is almost exclusively parenterally in Africa; while the risk of infection from mother to child is about 5%, but it is possible only when the mother has chronic hepatitis C viremia [9]. The treatment of viral diseases in children remains a real problem in the context of our African countries with limited resources [7]. The point on which we can act effectively remains prevention. This can only be effective if the magnitude of the problem is known in our context. We conducted this study to make an inventory of the seroprevalence of hepatitis B, C and HIV in children 6 to 59 months and to assess the risk of transmission of these viruses in the child by blood products.

2. Methodology

2.1. Part of the Study

This is a descriptive and analytical cross-sectional study of children aged 6 to 59 months, from the period of 24 June to 24 July 2013 and conducted in two health zones of the city of Kindu (Kindu area and area health Alunguli), as well as in rural areas 2 (Kasongo and Kunda). These four health areas include 46 health areas in total but 38 easily accessible health areas were the subject of the investigation. A reasoned choice of four zones was made given the presence in these areas of the program for the prevention of transmission from mother to child of HIV and geographical accessibility. Kindu is the capital of Maniema province, in the center-east of the Democratic Republic of Congo. This province is one of 11 provinces of the DRC. The province has an area equal to 132 250 km^2. It has 2,038,471 inhabitants, with a density of 15 inhabitants/km^2. Maniema is divided into 18 health zones responsible for providing primary health care to the population, with the health structures of the 1st and 2nd level. These areas have a total of 274 health areas. However, in general, the proportion of health centers offering a minimum package of comprehensive activities is low. The general referral hospitals are underequipped and quality of complementary package of activities offered by these hospitals does not meet national standards.

2.2. Study Population

We conducted a household survey after research project has been approved by ethics committee of our university. We made the calculation of the number of households to deduct approximately the number of children under 5 years hoping to have at least one child of that age per household. The calculated sample size of 324 was based on a proportion of pregnant women with HIV to 3.5% nationally [10] and an accuracy of 2%. After multiplication by the effect of sampling by two, a total of 648 households was included. Sampling was done in several stages: the first step was to divide the households in 33 clusters (health area), each cluster containing at least 20 households. A selection of health areas (cluster) on the basis of a list of all the health areas of the 4 health zones drawn up in alphabetical order was carried out using a random selection proportional to population size health areas. The second step was to make a selection of villages/streets in the health areas selected in the first stage. After drawing up an alphabetical list of villages or avenues, a random draw proportional to the size of the population of the villages/avenues has been achieved. Thus 138 villages were selected representing 12% of all villages/streets. The number of households to be surveyed in the villages/avenues selected was obtained by dividing the number of required households (20 households) by the number of avenues/villages selected. The investigation team consisted of 4 people per health area: the supervising physician, a nurse, a laboratory technician and a plot of reliever recruited in the community. The investigation team visited the village center/avenues selected and chose a direction at random following the pen tip tossed and applied a systematic sampling type: in the selected travel direction The first household was the one that matched the random number drawn between 1 and the sampling interval was determined by the number of households in the village (known in advance by the plot reliever) divided by the number of households to be surveyed. The selection thus increased from household to household by adding the sampling interval k in the household corresponding number last visited up to the number of households required for this village/this avenue. From this set we selected the households that had a child from 6 to 59 months and who have freely agreed to participate in the survey. Thus we have reached 781 children aged 6 to 59 months. We studied the following parameters: the age of the child, gender, MUAC, fever defined by an axillary temperature above 38°C, anemia defined by hemoglobin levels below 11 g/dl. The value of hemoglobin was obtained by the HemoCueR device. We also noted the state of conjunctiva, the presence of edema, blood transfusion history in the past 12 months, the level of education of the mother, the maternal age, the antecedent of transfusion in the mother during pregnancy, HBV serology results, Anti-HIV and anti-HCV. Aspects ethics were complied in sens, the study participation was voluntary after a clear explanation and verbal approval was obtained.

2.3. Serology

Serodiagnosis on each sample was taken from the following reagents: a) Determine TM HBV HBsAg, Inverness Medical Japan Ltd.; b) HCV Orgenics Ltd., Medical Innovations Group, Israel c) HIV: HIV-Determine TM half Abbott.

2.4. Statistical Analysis

We encoded the data using SPSS 20. Some variables taken into account in the analysis were categorized age of the child in months in 3 categories (between 6 and 12 months, between 13 and 24 months and between 25 and 59 months) for the descriptive analysis but into two groups for the univariate analysis: less than 24 months and over 24 months, sex, social background in both rural and urban groups, the MUAC into 3 categories (less than 11 cm, between 11 and 12.5 cm and 12.5 cm), the mother's level of education into 4 categories (none, primary, secondary and higher) and then two groups in the univariate analysis: and without education, age of the mother in four categories for the description of the sample (20 years and under, 21 to 30 years, between 31 and 40 years and over 40 years) and then into two groups for the following analyzes: 30 years old, over 30 years. The usual descriptive statistical analysis consisted of proportions for categorical variables, median, minimum and maximum for the age of the child and the mother's age. To analyze the association between the presence of viral markers and potential risk factors the chi-square test of Pearson was applied, the odds ratios (OR) and their 95% confidence intervals (95% CIs) were were calculated. The Fisher exact test was used when the conditions for application of the chi-square test of Pearson were not met. The statistical significance chosen was $p < 0.05$.

3. Results

The median age of children in our sample was 34 months, more than half are found in the age group of 25 - 59 months. The proportion of girls is slightly higher than that of boys. 3/4 of the sample are from rural areas. Ten percent of the children had had a blood transfusion during the 12 months preceding the survey. When passing investigators 6.6% of children had fever, 64% were anemic and 9.2% had edema of the lower limbs (**Table 1**). Furthermore 9.3% of mothers of children were transfused during pregnancy of the child. The median age of the

Table 1. General children 6 to 59 months of Maniema province in 2013.

	n	%	Me (min-max)
Child's age (in months)	781		34 (6 - 59)
06 - 12		15.1	
13 - 24		33.2	
25 - 59		51.7	
Sex of child	781		
male		49.0	
female		51.0	
Original middle	781		
urban		28.4	
rural		71.6	
Arm circumference (cm)	699		
<11.0		72.1	
11.0 to 12.5		4.3	
>12.5		23.6	
Mother Study level	781		
primary		20.2	
secondary		51.0	
University		14.1	
without		14.7	
Age of mother (in years)	781		31.0 (16 - 50)
≤20		14.2	
21 - 30		47.0	
31 - 40		26.2	
> 40		12.6	
fever	707	6.6	
anemia	644	63.6	
Conjunctiva pale eyelid	778	7.5	
Swelling of lower limbs	723	9.2	
Transfusion history of the last 12 months	781	10.3	
History of transfusion for the mother when the child's pregnancy	781	9.3	

Me = median, Min = Minimum and max = maximum.

mothers was 31 years, 14% were under 20 years old while 15% had not studied and 51% had a secondary level of study as shown in **Table 1**.

The seroprevalence of hepatitis B in children 6 to 59 months was 3.6% (95% CI 2.6 to 5.3). The seroprevalence of HBV surface antigen differed statistically significantly by gender (p = 0.001) and the place of origin (p = 0.01). It was observed a higher proportion of presence of the surface antigen of hepatitis B among male children (OR = 2.8) and among rural children (5.0%). The risk of the hepatitis B antigen was also increased for children with a history of blood transfusion and those whose mothers had been transfused during pregnancy (**Table 2**).

The presence of blood transfusion history in the mother and in children is associated with a statistically significant risk of positivity of antibodies to hepatitis C. The overall seroprevalence of HCV was 2.8% (95% 1.8 to 4.3) (**Table 3**). The seroprevalence of anti-HCV was 7.6% in children who were transfused against 2.5% in those who did not. The proportion of children with antibodies against hepatitis C was 11% in children whose mothers had been transfused against 2.2% in children without transfusion history in their mothers. Strong but not statistically significant association (p = 0.08) was observed between the mid and hepatitis C.

We found a child with a co-infection of HIV-HCV three viruses HBV, two had co-infected hepatitis B and C, a child had HIV and hepatitis B co-infection and another child had a co-infection HIV and hepatitis C. HIV seroprevalence was 3.7% (95% CI 2.6 to 5.3) (**Table 4**).

We did not observe significant difference in HIV prevalence in children based on the following variables: age and sex of the child; the place of origin, age and level of mother study. As against the proportion of HIV was statistically significantly higher in children with a history of blood transfusion or for either himself or with his mother (**Table 4**).

Table 2. Seroprevalence of hepatitis B and its determinants in children 6 to 59 months.

	HBV + %	OR (IC à 95%)	p
Total (776)	3.6		
Child's age (in months)			0.58
≤24 (n = 359)	3.3	0.8 (0.0 - 1.7)	
>24 (n = 390)	4.1	1	
Sex of child			0.001
Male (n = 361)	5.5	2.8 (1.3 - 6.9)	
Female (n = 398)	2.0	1	
Original environment			0.01
Urban (n = 197)	0.5	0.1 (0.01 - 0.72)	
Rural (n = 541)	5.0	1	
Mother Study level			0.70[*]
Without (n = 113)	2.6	0.6 (0.1 - 2.0)	
Instruction (n = 624)	4.0	1	
Age of mother (in years)			0.70
≤30 (n = 468)	4.0	1.2 (0.5 - 2.7)	
>30 (n = 258)	3.5	1	
Transfusion of the child the last 12 months			0.34[*]
Yes (n = 76)	6.6	1.9 (0.6 - 4.8)	
No (n = 608)	3.6	1	
Transfusion of the parent on the child's pregnancy			0.63[*]
Yes (n = 70)	5.7	1.5 (0.4 - 4.2)	
No (n = 614)	3.9	1	

[*]Fisher exact.

Table 3. Seroprevalence of hepatitis C and its determinants in children 6 to 59 months.

	HCV + %	OR (IC à 95%)	p
Total (744)	2.8		
Child's age (in months)			0.65
≤24 (n = 299)	2.7	0.8 (0.3 - 1.9)	
>24 (n = 399)	3.3	1	
Sex of child			0.41
Male (n = 366)	3.3	1.4 (0.5 - 3.5)	
Female (n = 383)	2.3	1	
Original environment			0.08
Urban (n = 208)	4.8	2.3 (0.9 - 5.4)	
Rural (n = 508)	2.2	1	
Mother Study level			0.75*
Without (n = 111)	1.8	0.6 (0.1 - 2.5)	
Instruction (n = 603)	3.2	1	
Age of mother (in years)			0.79
≤30 (n = 402)	2.9	0.9 (0.4 - 2.2)	
>30 (n = 270)	3.3	1	
Transfusion of the child the last 12 months			0.05*
Yes (n = 79)	7.6	3.2 (1.1 - 8.5)	
No (n = 610)	2.5	1	
Transfusion of the parent on the child's pregnancy			0.001*
Yes (n = 72)	11.1	5.6 (2.1 - 14.1)	
No (n = 602)	2.2	1	

*Fisher exact.

Table 4. Prevalence of HIV infection and its determinants in children 6 to 59 months.

	HIV + %	OR (IC à 95%)	p
Total (778)	3.7		
Child's age (in months)			0.97
≤24 (n = 328)	3.9	1.0 (0.5 - 2.1)	
>24 (n = 399)	4.0	1	
Sex of child			0.26
Male (n = 361)	4.7	1.5 (0.7 - 3.3)	
Female (n = 383)	3.1	1	
Original environment			0.22
Urban (n = 201)	2.5	0.5 (0.2 - 1.4)	
Rural (n = 541)	4.4	1	
Mother Study level			0.99*
Without (n = 114)	3.5	0.8 (0.3 - 2.6)	
Instruction (n = 636)	3.9	1	
Age of mother (in years)			0.3
≤30 (n = 411)	3.6	0.7 (0.3 - 1.4)	
>30 (n = 264)	5.3	1	
Transfusion of the child the last 12 months			0.005*
Yes (n = 79)	11.4	3.8 (1.6 - 8.7)	
No (n = 618)	3.2	1	
Transfusion of the parent on the child's pregnancy			0.04*
Yes (n = 71)	9.8	2.9 (1.1 - 7.1)	
No (n = 625)	3.5	1	

*Fisher exact.

4. Discussion

In our study on hepatitis B, C and HIV in children between 6 and 59 months, the prevalence of hepatitis B was 3.6%, hepatitis C and HIV 2.8% and 3.7%. This study has some methodological limitations. Indeed, our study population was taken from the community and the calculation of proportions ignored vaccinations against hepatitis previously received by the children. These two reasons might be that there under-or overestimation of different prevalences. In addition the calculation of proportion did not take into account the effect of cluster sampling which may impact on confidence intervals and p-values. However, despite these reservations, this study has achieved its objectives: to estimate the prevalence of the three viruses in the age group 6 to 59 months and identify risk factors in our context.

The frequency of chronic carriers of hepatitis B surface antigen found in our study is higher than that found in Egypt 0.38% [11] but lower than projected estimates for the age group 0 to 4 years Central Africa [3] which were between 4% and 5%. The male children (OR 2.8) and children from rural areas (OR = 10) were more exposed respectively from the female children and those from urban areas. For sex the result is different from that found in Egypt but the result is similar to that found in Laos. [12] Regarding the environment from Mao et al. in Cambodia [13] and in Egypt Iman et al. [14] found similar results to ours. We did not find any plausible explanation in the literature for this. However, in rural areas the viral infection prevention measures are less present than in urban areas. Our study found no statistically significant association between seropositivity to HBsAg and blood transfusion history, this differs results of other studies in Egypt and Brazil [14] [15]. Indeed the infectivity of HBV is related to the presence of virus in most biological liquids infectious titers often very high, up to 109 virus/ml (blood, exudates, genital secretions mainly) [6] [7] for the three contamination routes: blood, sex and mother to child. The first route (blood) became less and less common in developed countries through the rigorous screening for all blood but in the countries of sub-Saharan Africa the risk remains high.

The main risk factors for viral hepatitis C identified in our study are the history of blood transfusion in the child and the mother. Egypt Gamal et al. [11] also found blood transfusion as a risk factor for HCV as Fafri Pakistan et al. [16] Apart from that, Gamal et al. also observed that the tattoo and surgery were risk factors for hepatitis C. But be aware that HCV infection is less common in children than in adults , and natural history, prognosis and clinical significance of HCV infection in childhood is based on estimates [11] [17] [18]. It is recognized that spontaneous clearance of the virus is possible but curing date is not determinable and prognostic factors are currently not known. [9] In children infected with HCV vertical transmission by up to 24% of spontaneous resolutions have been described before age 2 years but less than 2.5% after that age. [19] The spontaneous resolution rate the highest (up to 45%) is described in children who received postnatal transfusion [19] [20]. Anyway, the treatment of a viral infection with hepatitis C is not within the reach of people in sub-Saharan Africa or in cost or monitoring. Mortada et al. [21] estimated the cost at 7500 Euros per year to control infection and improve the quality of life of patients who suffer.

HIV prevalence observed in our study is similar to that of the general population of the country [10] and slightly higher than that observed in the population of blood donors 2.9% [22]. As for hepatitis C, the risk factors of HIV in children is the history of blood transfusion in the child and the mother. The mother-child transmission of HIV (HIV) has become a rare event in the most economically advantaged countries [4] and low frequency in countries with lower income. The weakness of the transmission of HIV from mother to child is achieved by routine screening in all pregnant women, monitoring and medical care for mothers and newborns. In all these measures, there are the strategies related to the mode of feeding among women living with HIV as they aim to reduce the risk of HIV transmission from mother to child as [5].

5. Conclusion

The seroprevalence of viral markers is a reflection of the prevalence gives an idea about the problem state. The weight of infections of hepatitis B, C and HIV are real in children as in adults. Blood transfusion remains a means of transmission of hepatitis and HIV in our midst. These infections are preventable, should be put in place for all vaccination against HBV, education of the population and screening of pregnant mothers hope for reducing the incidence of hepatitis in children. It should also strengthen the blood donor selection and qualification measures of all blood unit for secure blood products.

References

[1]   Debbeche, R., Said, Y., Ben Temime, H., El Jery, K., Salem, S.B.M. and Najjar, T. (2013) Epidemiology of Hepatitis C in Tunisia. *The Tunisia Medicale*, **91**, 86-91.

[2]   Hanafiah, K.M., Groeger, J., Flaxman, D.A. and Wiersma, S.T. (2013) Global Epidemiology of Hepatitis C Virus Infection: New Estimates of Age Specific-Antibody to HCV Seroprevalence. *Hepatology*, **57**, 1333-1342.

[3]   Otta, J.J., Stevensa, G.A., Groegerb, J. and Wiersmaa, S.T. (2012) Global Epidemiology of Hepatitis B Virus Infection: New Estimates of Age-Specific and HBsAg Seroprevalence Endemicity. *Vaccine*, **30**, 2212-2219. http://dx.doi.org/10.1016/j.vaccine.2011.12.116

[4]   Becquet, R. and Leroy, G. (2007) The Challenges Raised by the Prevention of Mother-Child Transmission of HIV in Africa. *Medical Press*, **36**, 1947-1957. http://dx.doi.org/10.1016/j.lpm.2007.02.031

[5]   Tabone, M.D., Vaudre, G., Dehée, A. and Dollfus, C. (2005) Maternal-Fetal Transmission of HIV: Progress and Prospects. *Archives of Pediatrics*, **12**, 1-3. http://dx.doi.org/10.1016/j.arcped.2004.11.007

[6]   Cadranel, J.F., Caron, C., Collot, G., Van Batten, C. and Dumouchel, P. (1999) Hepatitis B Epidemiology, Natural History, Biology, Treatment Monitoring. *Biology Pathology*, **47**, 917-927.

[7]   Ranger Rogez, S., Alain, S. and Denis, F. (2002) Hepatitis Viruses: MTCT. *Pathology Biology*, **50**, 568-575.

[8]   Singh, A.E., Plitt, S.S., Osiowy, C., Surynicz, K. and Kouadjo, E. (2011) Factors Associated with Vaccine Failure and Vertical Transmission of Hepatitis B among a Cohort of Mothers and Infants Canadian. *Journal of Viral Hepatitis*, **18**, 468-473. http://dx.doi.org/10.1111/j.1365-2893.2010.01333.x

[9]   Lacaille, F. (2002) Chronic Hepatitis C in Children. *Pediatrics Archive*, **9**, 539-542.

[10] National Plan to Combat AIDS (NSP) 2014-2017, Ministry of Health, DRC, Kinshasa 2013.

[11] Esmat, G., Hashem, M., El-Raziky, M., El-Akel, W., El-Naghy, S., El-Koofy, N., *et al.* (2012) Risk Factors for Hepatitis C Virus Acquisition and Predictors of Persistence among Egyptian Children. *Liver International*, **32**, 449-456.

[12] Xeuatvongsa, A., Komada, K., Kitamura, T., Vongphrachanh, P., Pathammavong, C., Phounphenghak, K., *et al.* (2014) Chronic Hepatitis B Prevalence among Children and Mothers: Results from a Nationwide, Population-Based Survey in Lao People's Democratic Republic. *PLoS ONE*, **9**, e88829.

[13] Mao, B., Patel, M.K., Hennessey, K., Duncan, R.J., Wannemuehler, K. and Soeung, S.C. (2013) Prevalence of Chronic Hepatitis B Virus Infection after Implementation of a Hepatitis B Vaccination Program among Children in Three Provinces in Cambodia. *Vaccine*, **31**, 4459-4464.

[14] Salama, I.I., Sami, S.M., Salama, S.I., Said, Z.N., Rabah, T.M. and Abdel-Mohsin, A.M. (2013) Hepatitis B Virus Infection among Egyptian Children Vaccinated during Infancy. *International Journal of Medical, Health, Biomedical and Pharmaceutical Engineering*, **7**, 554-561.

[15] Compri, A.P., Miura, I., Porta, G., Lemos, M.F., Saraceni, C.P. and Moreira, R.C. (2012) Hepatitis B Virus Infection in Children, Adolescents, and Their Relatives: Genotype Distribution and Precore and Core Gene Mutations. *Revista da Sociedade Brasileira de Medicina Tropical*, **45**, 301-304. http://dx.doi.org/10.1590/S0037-86822012000300004

[16] Jafri, W., Jafri, N., Yakoob, J., Islam, M., Tirmizi, S.F.A., Jafar, T., *et al.* (2006) Hepatitis B and C: Prevalence and Risk Associated with Seropositivity Factoring among Children in Karachi, Pakistan. *BMC Infectious Diseases*, **6**, 101. http://dx.doi.org/10.1186/1471-2334-6-101

[17] Kelly, D. and Skidmore, S. (2002) Hepatitis C-Z: Recent Advances. *Archives of Disease in Childhood*, **86**, 339-343. http://dx.doi.org/10.1136/adc.86.5.339

[18] Zein, N.N. (2007) Hepatitis C in Children: Recent Advances. *Current Opinion in Pediatrics*, **19**, 570-574. http://dx.doi.org/10.1097/MOP.0b013e3282f04ea8

[19] Martin, S.R. (2009) Hepatitis C in Children. *Pediatrics Archive*, **16**, 715-716.

[20] Vogt, M., Lang, T., Frösner, G., Klingler, C., Sendl, A.F., Zeller, A., *et al.* (1999) Prevalence and Clinical Outcome of Hepatitis C Infection in Children Who Underwent Cardiac Surgery before the Implementation of Blood-Donor Screening. *New England Journal of Medicine*, **341**, 866-870. http://dx.doi.org/10.1056/NEJM199909163411202

[21] El-Shabrawi, M.H. and Kamal, N.M. (2013) Burden of Pediatric Hepatitis C. *World Journal of Gastroenterology*, **19**, 7880-7888. http://dx.doi.org/10.3748/wjg.v19.i44.7880

[22] Nzaji, M.K. and Ilunga, B.K. (2013) A Study of the Prevalence of Infectious Markers in Blood Donors in Rural Areas. The Case of Kamina Hospital. *Santé Publique*, **25**, 213-217.

23

Association of Body Mass Index and Lipid Profiles in Children

Gülsen Meral[1]*, Ayşegül Uslu[1], Ali Ünsal Yozgatli[2], Faruk Akçay[1]

[1]Department of Children Health and Disease, Kagithane State Hospital, Istanbul, Turkey
[2]Department of Obstetrics & Gynecology, Kagithane State Hospital, Istanbul, Turkey
Email: [*]gulsenmeral@drgulsenmeral.com, ayseguluslu1@yahoo.com.tr, unsalyoz@hotmail.com, farukakcay@mynet.com

Abstract

We examined the lipid values of obese and normal-weight children, to look if there is an association between Body Mass Index (BMI) and lipid profiles. Our study group included 100 volunteers (50 children with normal BMI and 50 with high BMI) who were admitted to Kagithane State Hospital Pediatrics Clinic for various reasons between July 2010 and May 2011. The inclusion criteria were as follows: age between 2 and 14 years, no chronic disease and no developmental defects. The high BMI group had significantly higher Low Density Lipoprotein (LDL) levels in comparison to the normal BMI group ($p < 0.05$). We also found that the high BMI group had higher cholesterol levels close to upper limit than the normal BMI group. We found high triglyceride levels not only in the high BMI group but also in the normal BMI group with a rate of 26% and 24% respectively. The difference of 2% was not significant. We advise that identification and treatment of elevated LDL cholesterol levels is of tremendous significance for obese children or adolescents for future cardiovascular disease risk in adulthood. In the light of these findings, we must not overlook cardiovascular risk in the normal BMI group children. We believe that necessary precautions must be taken for preventing overweight and dyslipidemia in early childhood. Accordingly, it is of paramount importance not only to reduce obesity in children and adolescents but also to monitor dyslipidemia in normal BMI children to avoid the subsequent risk for cardiovascular disease.

Keywords

Body Mass Index, Children, Cholesterol, Dyslipidemia

1. Introduction

Overall the global prevalence rate of obesity is 3.3% reportedly. Some countries especially in Middle East, Latin

---

[*]Corresponding author.

America and North America have higher rates. Overweight is showing an increasing global trend [1].

Current estimates suggest that up to 1.7 billion people are overweight or obese workdwide. Obesity is increasing all over the word. Over 115 million people are obese and have problems associated with obesity in developing countries [2]. Overweight problem is increasing continuously in children and adolescents at an alarming pace [2] [3].

Cardiovascular diseases are associated with risk factors such as obesity and dyslipidemia, which, if present during infancy, could continue throughout adult life [1] [4] [5].

High serum cholesterol HDL level is associated with longevity as evidence suggest. Low HDL cholesterol level is associated with an increased cardiovascular risk particularly if serum cholesterol and triglycerides are also elevated.

The most common primary lipid disorder familial combined hyperlipidemia which is an autosomal dominant condition occurring in 1/200 people could not affect the results of our study with its low incidence.

The most common dyslipidemia of obesity is associated with increased triglyceride levels, decreased HDL levels and abnormal LDL cholesterol composition .Accepted risk factors for CVD are elevated LDL and decreased HDL [5] [6].

In this research, BMI and lipid profiles in children were examined to look for the association of obesity and dyslipidemia as was the case in adults.

2. Material and Method

Our study group enrolled 100 volunteers (50 children with normal BMI and 50 children with high BMI) who were admitted to Kagithane State Hospital Pediatrics Clinic consecutively for various reasons during July 2010-May 2011 and met the criteria of our research and accepted to participate. The inclusion criteria were as follows: the age between 2 and 14 years, no chronic disease and no developmental defects.

The Ethics Committee of Şişli Etfal Education and Research Hospital approved the study protocol used for all participants.

Social and lifestyle issues were investigated with the help of a questionnaire.

BMI is calculated with weight/height^2 formula. Obese, overweight and underweight are defined using BMI percentiles; children > 2 years old with a BMI > 95th percentile meet the criterion for obesity, between 85th and 95th percentiles fall in the overweight range and a BMI < 5th percentile meet criterion for underweight (7).

Descriptive and observational study of 100 children and adolescents stratified BMI into two groups. They were classified as either normal weight or obese. Total cholesterol (T-chol), HDL and triglycerides (TG) were determined and LDL was calculated.

Acceptable total cholesterol level among children and adolescents is <170 mg/dL; borderline 170 - 199 mg/dL; and high >200 mg/dL. Acceptable LDL cholesterol value is <110 mg/dL; borderline 110 - 129 mg/dL; and high >130 mg/dL. HDL cholesterol value should be >40 mg/dL ideally; the higher the better. We accept normal triglycerides levels for 2 and 5 year-olds to be 30 - 86 mg/dL (boys) and 32 - 99 mg/dL (girls), for the 6 - 11-year-olds 31 - 108 mg/dL (boys) and 35 - 114 mg/dL (girls), for the 12 - 14 year-olds 36 - 138 mg/dL (boys) and 41 - 138 mg/dL (girls) [7].

After taking the blood into a vacuum tube including an activator & gel, the sample was centrifuged at 4,000 rpm for 10 minutes and rested for 10 - 15 minutes. The serum was separated into the Beckmann couture LX20 analyzer. Cholesterol and lipid profile values were studied with auto analyzer by the photometric method.

For low levels of triglyceride below 400 mg/dL, serum LDL cholesterol level was calculated by the following method.

LDL Cholesterol = Total Cholesterol-Triglycerides/5-HDL Cholesterol.

For Triglyceride levels above 400 mg/dL. LDL Cholesterol levels were assessed photometrically.

Statistical Analysis

For Statistical Analysis, NCSS (Number Cruncher Statistical System) 2007 & PASS (Power Analysis and Sample Size) 2008 Statistical Software (Utah, USA) was used. Descriptive statistical methods (mean, standard deviation, median, frequency and ratio) were used along with Independent samples t test, for analyzing the differences of normally distributed variables between groups whereas Mann Whitney U test was used to analyze the differences of non-normally distributed variables. Pearson Chi-square test, Fisher's exact test and Yates' Chi-Square test were used to analyze the distribution of categorical variables among groups. The results were evaluated at 95%

confidence interval and $p < 0.05$ was accepted as statistically significant.

3. Results

Lipid profile of 50 children with normal BMI and 50 with high BMI were evaluated presenting to Kagithane State Hospital between 1 July 2010 and 1 May 2011.

The mean age of children with normal BMI were 7.8 ± 2.65 yrs, and those with high BMI were 10.73 ± 2.78 yrs. There were 23 (46.0%) girls and 27 (54.0%) boys in the normal BMI group and 21 (42.0%) girls and 29 (58.0%) boys in the high BMI group. No statistically significant difference with respect to gender was found between the two groups ($p > 0.05$) (**Table 1**).

No statistically significant difference was observed between the groups regarding monthly income ($p > 0.05$) families' education levels and as to the rank among siblings (**Table 2**).

There was no statistically significant difference between normal BMI group and high BMI group as to HDL levels (**Table 3**).

A statistically significant difference was found as to LDL levels ($p < 0.01$). The high BMI group had significantly higher LDL levels compared to the normal BMI group ($p < 0.05$) (**Table 4**).

We found that high BMI group had higher cholesterol levels close to upper limit in comparison to the normal BMI group (**Table 5**).

There was no significant difference in the triglyceride levels between the high and normal BMI groups ($p >$

Table 1. Descriptive information.

		Normal BMI (n = 50)	Obes BMI (n = 50)	p
		N (%)	N (%)	
Sex	Girl	23 (46.0%)	21 (42.0%)	
	Boy	27 (54.0%)	29 (58.0%)	0.687

Pearson Chi-Square test.

Table 2. Evaluation of characteristics of family.

	Obese BMI (n = 50)	Normal BMI (n = 50)	p
	Mean ± SD	Mean ± SD	
Income (TL)	1363.14 ± 543.56	1411.63 ± 676.37	0.715

Independent samples t test.

Table 3. The assessment of HDL measurement.

		Normal BMI (N = 50)	Obese BMI (N = 50)	p
		N (%)	N (%)	
+HDL	Low	15 (30.0%)	21 (42.0%)	
	Normal	35 (70.0%)	29 (58.0%)	0.21

+Fisher's exact test.

Table 4. The assessment of LDL measurement.

		Normal BMI (n = 50)	Obes BMI (n = 50)	p
		N (%)	N (%)	
LDL	++Normal	43 (86.0%)	28 (56.0%)	0.002**
	++Borderline	6 (12.0%)	13 (26.0%)	0.126
	High	1 (2.0%)	9 (18.0%)	0.016*

Pearson Chi-Square test; ++Yates Chi-Square test; *$p < 0.05$; **$p < 0.01$.

Table 5. Evaluation of cholesterol measurements.

		Normal BMI (n = 50)	Obese BMI (n = 50)	p
		N (%)	N (%)	
Cholesterol	+Normal	45 (90.0%)	26 (52.0%)	0.001**
	+Borderline	4 (8.0%)	18 (36.0%)	0.001**
	+High	1 (2.0%)	6 (12.0%)	0.112

+Fisher's exact test; **$p < 0.01$.

0.05). Contrary to expectations significant elevations were not found in triglyceride levels in children with increased BMI. Triglyceride values showed no significant difference with respect to gender in either groups ($p > 0.05$) (**Table 6**).

No significant difference was detected in behavior with respect to doing regular exercise between the two groups ($p > 0.05$). Both groups were not very much active in sports. There were significantly great differences with respect to sedentary activities like mean time of TV watch/ computer usage between the groups ($p < 0.01$). Obese children seemed to spend much longer time watching TV/using computer compared to normal-weight children ($p = 0.013$; $p < 0.05$) (**Table 7**).

4. Discussion

Cardiovascular disease (CVD) seems to be the primary cause of mortality in developed countries and is laden with considerable morbidity. It ranks high on the list of causes of deaths in developing countries also. A variety of studies demonstrated that CVD risk factors such as obesity, high lipid profile, malnutrition and passive lifestyle begins in childhood and progress into adult life. Thus, it is of crucial importance to recognize and appreciate behavioral and physiological variables associated with CVD, early in life in order to save lives of children at risk [4] [8].

Recently, studies of overweight patients have observed a correlation between BMI and dyslipidemia. A study by Suarez et al. found that values of cholesterol close to potential risk level were found in 30% of the population, 16% for triglycerides, 28% for LDL cholesterol. Lipid values were shown to be significantly different in overweight from those of general population [1]. Similar studies show that obesity is associated with abnormal values for cholesterol, triglycerides, LDL, HDL. Significant abnormalities were observed in lipid values of overweight children [8]-[10]. Overweight children have the higher LDL, triglyceride and cholesterol levels and the lower HDL in comparison to normal weight children [9]-[12].

Reck *et al.*'s study showed that abnormal lipid profiles were seen in 45.8% of overweight children [13]. A similar study showed that LDL cholesterol of obese children is 9 times high when compared to the normal weight children [14]. Yet there is a study showing no association between BMI and LDL levels [15].

Our result are in agreement with the findings of former studies demonstrating higher dyslipidemia values in obese children with LDL cholesterol concentrations significantly higher in the overweight children in comparison to normal weight children.

The study by Shamai *et al.* demonstrated that higher BMI was inversely associated with HDL [15]. Similar studies showed that HDL cholesterol is negatively associated with BMI level [16]-[18]. Sanlier observed that overweight students had significantly higher TG/HDL ratio and LDL/HDL ratio when compared to the normal and underweight students [19]. Similar to our study, there was no difference in HDL cholesterol between the normal and the high BMI group, either.

The study by Friedemann *et al.* pointed out that concentration of total cholesterol of obese children was 7.5 times as high as that of the normal weight children [14]. Other similar studies indicated that obese children have higher total cholesterol values in comparison to the normal children [16]-[18]. We also observed that the high BMI group had higher cholesterol levels close upper limit when compared to the normal BMI group. But there was no significant difference with respect to cholesterol levels between the two groups.

Recent studies have shown that high BMI is closely related with abnormal triglyceride levels [15]-[18]. Overweight students had significantly higher level triglyceride (TG) rates than normal and underweight students [19]. However, we found that there was no significant difference in the triglyceride levels between the high and

Table 6. Evaluation of triglyceride measurements.

		Normal BMI (n = 50)	Obese BMI (n = 50)	p
		N (%)	N (%)	
[++]Triglyceride	Normal	38 (76.0%)	37 (74.0%)	0.999
	High	12 (24.0%)	13 (26.0%)	

[++]Yates Chi-Square test.

Table 7. Evaluation of Time of doing exercise and TV watch/computer usage.

		Normal BMI (n = 50)	Obes BMI (n = 50)	p
		n (%)	n (%)	
Doing exercise	Yes	4 (8%)	7 (14%)	0.613
	No	46 (92%)	43 (86%)	
		Mean ± SD (Median)	Mean ± SD (Median)	[+]p
TV watch /Computer usage time (hour)		3.90 ± 2.07 (3.00)	5.02 ± 2.46 (3.00)	0.004[**]

[+]Kruskal wallis; [**]$p < 0.01$.

the normal BMI group.

Various studies have pointed out that obese patients with enlarged livers present with increased cholesterol synthesis, which may result from higher activity of the enzymes involved in cholesterol synthesis [20] [21].

In the light of our research, follow-up of lipid values provide an insight into future difficulties. Specialists should strongly urge their obese patients to have their lipid levels measured, enabling intervention at an early stage.

Given our results, we propose that obese children or adolescents with elevated LDL cholesterol levels be identified who will be at risk for cardiovascular diseases in adulthood. It is necessary to prevent obesity and dyslipidemias in an early age. Reducing obesity in children and adolescents precludes subsequent cardiovascular disease.

Authors' Contribution and Background

G.M, AU, FA, EE, AUY have made contributions in the conception and design of study and also in the acquisition, analysis and interpretation of data. They also have been involved in drafting and revision of the manuscript. All authors gave final approval of the version to be published.

All authors are actively practicing medicine in their branches for almost 7 years in this Institution (Kağıthane State Hospital) in a densely populated district of Istanbul.

References

[1]   Suárez, N.P., Prin, M.C., Luciani, S.L., Pilottó, M.T., Dri, M.D. and Politti, I.R. (2008) Prevalencia de factores de riesgo de enfermedad cardiovascular: Obesidad y perfil lipídico. *Anales de Pediatría*, 68257-68263.

[2]   de Onis, M. and Blössner, M. (2000) Prevelance and Trends of Overweight among Preschool Children in Developing Countries. *American Journal of Clinical Nutrition*, **72**, 1032-1039.

[3]   Li, Y., Dai, Q., Jackson, J.C. and Zhang, J. (2008) Overweight Is Associated with Decreased Cognitive Functioning among School-Age Children and Adolescents. *Obesity*, **16**, 1809-1815. http://dx.doi.org/10.1038/oby.2008.296

[4]   Nascimento, H., Costa, E., Rocha-Pereira, P., Rego, C., Mansilha, H.F., Quintanilha, A., *et al.* (2012) Cardiovascular Risk Factors in Portuguese Obese Children and Adolescents: Impact of Small Reductions in Body Mass Index Imposed by Lifestyle Modifications. *The Open Biochemistry Journal*, **6**, 43-50. http://dx.doi.org/10.2174/1874091X01206010043

[5]   Committee on Nutrition (1998) Cholesterol in Childhood. *Pediatrics*, **101**, 141-147.

[6]   Pinhas-Hamiel, O., Lerner-Geva, L., Copperman, N.M. and Jacobson, M.S. (2007) Lipid and Insulin Levels in Obese

Children: Changes with Age and Puberty. *Obesity*, **15**, 2825-2831. http://dx.doi.org/10.1038/oby.2007.335

[7]   Kliegman, R.M., Stanton, B.F., Schor, N.F., Geme, J.W. and Behrman, R.E. (2011) Nelson Textbook of Pediatrics. 19th Edition, Elsevier Saunders, USA, 589.

[8]   Manios, Y., Dimitriou, M., Moschonis, G., Kocaoglu, B., Sur, H., Keskin, Y., *et al.* (2004) Cardiovascular Disease Risk Factors among Children of Different Socioeconomic Status in Istanbul, Turkey: Directions for Public Health and Nutrition Policy. *Lipids in Health and Disease*, **3**, 11-18. http://dx.doi.org/10.1186/1476-511X-3-11

[9]   Romero-Velarde, E., Campollo-Rivas, O., Celis de la Rosa, A., Vásquez-Garibay, E.M., Castro-Hernández, J.F. and Cruz-Osorio, R.M. (2007) Factores de riesgo de dislipidemia en niños y adolescentes con obesidad. *Salud Publica Mex*, **49**, 103-108. http://dx.doi.org/10.1590/S0036-36342007000200005

[10]   Denke, M.A., Sempos, C.T. and Grundy, S.M. (1993) Excess Body Weight. An Underrecognized Contributor to High Blood Cholesterol Levels in White American Men. *Archives of Internal Medicine*, **153**, 1093-1103. http://dx.doi.org/10.1001/archinte.1993.00410090045006

[11]   Krauss, R.M., Winston, M., Fletcher, B.J. and Grundy, S.M. (1998) Obesity: Impact on Cardiovascular Disease. *American Heart Association*, **98**, 1472-1476.

[12]   Kouda, K., Fujita, Y., Nakamura, H., Takeuchi, H., Iki, M. (2011) Effect of Recovery from Obesity on Cardiovascular Risk Factors among Japanese Schoolchildren: The Iwata Population-Based Follow-Up Study. *Journal of Epidemiology*, **21**, 370-375. http://dx.doi.org/10.2188/jea.JE20100140

[13]   Korsten-Reck, U., Kromeyer-Hauschild, K., Korsten, K., Baumstark, M.W., Dickhuth, H.H. and Berg, A. (2008) Frequency of Secondary Dyslipidemia in Obese Children. *Vascular Health and Risk Management*, **4**, 1089-1094.

[14]   Friedemann, C., Heneghan, C., Mahtani, K., Thompson, M., Perera, R., Alison, M. and Ward, A.M. (2012) Cardiovascular Disease Risk in Healthy Children and Its Association with Body Mass Index: Systematic Review and Meta-Analysis. *BMJ*, **345**, e4759. http://dx.doi.org/10.1136/bmj.e4759

[15]   Shamai, L., Lurix, E., Shen, M., Novaro, G.M., Szomstein, S., Rosenthal, R., *et al.* (2011) Association of Body Mass Index and Lipid Profiles: Evaluation of a Broad Spectrum of Body Mass Index Patients Including the Morbidly Obese. *Obesity Surgery*, **21**, 42-47. http://dx.doi.org/10.1007/s11695-010-0170-7

[16]   Horta, B.L., Victora, C.G., Lima, R.C. and Post, P. (2009) Weight Gain in Childhood and Blood Lipids in Adolescence. *Acta Paediatrica*, **98**, 1024-1028. http://dx.doi.org/10.1111/j.1651-2227.2009.01247.x

[17]   Sánchez Bayle, M., Sánchez Bernardo, A., Peláez Gómez de Salazar, M.J., González Requejo, A., Martinoli Rubino, C. and Díaz Cirujano, A. (2006) Relationship between Lipid Profile and Body Mass Index. Five-Year Follow-Up in Children Aged 6-11 Years Old. The Rivas-Vaciamadrid Study. *Anales de Pediatría*, **65**, 229-2933. http://dx.doi.org/10.1157/13092159

[18]   Sarni, R.S., Suano de Souza, F.I., de Oliveira Schoeps, D., Catherino, P., Pires de Oliveira, M.C.C., Pessotti, C.F.X., *et al.* (2006) Relationship between Waist Circumference and Nutritional Status, Lipid Profile and Blood Pressure in Low Socioeconomic Level Pre-School Children. *Arquivos Brasileiros de Cardiologia*, **87**, 153-158. http://dx.doi.org/10.1590/S0066-782X2006001500013

[19]   Sanlier, N. and Yabanci, N. (2007) Relationship between Body Mass Index, Lipids and Homocysteine Levels in University Students. *Journal of Pakistan Medical Association*, **57**, 491-495.

[20]   Miettinen, T.A. and Gylling, H. (2000) Cholesterol Absorption Efficiency and Sterol Metabolism in Obesity. *Atherosclerosis*, **153**, 241-248. http://dx.doi.org/10.1016/S0021-9150(00)00404-4

[21]   Santosa, S., Varady, K.A., AbuMweis, S. and Jones, P.J. (2007) Physiological and Therapeutic Factors Affecting Cholesterol Metabolism: Does a Reciprocal Relationship between Cholesterol Absorption and Synthesis Really Exist? *Life Sciences*, **80**, 505-514. http://dx.doi.org/10.1016/j.lfs.2006.10.006

24

The Correlation of Urine Retinol Binding Protein-4 and Serum HbA$_{1c}$ with Glomerular Filtration Rate in Type 1 (Insulin-Dependent) Diabetic Children: A Perspective on the Duration of Diabetes

Edy Novery*, Susi Susanah, Dedi Rachmadi

Department of Child Health, Faculty of Medicine, Universitas Padjadjaran, Bandung, Indonesia
Email: *novery_fk02@yahoo.co.id

Abstract

Objective: To analyze the correlation between urine retinol binding protein-4 (RBP-4) and serum HbA$_{1c}$ with glomerular filtration rate (GFR) in type 1 diabetic children. Methods: This was a cross-sectional observational analytic study. The subjects were type 1 diabetic children aged 2 - 14 years. Sample collection was conducted from October to November 2014. Exclusion criteria were patients with obesity, renal insufficiency that was not caused by diabetes, history of hepatic diseases, and history of blood cell disorders. We performed anamnesis, physical examination, and blood sampling for serum HbA$_{1c}$ and serum cystatin-C, and urine sampling for RBP-4 on all subjects. Glomerular filtration rate was calculated from the concentration level of cystatin-C using Filler formula. Data analysis was performed by Spearman test to determine the correlation between urine RBP-4 and serum HbA$_{1c}$ with GFR. The Fisher's exact test was used to determine the correlation between duration of diabetes and RBP-4, HbA$_{1c}$, and also GFR. Results: Twelve females (60%) and 8 males (40%) participated in the study. The mean age of the subjects with 95% CI was: 10.5 (2 - 14) years while the mean age of duration diabetes with 95% CI: 3.8 (0.5 - 10) years. Twelve (60%) subjects had <5 years duration of diabetes, while eight (40%) subjects had ≥5 years duration of diabetes. Twelve (60%) subjects had normal RBP-4 level, while eight (40%) subjects had elevated RBP-4 level. The mean level of HbA$_{1c}$ with 95% CI: 8.9 (5.1 - 15.2)%. Thirteen (65%) subjects had poor metabolic. The mean GFR of the subjects with 95% CI: 99.3 (35.2 - 147.4) mL/1.73/m². Nineteen (95%) subjects had normal GFR, while 1 (5%) had renal insufficiency. The results of data analysis using Spearman test on the correlation between urine RBP-4 and serum

---

*Corresponding author.

HbA$_{1c}$ with GFR were not significant. The result of correlation between duration of diabetes and urine RBP-4 was significant using Fischer's test. Conclusion: The results showed no correlation between urine RBP-4 and serum HbA$_{1c}$ with GFR. Urine RBP-4 could be considered to assess renal function in type 1 diabetic patients with a duration of diabetes of more than 5 years.

Keywords

RBP-4, HbA$_{1c}$, Glomerular Filtration Rate, Diabetes, Children

1. Introduction

Diabetes mellitus (DM) is a world health problem affecting all age groups. Diabetic nephropathy (DN) is a serious major microvascular diabetic complication in type1 diabetic patients [1]. About 30% - 40% of diabetic patients develop an end-stage renal disease and require either dialysis or renal transplantation [2]. Recent studies demonstrated that there was a tubular component in renal complications of diabetes as shown by the detection of renal tubular enzymes and low molecular weight (LMW) proteins (e.g. RBP-4) in the urine. In fact, tubular involvement may precede glomerular involvement in DN [3] [4]. Declined GFR often occurs in type 1 diabetic patients with poor metabolic control, which is characterized by elevated serum HbA$_{1c}$ level [5]. Glomerular filtration rate by measuring the level of cystatin-C would be better compared to creatinine which is commom for measuring GFR [6].

Retinol binding protein-4 is an LMW protein that filtrated by glomerulus and then re-absorbed by proximal tubules. Elevated level of RBP-4 occurs when tubules function decreases and re-absorption function of proximal tubules does not run properly [7]. The progression of nephropathy in type 1 diabetes has classically been described as a series of stages in relentlessly deteriorating course from normal renal function to end stage renal disease marked by increasing amounts of albuminuria. At the time of initial diagnosing, there are no significant renal histologic abnormalities, renal plasma flow and GFR. Within 3 years of duration diabetes, minimize changes of the renal will be seen [8] [9]. But some studies reported that renal changes will be happened at least 5 years duration of diabetes and tubular involvement may precede glomerular involvement in ND [10]-[12]. This is evidenced by the increase preceded RBP-4 before going on condition of albuminuria [4]. Poor metabolic control causes early renal function decrease which is characterized by declined GFR [5]. Therefore, We decided to analyze the correlation between urine RBP-4 and serum HbA$_{1c}$ with GFR in type 1 diabetic children.

2. Materials and Methods

Subjects were patients with type 1 diabetic children aged between 2 - 14 years who visited the pediatric endocrinology division of Dr. Hasan Sadikin General Hospital, a tertiary level university teaching hospital with total of 554,000 inpatients and outpatients per year in West Java, Indonesia. The exclusion criteria were patients with obesity, renal disease that was not caused by diabetes, history of hepatic diseases, and history of blood cell disorders. This was a cross-sectional observational analytic study. Sample collection was conducted from October to November 2014 by inviting these patients to participate in this study. This study was approved by the ethical committee of the Faculty of Medicine, Universitas Padjadjaran/Dr. Hasan Sadikin General Hospital Bandung, Indonesia.

Urine RBP-4 were collected after informed consent the patient's parents were obtained in accordance with the standard protocol.This assay employs the quantitative sandwich enzymes immunoassay technique [13]. Serum HbA$_{1c}$ was collected after informed consent. This assay employs chromatography technique [14]. Serum cystatin-C was used as a marker for GFR. Serum cystatin-C employs the particle enhanced turbidimetric immunoassay (PETIA) [15] and then the GFR value was gained through Filler formula [16].

Data were presented as means, standard deviations, and medians with range. Statistical parameters were calculated using SPSS^{TM} version 20.0. Due to unnormally distributed data, the nonparametric Shapiro-Wilk test was used to test the significant differences between the groups. Data analysis was performed using Spearman's rho correlation to determine the correlation between urine RBP-4 and serum HbA$_{1c}$ with GFR. The Fisher's exact test was used to determine the correlation between the duration of diabetes and RBP-4, HbA$_{1c}$, and also GFR. p Values < 0.05 were considered as significant.

3. Results

The study population consisted of 20 pediatric patients with type 1 DM. Subjects were recruited from patients who visited the pediatric endocrinology division of Dr. Hasan Sadikin General Hospital in Bandung, Indonesia. The 20 subjects consisted of 12 females (60%) and 8 males (40%). The mean age of the subjects with 95% CI: 10.5 (2 - 14) years while the mean age of duration of diabetes with 95% CI: 3.8 (0.5 - 10) years. Twelve (60%) subjects had had diabetes for <5 years, while eight (40%) subjects had had diabetes for ≥5 years. Twelve (60%) subjects had normal RBP-4 (<100 ng/mL), while eight (40%) subjects had elevated RBP-4 level (all of them with a duration of diabetes of ≥5 years). The mean level of HbA_{1c} with 95% CI: 8.9 (5.1 - 15.2)%. Thirteen (65%) subjects had poor metabolic ($HbA_{1c} > 8$%). The mean GFR of the subjects with 95% CI: 99.3 (35.2 - 147.4) $mL/1.73/m^2$. Nineteen (95%) subjects had normal GFR, while 1 (5%) had renal insufficiency (GFR < 80 $mL/1.73/m^2$). The clinical characteristics of the subjects are presented in **Table 1**, while biochemical parameters of the subjects are presented in **Table 2**.

Table 1. Characteristics of the subjects (n = 20).

Characteristics	n	
Sex		
Male	8	
Female	12	
Age (years)		
Mean (SD)		10.5 (3.3)
Median		12
Range		2 - 14
Duration of Diabetes (years)		
<5 years	12	
≥5 years	8	
Mean (SD)		3.8 (2.6)
Median		4
Range		5 - 10

SD, standard deviation.

Table 2. Biochemical parameters of the subjects.

Variables	n = 20
RBP-4 (ng/mL)	
Mean (SD)	163.6 (238.6)
Median	58.3
Range	2.4 - 881.9
HbA_{1c} (%)	
Mean (SD)	8.9 (3)
Median	9.1
Range	5.1 - 15.2
Cystatin-C (mg/L)	
Mean(SD)	0.7 (0.4)
Median	0.6
Range	0.3 - 2.3
GFR ($mL/1.73/m^2$)	
Mean (SD)	99.3 (21.1)
Median	100.5
Range	35.2 - 147.4

RBP-4, retinol binding protein-4; HbA_{1c}, glicosated hemoglobin; GFR, glomerular filtration rate; SD, standard deviation.

The results of data analysis with Spearman test on the correlation between urine RBP-4 and serum HbA1c with GFR were not significant (**Table 3**). The result of correlation based on Fischer's test shows that the duration of diabetes was only significant with urine RBP-4 (**Table 4**).

The results showed that the correlation of RBP-4 and HbA1c with GFR had $p => 0.25$. Therefore, this result cannot be proceed to multiple regression analysis because it does not meet the criteria for this analysis.

4. Discussion

In our work we studied the excretion of LMW protein RBP-4. Hong and Chia stated that the detection of renal tubular proteins and enzymes may precede glomerular involvement as several of these tubular proteins and enzymes are detectable even before the appearance of microalbumunuria [1]. Within 5 years of the onset of albuminuria in DN, approximately half of the individuals will have experienced a 50% reduction in the GFR and doubling of their serum creatinine [9]. Jung *et al.* stated that the urinary excretion of renal tubular LMW were recommended as a useful marker for detection of minor changes in proximal tubules function long before the elevation of other markers like proteinuria and rised in serum creatinine [12]. This study has the strength because the assessment of GFR was performed by serum cystatin-C. Previous studies had shown that cystatin-C is more superior to measure GFR than creatinine [6]. Metabolic control in type 1 DM with measurement serum HbA$_{1c}$ level has a high risk of complication of DN if elevated level of serum HbA$_{1c}$ was found [17].

This study reported that the correlation between RBP-4 and HbA$_{1c}$ was not significant. This result is similar to Holm *et al.*'s statement that the correlation between RBP-4 and HbA$_{1c}$ was not significant [18]. However, this study reported that, in the average most of the subjects had poor metabolic control. However, Olsen *et al.* stated that poor metabolic control will take more than 5 years to cause changes in renal function in type 1 DM [19]. In type 1 diabetes, hyperglycemia starts in the first decades of life and is usually the only recognized cause of nephropathy. On the contrary, in type 2 diabetes hyperglycemia starts after the forties, usually when the kidneys have already suffered from the long-term consequences of ageing and of other recognized promoters of chronic renal injury, such as arterial hypertension, obesity, dyslipidemia, and smoking [20]. Tubular dysfunction appears to be correlated with the duration of type 1 diabetes. This study records that duration of diabetes ≥ 5 years is associated to the rise of RBP-4 ($p =< 0.01$) (**Figure 1**), but not to HbA$_{1c}$ and GFR ($p = 0.69$ and $p = 0.4$). This is similar to recent studies that renal changes need more than 5 years duration of diabetes [10]-[12]. Tubular involvement may precede glomerular involvement in DN [3] [4]. This study showed that duration of diabetes ≥ 5 years began to elevate RBP-4 value but it did not followed by declined GFR value. Most of the subjects still had normal GFR value. Actually, it is consistent to natural history of diabetic nephropathy in type 1 which needs at least 5 years to make changes in renal structure [21] [22].

This study showed that the correlation between urine RBP-4 and GFR was not significant. This results is similar to Fathy *et al.*'s statement that the correlation of urine RBP-4 and serum creatinine was not significant ($p =$

Table 3. Correlation between urine RBP-4 and serum HbA1c with GFR.

	r_s	p^* value
Correlation urine RBP-4 with GFR	0.18	0.45
Correlation serum HbA$_{1c}$ with GFR	−0.06	0.82

*Spearman's rho Test. RBP-4, retinol binding protein-4; HbA$_{1c}$, glicosated hemoglobin; GFR, Glomerular filtration rate; rs, correlation coefficient.

Table 4. Duration of diabetes with urine RBP-4.

Duration of Diabetes	RBP-4		Total	p^* value
	<100 ng/mL	≥100 ng/mL		
<5 years	12	0	12	
≥5 years	0	8	8	
Total	12	8	20	<0.01

*Fisher's Exact Test. RBP-4, retinol binding protein-4.

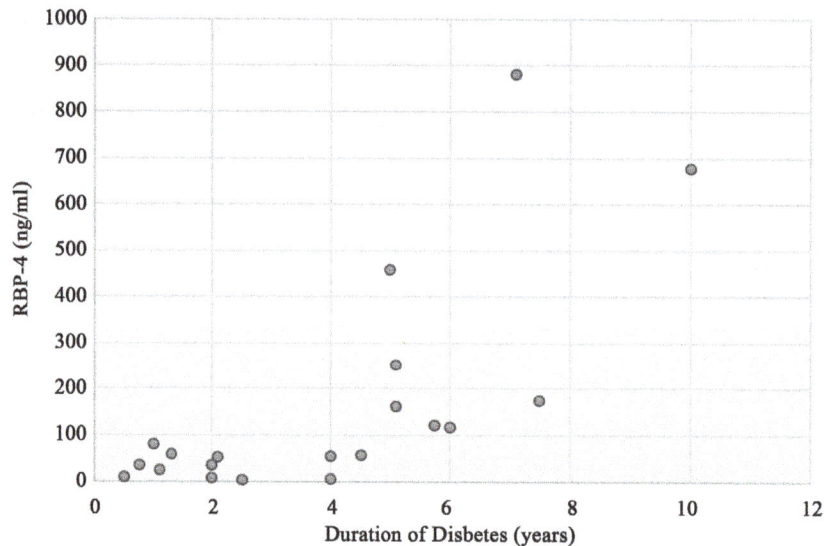

Figure 1. Urine concentrations of RBP-4 were significantly higher in type 1 diabetes children with duration of diabetes ≥5 years than <5 years (*p* =< 0.01). RBP-4, retinol binding protein-4.

0.32) [5]. This study, that used cystatin-C to measure GFR, showed that the correlation between urine RBP-4 and GFR was not significant (*p* = 0.45). The mean GFR of the subjects with 95% CI: 99.3 (35.2 - 147.4) mL/1.73/m^2. This result showed that most of the subjects has not declined GFR. This result is similar to recent studies demonstrated that, there is a tubular component in renal complications of diabetes as shown by the detection of renal tubular LMW proteins (RBP-4) in the urine. Tubular involvement may precede glomerular involvement in DN [3] [4]. This result showed there is a significant elevated RBP-4 in duration of diabetes ≥5 years than <5 years (*p* =< 0.01), but they do not have declined GFR. The early stage of DN is associated with greater than 18% - 26% increase in GFR. Hyperfiltration and the rise of glomerular filtration are believed to occur during the first five years of the disease [23]. At the time of initial diagnosis there are no significant renal histologic abnormalities, renal plasma flow, and GFR elevated. Within 3 - 5 years, histologic changes (increased measangial matrix and glomerular basement membrane thickening) of DN [8] [24]. In this study, according to Thomas *et al.* as normal reference for GFR aged 1 - 20 years is >80 ml/1.73/m^2 [25], GFR rises 24.1% of the baseline limit of the normal reference.

In our study, we could not find the correlation between urine RBP-4 and serum HbA$_{1c}$ with GFR when using Spearman's rho test. The result of the correlation between duration of diabetes ≥5 years and increased urine RBP-4 was significant with Fischer's test. The weakness of this study is that duration of diabetes in most of subjects was less than 5 years and this study is not associated a series of stages in ND. We realized that our small sample size of this study could not be the benchmark to explain actual condition in general population. We suggested making further studies, to find out the correlation between RBP-4 and HbA$_{1c}$ with GFR more than 5 years of diabetes duration.

5. Conclusion

In conclusion, no correlation was found between urine RBP-4 and serum HbA$_{1c}$ with GFR in type 1 diabetic children. We found increased urine RBP-4 with ≥5 years duration of type 1 diabetes. However, due to our limitations, more studies are needed.

Acknowledgements

Statistical analysis was performed together H. Sukandar (PhD) from the institute for Medical Informatics, Statistics, and Epidemiology (Universitas Padjadjaran, Bandung, Indonesia). We also thank the children and adolescents for their participitation in the present study.

References

[1] Hong, C.Y. and Chia, K.S. (1998) Markers of Diabetic Nephropathy. *Journal of Diabetes and Its Complications*, **12**, 43-60. http://dx.doi.org/10.1016/S1056-8727(97)00045-7

[2] Yagoob, M., Celland, P.M., Patrick, A.W., Stenensen, A., Mason, H. and Bell, G.M. (1994) Tubulopathy with Micro-albuminuria Due to Diabetic Nephropathy and Primary Glomerulonephritis. *Kidney International*, **46**, 101-104.

[3] Catalano, C., Winocour, P.H., Gillespie, S. and Gibb Alberti, K.G. (1993) Effect of Posture and Acute Glycaemic Conditions on the Excretion of Retinol Binding Protein in Normoalbumiuric Insulin Dependent Diabetic Patients. *Clinical Science*, **84**, 461-467.

[4] Uslu, S., Efe, B. and Alatas, O. (2005) Serum Cystatin-C and Urinary Enzymes as Screening Markers of Renal Dysfunction in Diabetic Patients. *Journal of Nephrology*, **18**, 559-567.

[5] Fathy, M.A., Elkady, N.N., Fathy, H.A., Award, S.A. and Elmenshawy, A.A. (2009) Estimation of Renal Tubulus Markers for Predicting Early Stage Diabetic Nephropathy in Egyptian Children with Type I Diabetic Mellitus. *Research Journal of Medical Sciences*, **4**, 207-211.

[6] Dharnidharka, V.R., Kwon, C. and Stevens, G. (2002) Serum Cystatin-C Is Superior to Serum Creatinine as a Marker of Kidney Function: A Meta-Analysis. *American Journal of Kidney Diseases*, **40**, 221-226. http://dx.doi.org/10.1053/ajkd.2002.34487

[7] Skalova, S. (2005) The Diagnostic Rote of Urinary N-Acetyl-Beta-D-Glucosaminidase Activity in Healthy Children. Nephrology (NSG) Activity in the Detection of Renal Tubulus Impairment. *Acta Medica*, **48**, 75-80.

[8] Parchwani, D.N. and Upadhyah, A.M. (2012) Diabetic Nephropathy: Progression and Pathophysiology. *International Journal of Medical Science and Public Health*, **1**, 59-70. http://dx.doi.org/10.5455/ijmsph.2012.1.59-70

[9] Marshall, R. (2004) Recent Advances in Diabetic Nephropathy. *Postgraduate Medical Journal*, **80**, 624-633. http://dx.doi.org/10.1136/pgmj.2004.021287

[10] Nelson, R.G. (2008) Kidney Disease in Childhood-Onset Diabetes. *American Journal of Kidney Diseases*, **58**, 407-411. http://dx.doi.org/10.1053/j.ajkd.2008.06.001

[11] Amin, R., Widmer, B., Prevost, A.T., Schwarze, P., Cooper, J., Edge, J., *et al.* (2008) Risk of Microalbuminuria and Progression to Macroalbuminuria in a Cohort with Childhood Onset Type 1 Diabetes: Prospective Observational Study. *BMJ*, **336**, 697-701.

[12] Jung, K., Pergande, M., Schinrte, E., Ratzmann, K.P. and Lius, A. (1988) Urinary Enzymes and Low Molecular Mass Proteins as Indicators of Diabetic Nephropathy. *Clinical Chemistry*, **34**, 544-547.

[13] Biovendor Research and Diagnostic (2013) A Sandwich Enzyme Immunoassay for the Quantitative Measurement of Human RBP-4 Protein. BioVendor R&D, 1-5.

[14] Rohlging, C., Wiedmeyer, H.M., Little, R., Grotzl, V.L., Tennill, A., England, J., *et al.* (2002) Biological Variation of Glycohemoglobin. *Clinical Chemistry*, **48**, 1116-1118.

[15] Hannemann, A., Friedriech, N., Dittmann, K., Spielhagen, C., Wallaschofski, H., Völzke, H., *et al.* (2012) Age- and Sex-Specific Reference Limits for Creatinine, Cystatin C and the Estimated Glomerulus Filtration Rate. *Clinical Chemistry and Laboratory Medicine*, **50**, 919-926. http://dx.doi.org/10.1515/cclm.2011.788

[16] Filler, G., Bokenhamp, A., Hofmann, W., Bricon, T.L., Martinez-Bru, C. and Grubb, A. (2005) Cystatin C as a Marker of GFR—History, Indications, and Future Research. *Clinical Biochemistry*, **38**, 1-8. http://dx.doi.org/10.1016/j.clinbiochem.2004.09.025

[17] McCarter, R.J., Hempe, J.M., Gomez, R. and Chalew, S.A. (2004) Biological Variation in HbA$_{1c}$ Predicts Risk Retinopathy and Nephropathy in Type 1 Diabetes. *Diabetes Care*, **27**, 1259-1264. http://dx.doi.org/10.2337/diacare.27.6.1259

[18] Holm, J., Hemmingsen, L. and Nielsen, N.V. (1988) Relationship between the Urinary Excretion of Albumin and Retinal-Binding Protein in Insulin-Dependent Diabetics. *Clinica Chimica Acta*, **177**, 101-105. http://dx.doi.org/10.1016/0009-8981(88)90312-9

[19] Olsen, B.S., Sjølie, A.-K., Hougaard, P., Johannesen, J., Borch-Johnsen, K., Marinelli, K., *et al.* (2000) A 6-Year Nationwide Cohort Study of Glycaemic Control in Young People Type 1 Diabetes: Risk Markers for the Development of Retinopathy, Nephropathy and Neuropathy. *Journal of Diabetes and its Complications*, **14**, 295-300. http://dx.doi.org/10.1016/S1056-8727(00)00078-7

[20] Ruggenenti, P. and Remuzzi, G. (2000) Nephropathy of Type 1 and Type 2 Diabetes: Diverse Pathophysiology, Same Treatment? *Nephrology Dialysis Transplantation*, **15**, 1900-1902. http://dx.doi.org/10.1093/ndt/15.12.1900

[21] Breyer, J.A. (1992) Diabetic Nephropathy in Insulin-Dependent Patients. *American Journal of Kidney Diseases*, **20**, 533-547. http://dx.doi.org/10.1016/S0272-6386(12)70215-9

[22] Steinke, J.M. and Mauer, M. (2008) Lessons Learned from Studies of the Natural History of Diabetic Nephropathy in

Young Type 1 Diabetic Patients. *Pediatric Endocrinology Reviews*, **5**, 958-963.

[23] Sabatini, S. and Kurtzman, N. (2010) Role of Hyperfiltration in the Pathogenesis of Diabetic Nephropathy. In: Sharma, S. and Prabhakar, P.P., Eds., *Advances in Pathophysiology of Diabetic Nephropathy*, Nova Science Publisher, New York, 1-10.

[24] Caramori, M.L., Fioretto, P. and Mauer, M. (2006) Enhancing the Predictive Value of Urinary Albumin for Diabetic Nephropathy. *Journal of the American Society of Nephrology*, **17**, 339-352. http://dx.doi.org/10.1681/ASN.2005101075

[25] Thomas, C. and Thomas, L. (2009) Renal Failure—Measuring the Glomerular Filtration Rate. *Deutsches Ärzteblatt International*, **106**, 849-854.

Neonatal Nutrition and Later Outcomes of Very Low Birth Weight and Preterm Infants <32 Gestational Age at a Tertiary Care Hospital of Portugal

Conceição Costa[1*], Teresa Torres[1], Andreia Teles[2]

[1]Departments of Pediatrics—Centro Hospitalar Vila Nova de Gaia/Espinho, Vila Nova de Gaia, Portugal
[2]Departments of Pediatrics, Neonatology Unit—Centro Hospitalar Vila Nova de Gaia/Espinho, Vila Nova de Gaia, Portugal
Email: *saocdcosta@gmail.com

Abstract

Premature infants, especially those born with less than 1500 g, often exhibit slow overall growth. Lack of early nutritional support is an important element. The present authors describe parenteral nutritional practices in a tertiary hospital and evaluate postnatal growth of preterm infants under 32 weeks of gestational age or with a birth weight < 1500 g. For population study, we examined 431 newborn files. Their median gestational age was 29.7 weeks. Of them, 25.4% were small for gestational age (SGA). 77.5% received parenteral nutrition (PN), 54.5% of which was provided on the first day. The average time was 14.7 days. The average weight gain by the 30th day was 425 g. At discharge, 37% were <P3 and 26% were P3 - P10. By the 3rd month 20% had their weight under P3, decreasing to 10% by the 12th month. Children who initiated PN in the first 24 hours of life had significantly better weight on the 30th day of their life (p < 0.001) and in the 6th month of corrected age (p = 0.038). And they had better Body Mass Index (BMI) in the 3rd (p = 0.012) and 12th (p = 0.023) months. Despite better feeding practices, there is still significant failure in post natal growth. Early introduction of PN was associated with an improved weight gain, which suggests that nutrition that included amino acids may be critical during the first 24 hours of life.

Keywords

Growth, Parenteral Nutrition, Preterm Infant, Very Low Birth Weight

---

*Corresponding author.

1. Introduction

Feeding preterm infants is a challenge because there is still much to learn. And nutrition is often limited by the management of the clinical problems of extreme prematurity. Although great efforts have been made to improve neonatal nutrition in very low birth weight (VLBW) infants, many do not receive adequate nutrient intake and thus develop extrauterine growth restriction. Parenteral nutrition (PN), which allows the infant's requirements for growth and development to be met, is indicated in infants for whom feeding via the enteral route is impossible, inadequate, or hazardous. Despite some recommendations, insufficient alimentation and postnatal growth restriction are still frequently observed these days [1].

Extensive research has established that infants with very low birth weight (VLBW) are particularly vulnerable to the effects of early nutritional deficiencies. Any insufficiency or delay in early nutritional support may be deleterious and contribute to both postnatal morbidities and impaired neurodevelopmental outcomes [2]. So a premature birth is a nutritional emergency!

The goal of nutrient supply for preterm infants is to achieve a pattern of growth that is similar to intra-uterine pattern [3]. The achievement of a postnatal growth at a rate approximating that of the third trimester of intrauterine life is considered the best means to facilitate later growth and development [2]-[4].

The history of neonatal feeding practices has undergone many modifications. In the last few years, great attention has been given to high amino acid supply in VLBW infants from the first day of life in order to avoid catabolism, establish anabolism, achieve in utero protein accretion rates, and promote linear growth. Current scientific evidence highlights the importance of supplementing the premature infant with sufficient nutrients not only to improve survival, growth and neurological development, but also to secure future health and quality of life [4] [5].

Although the association of an early PN and better growth in the first weeks of life has been studied by some authors, few studies report this benefit during the first year of life.

2. Objectives

The primary objectives were to describe alimentation of neonatal nutrition in a neonatal intensive unit in the last eleven years and determine the association between neonatal parenteral nutritional practices and infants' growth in the first year of life.

3. Material and Methods

We performed a retrospective cohort study. Our data were collected based on clinical records of infants admitted to the Neonatal Unit at a Tertiary Care Hospital of Portugal between January 2002 and December 2012 with less than 32 weeks of gestational age or birth weight less than 1500 g.

The data for each eligible infant were retrospectively collected. They include gender, birth, gestational age, hospitalization diagnosis, days with PN, PN start day, PN composition (proteins, lipids and carbohydrates) on the 1st day and maximum rate. Gestational age was based on obstetrical ultrasound; intrauterine growth restriction (IUGR) was considered if birth weight under P10. Weighing was routinely performed by nurses with digital electronic scales (reading to at least the nearest 10 g). Percentiles and Z-scores of growth were determined using Fenton and Kim curves of 2013 and growth curves from WHO 2006.

Statistical analysis was done using SPSS 20.0. Categorical variables were analyzed by using χ^2 for independent measures. Students' t test was used for continuous variables. P values of <0.05 were considered significant and confidence interval of 95% was used.

Permission to conduct the study was granted by the Hospital Ethics Committee.

4. Results

The study consisted 431 preterm infants admitted to the Neonatal Department between January 2002 and December 2012 with less than 32 weeks of gestational age or birth weight less than 1500 g. Baseline characteristics of the entire study population are displayed in **Table 1**. The median birth weight was 1216 g and the gestation age of 29.7 weeks. Those who had suffered intrauterine growth restriction took up 24.5%.

Table 2 characterizes the parenteral nutritional practices of the studied population. Of the total 431 infants, 334 (77.5%) received PN. Of the 92 infants who haven't received PN, 72 died and 6 were transferred to other

Table 1. Population characteristics.

Baseline characteristics	Observation
Median of gestational age in weeks	29.7
Infant Gender; N (%)	
Male	241 (55.9)
Female	190 (44.1)
Median of birth weight in grams	1216.3
Birth weight; N (%)	
<750	42 (9.9)
750 - 999	73 (17.2)
1000 - 1249	110 (25.9)
1250 - 1499	143 (33.6)
≥1500	57 (13.4)
IUGR[1]; N (%)	106 (24.6)

[1]IUGR = Intrauterine Growth Restriction.

Table 2. Characterization of parenteral nutrition.

Baseline characteristics	Observation
Total, N (%)	334 (77.5)
Beginning, N (%)	
First 24 hours	182 (54.5)
After 24 hours	152 (45.5)
Duration, average in days	14.7
Maximal doses of proteins, average in g/kg/day	
<28 weeks	3.3
[28 - 32] weeks	2.9
≥32 weeks	2.7
Maximal doses of lipids, average in g/kg/day	
<28 weeks	3
[28 - 32] weeks	2.6
≥32 weeks	2.4
Maximal doses of glucose, average in mg/kg/'	
<28 weeks	8.6
[28 - 32] weeks	8.6
≥32 weeks	7.7

hospitals during the first hours of life. Analyzing those who received PN, we found that 54.5% started during the first 24 hours. The average duration of PN was 14.7 days. The maximal dose of proteins, lipids and glucose was stratified according to gestational age.

These infants' average weight gain on the 30th day of their life was 425 g. Stratifying their weight on day 30 to their gestational age (**Figure 1**), 31% were under P3; 29% were between P3 and P10; 36% were between P10 and P50 and 4% between P50-P90. By the time of discharge, the average weight had become 2014 g with an average duration of 36.3 weeks. Stratifying the percentiles (**Figure 2**), 37% were under P3; 26% were between

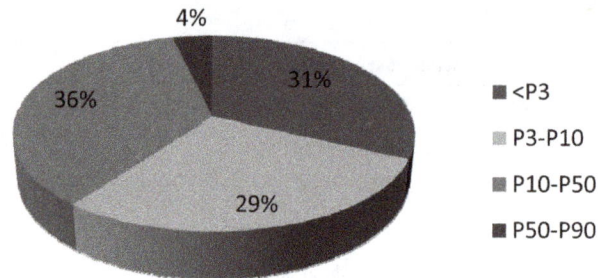

Figure 1. Weight stratified in percentiles at day 30 of life.

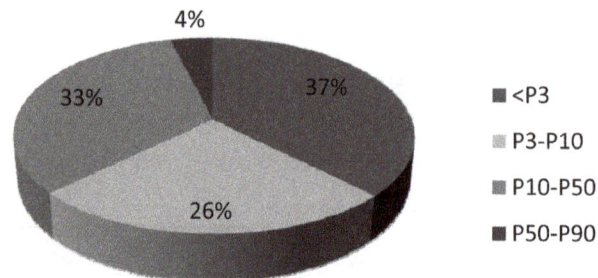

Figure 2. Weight stratified in percentiles at discharge.

P3 and P10; 33% were between P10 and P50 and 4% between P50 - P90.

Figure 3 and **Figure 4** show the evolution of weight and Body Mass Index (BMI) of the studied population's first year of life. The percentage of infants with weight under P3 is 20% in the 3rd month of corrected age, decreasing to 10% in the 12th month of corrected age. The proportion of infants with BMI under P3 is 8% and 4% in the 3rd and 12th months of corrected age. Of these children with weight under P3 in the 12th month, 40% were small for gestational age (SGA), and 23% were under 28 weeks at birth.

Comparing Parenteral Nutrition (PN) Started before and after the First 24 Hours of Live

According to the objectives of the study we compared infants who started parenteral nutrition in the first 24 hours of life (Group 1: N = 182) with those who started parenteral nutrition after 24 hours of life (Group 2: N = 152). Groups like these are naturally made. It is because our institution laboratory prepares PN one time per day, so infants born after PN preparation, will only start it on the 2nd day. **Table 3** compares the baseline characteristics of the two groups of the study. No differences were found in gestational age, birth weight, and the rate of SGA.

Analyzing the maximal doses of proteins, lipids and glucose achieved in parenteral nutrition of both groups (**Table 4**), we found no differences between the two groups. However, beginning of PN in the first 24 hours was associated with early achievement of maximal doses of proteins (6.6 days vs 9.2 days—p = 0.002), lipids (6.1 days vs 8.5 days—p = 0.003) and glucose (7.6 days vs 10.8 days—p = 0.003); and early start of enteral nutrition (2.8 days vs 3.9 days—p < 0.001).

The two groups under observation displayed different proportions of complications during hospitalization. Group 1, who started PN before 24 hours of life, had significantly less infants with necrotizing enterocolitis (NEC), 3.8% vs 16.1% (p < 0.001); intraventricular hemorrhage (IVH), 7.1% vs 13.4% (p = 0.013); sepsis, 25.0% vs 45.6%, (p < 0.001) and bronchopulmonary dysplasia (BPD), 3.3% vs 11.4% (p = 0.003).

Evaluating weight gain on the 30th day of life; we found that the 1st group was associated with better weight gain: 477 g (±214) vs 355 g (±200)—p < 0.001. At discharge there were no significant differences found between the groups during our evaluation of the percentiles of weight, length and head circumference.

The follow-up during the first year of life was possible for 85% of the population submitted to PN. In the 3, 6, 9 and 12 months infants' weight, length, head circumference, and BMI were evaluated. These records were converted to Z-score for corrected age (**Graphics 1-4**). In all the periods under study, the weight, length, and

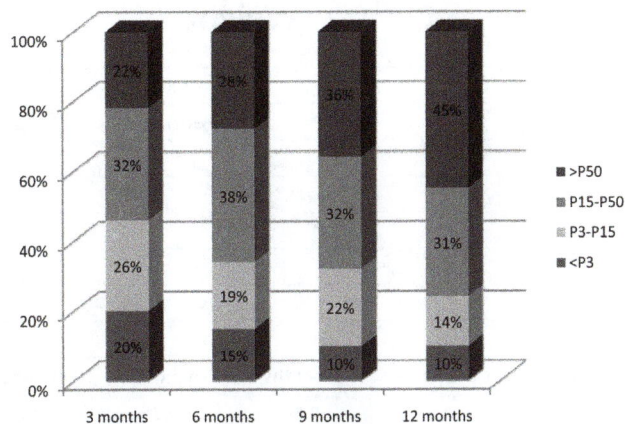

Figure 3. Weight evolution during the first year of life.

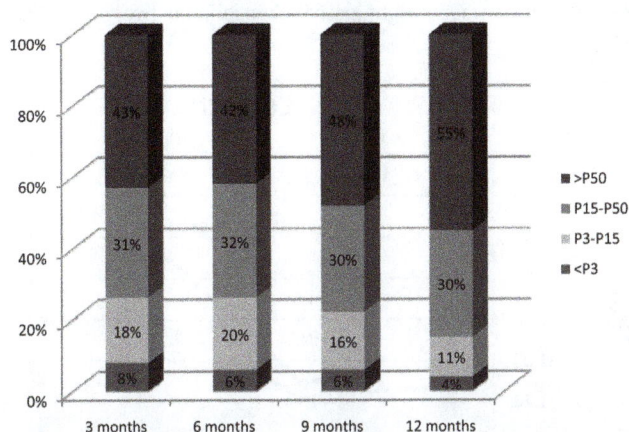

Figure 4. BMI evolution during the first year of life.

Table 3. Baseline characteristics of the two groups.

	PN before 24 h	PN after 24 h	p
Gestational age in weeks (average ± SD)	29.95 ± 2.19	29.50 ± 2.50	0.079
Birth weight in grams (average ± SD)	1240.97 ± 286	1188.74 ± 306	0.106
SGA[1] rate (%)	25.7%	24.5%	0.752

[1]SGA = Small for Gestational Age.

Table 4. Differences in parenteral nutrition (maximal doses of proteins, lipids and glucose) and enteral nutrition between two groups.

		PN before 24 h	PN after 24 h	p
Parenteral nutrition	Maximal dose of proteins (g/kg/d)	2.77 ± 0.52	2.74 ± 0.71	0.726
	Day of maximal dose	6.6 ± 5.2	9.2 ± 9.0	0.002
	Maximal dose of lipids (g/kg/d)	2.61 ± 0.55	2.64 ± 0.54	0.593
	Day of maximal dose	6.13 ± 4.4	8.53 ± 7.9	0.003
	Maximal dose of glucose (mg/kg/')	8.47 ± 4.9	8.38 ± 1.9	0.838
	Day of maximal dose	7.6 ± 6.4	10.8 ± 7.8	0.003
	Beginning of enteral nutrition	2.76 ± 1.3	3.9 ± 3.4	<0.001
	Day of exclusively enteral nutrition	27.2 ± 26.5	32.3 ± 30.5	0.074

Weight

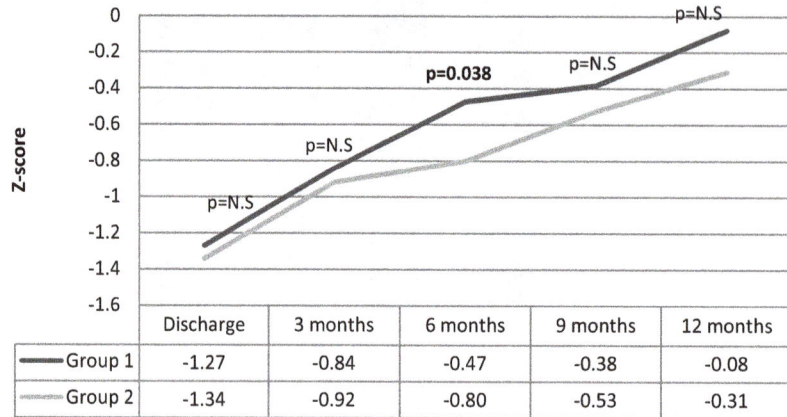

	Discharge	3 months	6 months	9 months	12 months
Group 1	-1.27	-0.84	-0.47	-0.38	-0.08
Group 2	-1.34	-0.92	-0.80	-0.53	-0.31

Graphic 1. Average weight z score change in the two groups from discharge to 12 months.

Length

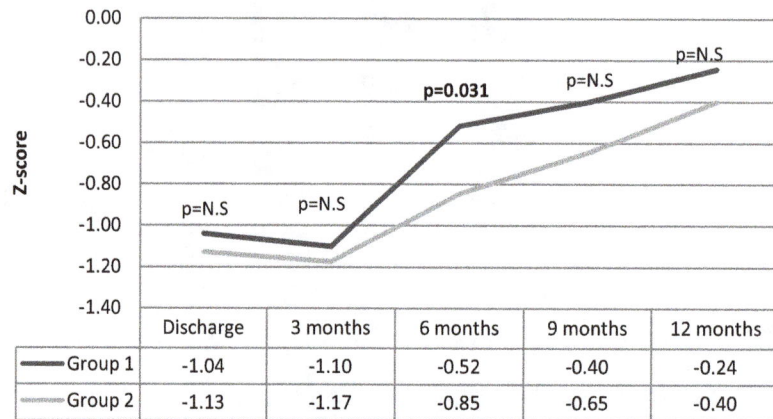

	Discharge	3 months	6 months	9 months	12 months
Group 1	-1.04	-1.10	-0.52	-0.40	-0.24
Group 2	-1.13	-1.17	-0.85	-0.65	-0.40

Graphic 2. Average length z score change in the two groups from discharge to 12 months.

Head circumference

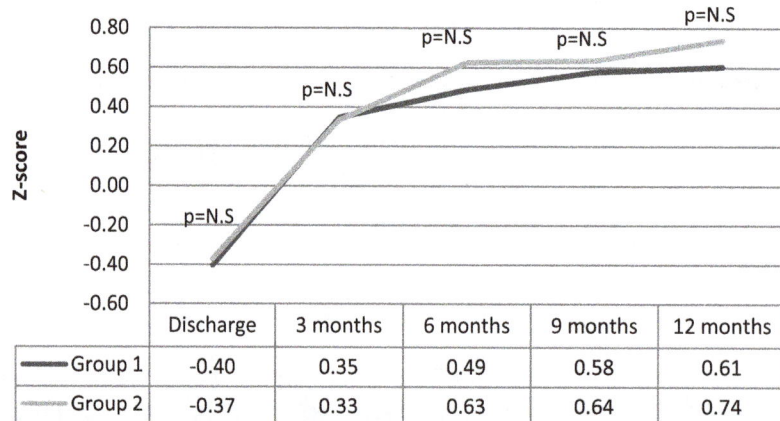

	Discharge	3 months	6 months	9 months	12 months
Group 1	-0.40	0.35	0.49	0.58	0.61
Group 2	-0.37	0.33	0.63	0.64	0.74

Graphic 3. Average head circumference z score change in the two groups from discharge to 12 months.

BMI

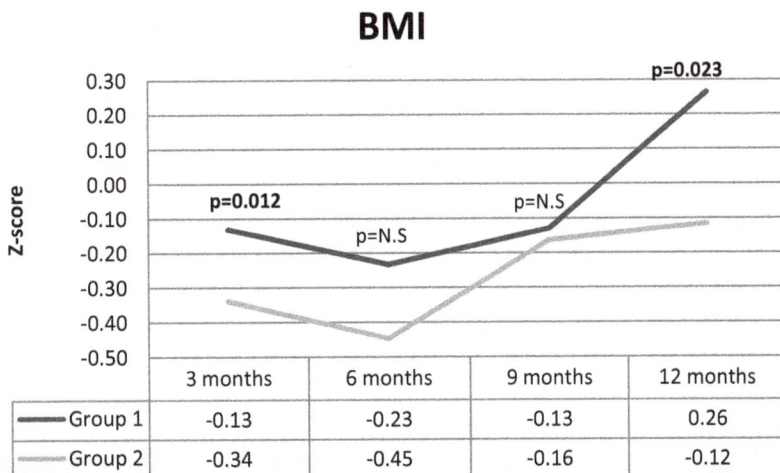

	3 months	6 months	9 months	12 months
Group 1	-0.13	-0.23	-0.13	0.26
Group 2	-0.34	-0.45	-0.16	-0.12

Graphic 4. Average BMI z score change in the two groups from 3 to 12 months.

BMI of the 1st group had a higher Z-score. These differences were statistically significant for the weight and length of 6-month-olds and for the BMI of 3- and 6-month-olds.

5. Discussion

The increasing survival of very low birth weight infant is still currently a challenge for the full medical team. As reported by some authors, "the chief variable in determining the weight curve of premature infant is the feeding policy" [6]. We conducted this study to determine postnatal growth in response to current nutritional practices and as a first step to improve post natal growth and nutritional status.

Of the total population only 54.5% started PN on the first day of life. In our Unit it was impossible to institute PN on the first day to all preterm infants who need it because, until now, there were no stock intravenous solutions with proteins.

The achieved maximal doses of proteins were high in preterm under 28 weeks. This was probably because these infants had prolonged PN with minimum enteral nutrition given the possibility to reach higher amounts of liquids, glucose and proteins with parenteral nutrition.

The weight growth of our population in the first 30 days of life (mean of 425 g) is according to relevant research literature [7]. VLBW preterm frequently suffers from extra-uterine growth restriction. And in our study, 60% of the infants were under P10 at 30 day of life, and 63% of the infants were under P10 at the time of discharge. These results are also similar to what is described in literature [8] [9]. However, these results are far from what is considered ideal, which means that the nutrition given to these infants cannot meet their needs.

This growth restriction observed in the first few weeks of life has consequences in the long term. As observed in **Figure 3**, 20% of the infants weighed <P3 in the 3rd month of corrected age. In the 12th months, only half (10%) recovered for a higher percentile.

The results of our study evidence the importance of early administration of proteins in the growth of these VLBW infants. The group who started PN on the first day (Group 1) achieved better weight in all periods studied. Another interesting observation was that the infants in the first group had shorter durations of PN administration, earlier start of enteral nutrition, and earlier achievement of full enteral feeding. The group who started parenteral nutrition earlier was also associated with fewer complications (NEC, IVH, sepsis and BPD). Although these data are not sufficient to assume a cause-effect relation, it is well recognized that poor nutrition is associated with more complications [10].

Previous studies have examined the relationship between amino-acid delivery and weight gain [4] [7] [10]. Early administration of amino acids has been shown to be safe, and it promotes nitrogen balance and glucose tolerance in preterm infants [4]. Recent studies support the importance not only of the amount and quality but also of a fast achievement of maximum nutrient levels [3]-[5]. A recent systematic review and meta-analysis [11] show that early PN provides benefit for some short-term growth outcomes with no evidence showing any increase of morbidity or mortality caused by early PN.

One limitation of the study was that conclusions are drawn on the basis of retrospectively collected data. Another limitation is that it did not evaluate the role of lipids and its influence in the growth of this preterm. Although studied and understood not as much as proteins, fatty acids play a critical role in postnatal brain development [12]. Current recommendations support that, in VLBW, the administration of parenteral amino acids combined with lipids from birth improves conditions for anabolism and growth, which is shown by improved nitrogen balance [13].

Finally it only evaluated growth. It could be argued that growth particularly that of weight might not be the best measure of clinical outcome in nutritional studies in preterm infants. Other criteria such as status of 2-year neurodevelopment or other morbidities may be preferred, especially because of the association between poor growth and these outcomes [14].

6. Conclusions

In conclusion, the results of this study, although subject to some limitations, show that the use of early PN is associated with better growth in the first few weeks of life and the first 12 months. Despite the changes in alimentation, it is still difficult to achieve an optimal extra-uterine growth. These facts highlight the importance of studying the underlying causes of postnatal growth failure. Therefore, additional research efforts should be directed to ascertaining the optimum composition and optimum use of PN in preterm infants in order to achieve nutritional strategies that both improve neurodevelopmental outcome and minimize long term metabolic and cardiovascular adverse effects.

Until better strategies arise, early start of the PN is critical. It is essential to maintain better nutritional care. As reported by some studies, adherence to these practices is still not totally ensured [1].

References

[1]   Lapillonne, A., Carnielli, V.P., Embleton, N.D., et al. (2013) Quality of Newborn Care: Adherence to Guidelines for Parenteral Nutrition in Preterm Infants in four European Countries. BMJ, 3, 1-8.
      http://dx.doi.org/10.1136/bmjopen-2013-003478

[2]   Latal-Hajnal, B., von Siebenthal, K., Kovari, H., et al. (2003) Postnatal Growth in VLBW Infants: Significant Association with Neurodevelopmental Outcome. Journal of Pediatrics, 143, 163-170.
      http://dx.doi.org/10.1067/S0022-3476(03)00243-9

[3]   Rigo, J. and Senterre, T. (2013) Intrauterine-Like Growth Rates Can Be Achieved with Premixed Parenteral Nutrition Solution in Preterm Infants. Journal of Nutrition, 143, 2066-2070. http://dx.doi.org/10.3945/jn.113.177006

[4]   Sánchez, A.R., Jiménez, R.M.R., Orgaz, M.C.S.G., et al. (2013) Agressive Parenteral Nutrition and Growth Velocity in Preterm Infants. Nutrición Hospitalaria, 38, 2128-2134.

[5]   Senterre, T. and Rigo, J. (2013) Parenteral Nutrition in Premature Infants: Practical Aspects to Optimize Postnatal Growth and Development. Archives de Pédiatrie, 20, 986-993. http://dx.doi.org/10.1016/j.arcped.2013.05.021

[6]   Dancis, J., O'Connel, J.R. and Holt Jr., L.E. (1948) A Grid for Recording the Weight of Premature Infants. The Journal of Pediatrics, 33, 570-572. http://dx.doi.org/10.1016/S0022-3476(48)80269-6

[7]   Garcia, L.V., Erroz, I.O., Freire, M.M., et al. (2012) Does Early Parenteral Protein Intake Improve Extrauterine Growth in Low Birth Weigth Preterm? Anales de pediatria (Barcelona, Spain), 76, 127-132.

[8]   Lima, P.A.T., Carvalho, M., Costa, A.C.C., et al. (2014) Variables Associated with Extra Uterine Growth Restriction in Very Low Birth Weight Infants. Jornal de Pediatria (Rio J), 90, 22-27. http://dx.doi.org/10.1016/j.jped.2013.05.007

[9]   Clark, R.H., Thomas, P. and Peabody, J. (2003) Extrauterine Growth Restriction Remains a Serious Problem in Prematurely Born Neonates. Pediatrics, 11, 986-990. http://dx.doi.org/10.1542/peds.111.5.986

[10] Valentine, C.J., Fernandez, S., Rogers, L.K., et al. (2009) Early Amino-Acid Administration Improves Preterm Infant Weight. Journal of Perinatology, 29, 428-432. http://dx.doi.org/10.1038/jp.2009.51

[11] Moyses, H.E., Johnson, M.J., Leaf, A.A., et al. (2013) Early Parenteral Nutrition and Growth Outcomes in Preterm Infants: A Systematic Review and Meta-Analysis. The American Journal of Clinical Nutrition, 97, 816-826.
      http://dx.doi.org/10.3945/ajcn.112.042028

[12] Vlaardingerbroek, H., Vermeulen, M.J., Carnielli, V.P., et al. (2014) Growth and Fatty Acid Profiles of VLBW Infants Receiving a Multicomponent Lipid Emulsion From Birth. Journal of Pediatric Gastroenterology and Nutrition, 58, 417-427. http://dx.doi.org/10.1097/MPG.0000000000000280

[13] Vlaardingerbroek, H., Vermeulen, M.J., Rook, D., et al. (2013) Safety and Efficacy of Early Parenteral Lipid and

Neonatal Nutrition and Later Outcomes of Very Low Birth Weight and Preterm Infants...

171

High-Dose Amino Acid Administration to Very Low Birth Weight Infants. *Journal of Pediatrics*, **163**, 638-644.
http://dx.doi.org/10.1016/j.jpeds.2013.03.059

[14] Ehrenkranz, R.A., Dusick, A.M., Vohr, B.R., *et al.* (2006) Growth in the Neonatal Intensive Care Unit Influences Neurodevelopmental and Growth Outcomes of Extremely Low Birth Weight Infants. *Pediatrics*, **117**, 1254-1261.
http://dx.doi.org/10.1542/peds.2005-1368

Abbreviations

BMI: Body Mass Index
BPD: bronchopulmonary dysplasia
GA: Gestational age
IUGR: Intrauterine growth restriction
IVH: Intraventricular hemorrhage
NEC: Necrotizating enterocolitis
PN: Parenteral nutrition
SGA: Small for gestational age
VLBW: Very low birth weight
WHO: World Health Organization

Neonatal Graves' Disease and Cholestatic Jaundice: Case Series and Review of the Literature

Osama Almadhoun[1*], Teresa Rivera-Penera[2], Lauren Lipeski[3]

[1]University of Kansas Medical Center, Kansas City, USA
[2]Division of Pediatric Gastroenterology, St. Joseph's Children Hospital, Paterson, USA
[3]Division of Pediatric Endocrinology, Upstate Medical Center, Golisano Children Hospital, Syracuse, USA
Email: [*]oalmadhoun@KUMC.edu, lipeskil@upstate.edu

Abstract

Cholestatic jaundice and elevated liver enzymes are uncommon, but recognized, manifestations of neonatal thyrotoxicosis. Current guidelines for evaluation of cholestatic jaundice and reviews in Neonatology literature do not discuss hyperthyroidism in the differential diagnosis of cholestatic jaundice. We report two cases of neonatal thyrotoxicosis secondary to neonatal Graves' disease that presented with cholestatic jaundice and elevated liver enzymes at birth. Early recognition of thyrotoxicosis as a cause of the hepatic disease in the neonate is crucial to prevent unnecessary diagnostic procedures and to initiate timely treatment.

Keywords

Neonate, Graves' Disease, Thyrotoxicosis, Hyperthyroidism, Cholestasis, Hepatitis, Jaundice, Conjugated Hyperbilirubinemia

1. Introduction

Cholestatic jaundice and elevated liver enzymes are uncommon, but recognized, manifestations of neonatal thyrotoxicosis. We report two neonates with cholestasis associated with neonatal thyrotoxicosis caused by maternal Graves' disease. The cause of liver disease in neonatal thyrotoxicosis has not been clearly established. Early recognition of thyrotoxicosis as a cause of the hepatic disease in the neonate is crucial to prevent unnecessary diagnostic procedures and to initiate timely treatment.

---
[*]Corresponding author.

2. Case 1

A 1285 g (50% percentile) female infant born by cesarean section at 29 weeks gestation to a 36-year-old mother, gravida 2 para 1, due to premature labor. The mother had a history of hypothyroidism and was treated with thyroid hormone replacement throughout the pregnancy.

Vital signs were within normal at birth except for tachypnea with a respiratory rate of 60 - 70/minute. The infant had respiratory distress secondary to hyaline membrane disease which required surfactant therapy and ventilator support for four days. Initial exam revealed jaundice and a diffuse rash with petichiae and macules distributed over the entire body but sparing palms and soles. Hepatosplenomegaly was present (liver 3.5 cm below costal margin, spleen 4 cm below costal margin). Facies were triangular with frontal bossing and both eyes were prominent with yellow sclera. A II/VI systolic murmur was noted.

Laboratory studies on the first day of life revealed thrombocytopenia with platelet count of 64,000/L, conjugated hyperbilirubinemia with a total bilirubin of 10.7 mg/dl and a direct of 7.8 mg/dl, and elevated liver enzymes with AST of 586 U/L (18 - 74), and ALT of 177 U/L (8 - 36). Based on the clinical picture, congenital infection was suspected and studies for toxoplasma, rubella, cytomegalovirus and herpes (TORCH) were performed and were normal. On day 2 of life, an echocardiogram revealed significant pulmonary hypertension with bidirectional shunt through a patent ductus arteriosus. Cranial ultrasound showed borderline enlargement of the lateral ventricles with no intracranial calcification or bleeding.

On day 4, the infant was extubated to CPAP but remained tachycardic with a heart rate of 180 - 200/minute and worsening of tachypnea with respiratory rate of 70 - 80/minute was noted. Nitric oxide (NO) was started for persistent pulmonary hypertension. NO was continued for 3 days and the pulmonary blood pressure normalized thereafter. Thrombocytopenia persisted and the conjugated hyperbilirubinemia continued to increase to a peak of 20.3 mg/dl total and 11.5 mg/dl conjugated on day 8 of life. Liver enzymes remained elevated and peaked on day 11 with AST of 771 U/L and ALT of 364 U/L. Abdominal ultrasound confirmed hepatosplenomegaly without a discrete mass lesion and no intrahepatic or extrahepatic biliary tree obstruction. Studies to evaluate the etiology of cholestatic jaundice including alpha-1-antitrypsin deficiency, tyrosinemia, and galactosemia were performed and were normal.

On day 11, mild exophthalmos of the mother was noted and further questioning revealed that she was diagnosed with Graves' disease 8 years previously and treated with radioactive iodine therapy resulting in hypothyroidism. Based on this history thyroid profile was obtained on the infant and revealed elevated T4 at 25.3 ug/dl (normal range 9.8 - 16.6) and suppressed TSH 0.011 uIU/ml (normal range 0.4 - 8.6). Antibody mediated Neonatal Grave' disease was confirmed by presence of TSH receptor antibodies which were significantly elevated at 302% (normal 0% - 129%). Careful examination of the infant revealed diffuse goiter. Treatment was initiated with methimazole on day 12 and resulted in gradual improvement of the thyroid profile as well as the conjugated bilirubinemia and liver function tests (**Table 1**). Treatment with methimazole continued for 2 months. A slight increase in AST and ALT was noted one month after Methimazole discontinuation but then gradually improved thereafter.

3. Case 2

An 1820 gm (75th percentile) male infant born by cesarean section at 32 weeks gestation to a 35-year-old mother, gravida 2 para 1, with a history of hypothyroidism treated with thyroid hormone replacement therapy.

Initial physical exam was remarkable for triangular facies, penoscrotal hypospadias, hepatosplenomegaly and jaundice. Vital signs were significant for tachypnea at birth with a respiratory rate of 50 - 60/minute. The baby required ventilatory support for 6 days by CPAP.

Laboratory studies on the first day of life revealed thrombocytopenia with platelets of 75,000/L, conjugated hyperbilirubinemia with a total bilirubin of 8.3 mg/dl and a direct bilirubin of 4.4mg/dl. On day 2, elevated liver enzymes were noted with ALT of 67 U/L and AST of 116 U/L. Cranial ultrasound showed mild lateral ventricular enlargement with no calcification or bleeding. Echocardiogram revealed mild pulmonary hypertension with tricuspid regurgitation and increased right ventricular pressure. Evaluation for congenital infection (toxoplasma, rubella, syphilis, CMV, and HSV), viral hepatitis, alpha-1-antitrypsin deficiency and tyrosinemia were normal.

Endocrinology evaluation was performed to evaluate the pituitary function as part of the diagnostic workup for penoscrotal hypospadias revealed neonatal hyperthyroidism. On day 6 of life, Total T3 was 688 ng/dl (normal range 0 - 256), free T4 > 12 ng/dl (normal range 1.71 - 6.6), total T4 28 ug/dl (normal range 10.1 - 20) and TSH was suppressed 0.006 uIU/ml (normal range 0.4 - 8.6). Antibody mediated neonatal Graves' disease was confirmed by presence of elevated TSH receptor antibodies at 49% (normal 0% - 14%). Additional history elicited after identification of neonatal Graves' disease revealed maternal history of Gravess' disease treated with radioactive iodine 5 years prior to this pregnancy with resultant hypothyroidism. The infant was started on propylthiouracil (PTU) and propanolol.

Thyroid profile improved within 48 hrs to T3 of 371 ng/dl, free T4 of 5.58 ng/dl, and total T4 of 22.3 ug/dl. Thyroid hormone levels normalized by 3 weeks of age (**Table 2**). The conjugated hyperbilirubinemia peaked on day 12 of life with a total bilirubin of 10.2 mg/dl and a direct of 6.2mg/dl and gradually improved with normalization by 8 weeks. Liver enzymes transiently increased after initiation of PTU treatment and peaked on day 12 of life (6 days on PTU treatment) with ALT 137 U/L and AST 230 U/L. Thereafter, there was gradual improvement in the ALT and AST with normalization by 8 months (**Table 2**).

Table 1. Case 1 laboratory studies.

Day of Life	AST (U/L)	ALT (U/L)	Bilirubin Total (mg/dl)	Bilirubin Direct (mg/dl)	Platelet × 10^3/ul	Total T4 (ug/dl)	TSH (uIU/ml)
1	586	177	10.7	7.8	64	-	-
3	342	197	15.9	9.8	98	-	-
8	405	234	20.7	12.1	84	-	-
11	771	364	15.4	9.0	60	25.3	0.011
20	430	199	10.6	6.3	76	13.1	0.014
30	369	237	9.4	5.8	169	9.9	0.012
40	220	145	5.8	3.7	187	3.7	0.012
60	301	273	-	-	-	7.6	0.223
120	195	299	2.0	1.3	-	9.7	0.89
200	89	145	0.3	0.12	-	6.4	0.59
230	71	138	0.3	0.08	-	-	-
Normal	(18 - 74)	(8 - 36)	0 - 3 d (2 - 10) >1 mo (0 - 1.5)	0 - 3d < 1.5 >1mo < 0.5	(250 - 450)	1 - 7 d (10.1 - 20) 8 - 14 d (9.8 - 16.6) 1 mo - 1y (5.5 - 16)	(0.4 - 8.6)

AST: Aspartate Amino-Transferase; ALT: Alanine Amino-Transferase, T4: Thyroxine; TSH: Thyroid Stimulating Hormone.

Table 2. Case 2 laboratory studies.

Day of Life	AST (U/L)	ALT (U/L)	Bilirubin Total (mg/dl)	Bilirubin Direct (mg/dl)	Platelet × 10^3/ul	Total T4 (ug/dl)	TSH (uIU/ml)
1-2	116	67	8.3	4.1	75	-	-
6	105	74	8.5	5.6	136	28	0.006
12	230	137	10.2	6.2	302	20	0.007
20	132	85	6.9	4.6	318	11	0.004
30	121	119	7.0	4.7	297	9.9	0.010
60	75	105	1.0	0.4	-	-	0.014
120	60	75	0.6	-	265	10.8	0.275
240	57	22	-	-	323	8.6	0.413
Normal (18 - 74)	(18 - 74)	(8 - 36)	0 - 3 d (2 - 10) >1 mo (0 - 1.5)	0 - 3 d < 1.5 >1 mo < 0.5	(250 - 450)	1 - 7 d (10.1 - 20) 8 - 14 d (9.8 - 16.6) 1 mo - 1 y (5.5 - 16)	(0.4 - 8.6)

4. Discussion

Neonatal Grave' disease affects 1% - 2% of infants born to mothers with a history of Graves' disease [1] [2]. The disease results from the transplacental passage of maternal Thyroid Stimulating Hormone Receptor Antibodies (TSHR-AB) [2]-[4]. While most infants are born to women with active Graves' hyperthyroidism, the disorder can also occur in infants of women with a history of Graves' hyperthyroidism treated with thyroidectomy or radioactive iodine in the past [5]. Our cases emphasize the importance of a thorough history in mothers who are on thyroid hormone replacement therapy during pregnancy to elucidate the etiology of the hypothyroidism. Recognition of the infants risk for neonatal Graves' is crucial for early diagnosis and treatment. Measurement of maternal serum TSHR-Ab is also helpful in predicting whether a newborn will be affected [6].

Neonatal Graves' disease has been reported to cause low birth weight for gestational age, premature birth, microcephaly, frontal bossing and triangular facies, warm, moist skin, irritability and hyperactivity [7] [8]. Tachycardia with a bounding pulse, pulmonary hypertension, high-output heart failure, fetal hydrops, hyperphagia, poor weight gain and diarrhea may also be present [8]. Thrombocytopenia, hepatosplenomegaly, jaundice, diffuse goiter, stare and occasionally exophthalmos may be evident [9]. Untreated neonatal hyperthyroidism has a high mortality rate and serious neurologic sequelae [10].

The time of onset is variable, depending upon whether the mother is receiving an antithyroid drug at the time of delivery and the presence of TSH receptor blocking antibodies. Infants of mothers taking an antithyroid drug may be euthyroid at birth, and become hyperthyroid several days later, as the antithyroid drug is metabolized or excreted [11]. The presence of blocking antibodies may delay the onset of clinical hyperthyroidism by weeks or months. The symptoms usually resolve spontaneously by 3 to 12 weeks as the maternal TSHR-Ab disappears from the infant's circulation. By 4 months of age, most infant are euthyroid and off antithyroid medication treatment [8] [9].

Hepatic manifestations of Graves' disease are recognized in both adults and neonates [12] [13]. The pathology of liver disease associated with hyperthyroidism was first reported in adults in the 1930s [13]. In a 1992 review of adults with hyperthyroidism in the *Journal of Clinical Gastroenterology*, the subset of patients without congestive heart failure presented with hepatosplenomegaly in 1/3 and cholestatic jaundice in 1/2 of the patients [13]. Two thirds of the patients had elevated liver enzymes, but only 5% of these had liver enzymes over 250 U/L.

Our two patients with neonatal hyperthyroidism presented with hepatosplenomegaly, conjugated hyperbilirubinemia and elevated liver enzymes. Hepatic manifestations of neonatal hyperthyroidism were reported as early as 1955 and are recognized, though less common, manifestations of neonatal Graves' disease [14]. Literature review identified 11 case reports discussing the hepatic manifestations of neonatal Graves' disease [14]-[24]. The majority had hepatosplenomegaly and early cholestatic jaundice presenting at birth or in the first week of life. Approximately half reported elevated liver enzymes with AST generally higher than ALT as was evident in our patients. The highest levels reported were AST 1111 U/L [24] and ALT 465 U/L [17]. Very limited information is available about the time course of recovery. In our patients, the time course to complete recovery was 6 - 9 months with the improvement in AST and ALT lagging behind resolution of conjugated hyperbilirubinemia.

Conjugated hyperbilirubinemia is estimated to occur in 1 of 2500 live birth [25]. The differential diagnosis of conjugated hyperbilirubinemia is extensive, but most affected infants present with progressive and prolonged jaundice. The early cholestasis seen in our patients was also evident in the cases reported in the literature and may also be seen in patients with congenital infection and embryonic biliary atresia. Despite the recognition of the hepatic manifestations of hyperthyroidism in the literature, this complication of neonatal Graves' disease is not listed in the differential diagnosis of cholestatic jaundice in recent guidelines for evaluation of cholestatic jaundice [25]-[27]. This lack of recognition may result in a delay in diagnosis and appropriate therapy or lead to unnecessary diagnostic procedures.

The cause of liver disease in neonatal thyrotoxicosis has not been clearly established but several possibilities have been suggested. The hypermetabolic state may result in increase hepatic oxygen consumption without increased hepatic blood flow, leading to hepatic dysfunction [28] [29]. Another possibility is that thyrotoxicosis causes high output congestive heart failure (CHF), which may result in hepatic dysfunction and hepatosplenomegaly [30]. However, in both the adult and pediatric literature, the hepatic manifestations occur in hyperthyroid patients without CHF [13]. Propylthiouracil (PTU) induced hepatitis is another possible mechanism [30] [31]. In three reported cases the fetus was exposed to PTU, however, these infants had a mild elevation in liver enzymes compared to the elevation reported in unexposed cases, including our two patients who were not exposed to PTU. Enlargement of the reticuloendothelial system seen in neonatal Graves' disease may disrupt hepatic architecture and cause cholestasis [32].

5. Conclusion

In summary, neonatal Graves' disease is a rare, but potentially fatal, condition. Cholestatic jaundice with hepatosplenomegaly and hepatitis are unusual, but recognized, complications of neonatal Graves' disease. Identification of an affected infant requires a careful maternal history, a high index of suspicion and an improved recognition of neonatal Graves' disease in the differential diagnosis of cholestasis.

Conflict of Interest

The authors of this manuscript report no conflicts of interest including, but not limited to, consulting fees, paid expert testimony, employment, grants, honoraria, patents, royalties, stocks, or other financial or material gain that may involve the subject matter of the manuscript.

References

[1]   Ramsay, I., Kaur, S. and Krassas, G. (1983) Thyrotoxicosis in Pregnancy: Results of Treatment by Antithyroid Drugs Combined with T4. *Clinical Endocrinology (Oxford)*, **18**, 73-85. http://dx.doi.org/10.1111/j.1365-2265.1983.tb03188.x

[2]   McKenzie, J.M. and Zakarija, M. (1992) Fetal and Neonatal Hyperthyroidism and Hypothyroidism Due to Maternal TSH Receptor Antibodies. *Thyroid*, **2**, 155-159. http://dx.doi.org/10.1089/thy.1992.2.155

[3]   Sunshine, P., Kusumoto, H. and Kriss, J.P. (1965) Survival Time of Circulating Long-Acting Thyroid Stimulator in Neonatal Thyrotoxicosis: Implications for Diagnosis and Therapy of the Disorder. *Pediatrics*, **36**, 869-876.

[4]   Smallridge, R.C., Wartofsky, L., Chopra, I.J., Marinelli, P.V., Broughton, R.E., Dimond, R.C., *et al.* (1978) Neonatal Thyrotoxicosis: Alterations in Serum Concentrations of LATS-Protector, T4, T3, Reverse T3, and 3, 3'T2. *Journal of Pediatrics*, **93**, 118-120. http://dx.doi.org/10.1016/S0022-3476(78)80620-9

[5]   Volpé, R., Ehrlich, R., Steiner, G. and Row, V.V. (1984) Graves' Disease in Pregnancy Years after Hyperthyroidism with Recurrent Passive-Transfer Neonatal Graves' Disease in Offspring. Therapeutic Considerations. *American Journal of Medicine*, **77**, 572-578. http://dx.doi.org/10.1016/0002-9343(84)90125-6

[6]   Peleg, D., Cada, S., Peleg, A. and Ben-Ami, M. (2002) The Relationship between Maternal Serum Thyroid-Stimulating Immunoglobulin and Fetal and Neonatal Thyrotoxicosis. *Obstetrics Gynecology*, **99**, 1040-1043. http://dx.doi.org/10.1016/S0029-7844(02)01961-0

[7]   Farrehi, C. (1968) Accelerated Maturity in Fetal Thyrotoxicosis. *Clinical Pediatrics*, **7**, 134-137. http://dx.doi.org/10.1177/000992286800700304

[8]   Radetti, G., Zavallone, A., Gentili, L., Beck-Peccoz, P. and Bona, G. (2002) Foetal and Neonatal Thyroid Disorders. *Minerva Pediatrica*, **54**, 383-400.

[9]   Zimmerman, D. (1999) Fetal and Neonatal Hyperthyroidism. *Thyroid*, **9**, 727-733. http://dx.doi.org/10.1089/thy.1999.9.727

[10]   Daneman, D. and Howard, N.J. (1980) Neonatal Thyrotoxicosis: Intellectual Impairment and Craniosynostosis in Later Years. *Journal of Pediatrics*, **97**, 257-259. http://dx.doi.org/10.1016/S0022-3476(80)80487-2

[11]   Zakarija, M., McKenzie, J.M. and Hoffman, W.H. (1986) Prediction and Therapy of Intrauterine and Late-Onset Neonatal Hyperthyroidism. *The Journal of Clinical Endocrinology & Metabolism*, **62**, 368-71. http://dx.doi.org/10.1210/jcem-62-2-368

[12]   Hung, W. and Sarlis, N. (2004) Autoimmune and Non-Autoimmune Hyperthyroidism in Pediatric Patients. *Pediatric Endocrinology Reviews*, **2**, 21-38.

[13]   Fong, T.L., McHutchison, J.G. and Reynolds, T.B. (1992) Hyperthyroidism and Hepatic Dysfunction. A Case Series Analysis. *Journal of Clinical Gastroenterology*, **14**, 240-244. http://dx.doi.org/10.1097/00004836-199204000-00010

[14]   Skelton, M. (1955) Congenital Thyrotoxicosis, Hepatosplenomegaly and Jaundice in Two Infants of Exophthalmic Mothers. *Archives of Disease in Childhood*, **30**, 460-464. http://dx.doi.org/10.1136/adc.30.153.460

[15]   Farber, S. and Craig, J. (1959) Clinical Pathological Conference: The Children's Medical Center Boston, Mass. *Journal of Pediatrics*, **54**, 829-837. http://dx.doi.org/10.1016/S0022-3476(59)80154-2

[16]   Hollinsworth, D. and Mabry, C.C. (1976) Congenital Graves Disease. Four Familial Cases with Long-Term Follow-Up and Perspective. *American Journal of Diseases of Children*, **130**, 148-155.

http://dx.doi.org/10.1001/archpedi.1976.02120030038008

[17] Neal, P.R., Jansen, R.D., Lemons, J.A., Mirkin, L.D. and Schreiner, R.L. (1985) Unusual Manifestation of Neonatal Hyperthyroidism. *American Journal of Perinatology*, **2**, 231-235. http://dx.doi.org/10.1055/s-2007-999957

[18] Cove, D. and Johnston, P. (1985) Fetal Hyperthroidim: Experience of Treatment in Four Siblings. *The Lancet*, **1**, 430-432. http://dx.doi.org/10.1016/S0140-6736(85)91148-1

[19] Singer, J. (1977) Neonatal Thyrotoxicosis. *Journal of Pediatrics*, **91**, 749-751. http://dx.doi.org/10.1016/S0022-3476(77)81028-7

[20] Polak, M. (1998) Hyperthyroidism in Early Infancy: Pathogenesis, Clinical Features and Diagnosis with a Focus on Neonatal Hyperthyroidism. *Thyroid*, **12**, 1171-1177. http://dx.doi.org/10.1089/thy.1998.8.1171

[21] Page, D.V., Brady, K., Mitchell, J., Pehrson, J. and Wade, G. (1988) The Pathology of Intrauterine Thyrotoxicosis: Two Case reports. *Obstetrics & Gynecology*, **72**, 479-481.

[22] Beroukhim, R.S., Moon, T.D. and Felner, E.I. (2003) Neonatal Thyrotoxicosis and Conjugated Hyperbilirubinemia. *Journal of Maternal-Fetal and Neonatal Medicine*, **13**, 426-428. http://dx.doi.org/10.1080/jmf.13.6.426.428

[23] Dryden, C., Simpson, J.H., Hunter, L.E. and Jackson, L. (2007) An Unusual Cause of Neonatal Coagulopathy and Liver Disease. *Journal of Perinatology*, **27**, 320-322. http://dx.doi.org/10.1038/sj.jp.7211687

[24] Loomba-Albrecht, L.A., Bremer, A.A., Wong, A. and Philipps, A.F. (2012) Neonatal Cholestasis Caused by Hyperthyroidism. *Journal of Pediatric Gastroenterology and Nutrition*, **54**, 433-434. http://dx.doi.org/10.1097/MPG.0b013e318228f9a8

[25] Karpen, S.J. (2002) Update on the Etiologies and Management of Neonatal Cholestasis. *Clinics in Perinatology*, **29**,159-180. http://dx.doi.org/10.1016/S0095-5108(03)00069-1

[26] Venigalla, S. and Gourley, G.R. (2004) Neonatal Cholestasis. *Seminars in Perinatology*, **28**, 348-355. http://dx.doi.org/10.1053/j.semperi.2004.09.008

[27] Moyer, V., Freese, D.K., Whitington, P.F., Olson, A.D., Brewer, F., Colletti, R.B., *et al.* (2004) North American Society for Pediatric Gastroenterology, Hepatology and Nutrition.Guideline for the Evaluation of Cholestatic Jaundice in infants: Recommendations of the North American Society for Pediatric Gastroenterology, Hepatology and Nutrition. *Journal of Pediatric Gastroenterology and Nutrition*, **39**, 115-128. http://dx.doi.org/10.1097/00005176-200408000-00001

[28] Myers, J.D., Brannon, E.S. and Holland, B.C. (1950) Correlative Study of the Cardiac Output and the Hepatic Circulation in Hyperthyroidism. *Journal of Clinical Investigation*, **29**, 1069-1077. http://dx.doi.org/10.1172/JCI102338

[29] Yao, J.D., Gross Jr., J.B., Ludwig, J. and Purnell, D.C. (1989) Cholestatic Jaundice and Hyperthyroidism. *American Journal of Medicine*, **86**, 619-620. http://dx.doi.org/10.1016/0002-9343(89)90398-7

[30] Hayashida, C.Y., Duarte, A.J.S., Sato, A.E. and E Yamashiro-Kanashiro.H. (1990) Neonatal Hepatitis and Lymphocyte Sensitization by Placental Transfer of Prpylthiouracil. *Journal of Endocrinological Investigation*, **13**, 937-941. http://dx.doi.org/10.1007/BF03349663

[31] Deidiker, R. and de Mello, D.E. (1996) Propythiouracil-Induced Fulminant Hepatitis: Case Report Review of the Literature. *Pediatric Pathology & Laboratory Medicine*, **16**, 845-852. http://dx.doi.org/10.3109/15513819609169310

[32] Foley, T. (1991) Maternally Transferred Thyroid Disease in the Infant: Recognition and Treatment. *Advances in Perinatal Thyroidology*, **299**, 209-226. http://dx.doi.org/10.1007/978-1-4684-5973-9_12

Preventative Strategies in the Management of ROP: A Review of Literature

Irina Livshitz

University Hospitals Case Medical Center, Cleveland, USA
Email: irina.livshitz@uhhospitals.org

Abstract

Retinopathy of prematurity (ROP) is a potentially blinding eye disorder that primarily affects premature infants weighing 1250 grams or less that are born before 31 weeks of gestation. It is one of the most common causes of visual loss in childhood and can lead to lifelong vision impairment and blindness. Certain strategies for prevention have been confirmed by numerous trials, namely the role of oxygen therapy as an independent risk factor for the development of ROP and the benefits of strict control of premature infant oxygen saturations in the NICU. There is valuable data that supports use of other approaches, such as beta adrenergic blockade and IGF-1 supplementation, for which clinical trials are still in the works to establish clear protocols for their clinical use. Supplementation with vitamin A, omega-3 fatty acids, and inositol are all exciting arenas for further trials as preliminary data shows promising results in ROP prevention. It has also been shown that the benefit of vitamin E is not worth the increased incidence of NEC and sepsis as potential side effects. Furthermore, while it was an interesting idea to use the chelator D-penicillamine as a preventative strategy for ROP, the results of multiple trials seemed to be equivocal. This brief review is not all-inclusive, as there are many more modes of prevention currently being studied.

Keywords

Retinopathy of Prematurity (ROP), Proliferative Retinopathy, Neonatology

1. Introduction

Retinopathy of prematurity (ROP) is a potentially blinding eye disorder that primarily affects premature infants weighing 1250 grams or less that are born before 31 weeks of gestation. It is one of the most common causes of visual loss in childhood and can lead to lifelong vision impairment and blindness [1]. We have progressed leaps and bounds in the realm of treatment for the proliferative phase of ROP. The standard of care at most institutions today is laser or cryo ablative therapy, which is unfortunately not always effective at preventing the sequelae of ROP and can lead to the loss of peripheral vision. This has sparked a new focus on anti-VEGF treatment, which itself carries a host of reservations because no one can yet be sure of the systemic effects of anti-VEGF in the neonate. For years, researchers have postulated that in order to tackle ROP and its potentially devastating consequences, we must consider preventative strategies rather than treatment alone. Such an approach could be of enormous benefit in providing a cheap, effective means to halt the disease in its tracks. What follows is a non-comprehensive review of modes of prevention that have already been addressed in the scientific community. It will also illustrate the direction that continued research will take us in the treatment and prevention of ROP.

2. Pathogenesis of ROP

It is necessary to understand the pathogenesis of ROP prior to exploring strategies for its prevention. ROP occurs when premature birth interrupts normal retinal vascular development [2]. In humans, normal retinal vasculature occurs in two phases: vasculogenesis and angiogenesis. Vasculogenesis is the *de novo* formation of blood vessels from endothelial precursor cells. Angiogenesis is the development of new blood vessels from existing blood vessels, which occurs from 17 - 18 weeks postmenstrual age, and is characterized by tissue hypoxia-driven blood vessel development mediated by Vascular Endothelial Growth Factor (VEGF) [2]. Given that physiologic hypoxia is the normal fetal state, ROP represents defective development of vasculature when the tissue environment is hyperoxic as compared to the in utero environment [2]. ROP itself is divided into two phases.

The first phase of ROP is a vaso-obliterative phase in which, due to the hyperoxic state of the premature infant, hypoxic stimulus for the secretion of VEGF by retinal astrocytes and Muller cells is stunted. This leads to a significant delay in endothelial cell angiogenesis and blood vessel development [2]. The second phase of ROP is a proliferative phase and begins at 32 - 34 weeks of postmenstrual age. It is characterized by a hypoxia-induced retinal neovascularization which can be explained by an imbalance between the poorly developed blood vessels and the increasing metabolic demands of developing neural retina [3]. Retinal hypoxia induces a molecular cascade that culminates in the expression of a variety of genes that encode for angiogenic growth factors, namely VEGF and IGF-1. These growth factors then participate in the pathological formation of blood vessels at the junction between the vascularized and nonvascularized retina. As is common in other proliferative retinopathies, pathological neovascularization can produce fibrous contraction which ultimately results in retinal traction, detachment, and possibly blindness [4].

3. Oxygen

We now know a great deal about the importance of physiologic hypoxia as a vital stimulus for VEGF in retinal vessel formation. It is thus not surprising that prolonged respiratory support and high pulse oximetry oxygen saturations have been associated with an increased risk of ROP [5]. It is important to note that the ideal target for oxygen saturation, in so far as it relates to the progression of ROP, varies depending on which phase of ROP is being studied. In phase I ROP, multiple studies have shown that keeping oxygen saturation lower than previously expected, resulted in a decreased incidence of ROP progression [5] [6]. The question that naturally follows is how low? In 2003 Chow et al implemented what was deemed an "oxygen management policy" with strict guidelines for use of FIO2 and monitoring oxygen saturation of neonates from the delivery room and throughout hospitalization. The researchers found the incidence of ROP progression from stage 3 to stage 4 to decrease from 12.5% to 2.5% in 4 years [7]. Wright et al. in 2006 published their results after implementation of a physiologic reduced oxygen protocol (PROP) in 3 NICUs across the country. They proposed that maintaining SpO_2 values between 83% and 93% in the immediate postgestation life, combined with strict control of oxygen fluctuations, prevents the early vaso-obliterative phase of ROP [8]. A number of studies have since followed that have confirmed this trend in strict oxygen control, and have culminated in the Oxygen with Love (OWL) protocol first introduced by Sink et al in 2012 [9]. The protocol proposes several methods in maintaining the target O2 saturation of 85% - 93% in very low birth weight infants from birth to 36 weeks post-menstrual age and then presents data showing a significant decline of ROP in their NICU. After education of neonatal physicians, nurses, and respiratory therapists on risks of hyperoxemia in neonatal infants and the use of standardized bedside oximeter alarm setting, the incidence of any ROP in this NICU dropped from 35% to 12%. Furthermore, the incidence of ROP requiring ablative procedures dropped from 11% to 0% [9].

With regards to phase II ROP, the studies have been concerned with treating retinal hypoxia produced by the metabolic demand of growing the neural retina not met due to impaired vasculogenesis of phase I. Researchers proposed that treating retinal hypoxia in a premature infant in phase II with supplemental oxygen could prevent the continued increase in retinal VEGF and may help prevent the progression of proliferative neovascularization [10]. In 2000, the STOP-ROP trial was published looking at the rate of progression from prethreshold to threshold ROP in premature infants that were randomized to a conventional arm with pulse oximetry targeted at 89% to 94% saturation versus a supplemental arm with pulse oximetry targeted at 96% to 99% saturation. The rate of progression to threshold in at least 1 eye was 48% in the conventional arm and 41% in the supplemental arm [11]. Although low oxygen saturation appears to reduce the risk of severe ROP when carefully controlled within the first few weeks of life, the optimal level of saturation still remains uncertain [12]. This necessarily begs the question what other preventative measures can be implemented to prevent or at least modify the progression of ROP in premature births?

4. Beta Blockers

Beta$_2$-adrenergic receptors (beta$_2$-ARs) are expressed on vascular endothelial cells, and there has been evidence that the stimulation of beta$_2$-ARs can upregulate VEGF and subsequently promote neoangiogenesis in response to chronic ischemia [4]. In 2010, Filippi et al published a pilot study describing a protocol, PROP-ROP, to explore the possible therapeutic role of beta blockers in ROP. They demonstrated that in oxygen induced retinopathy (OIR) mice, proangiogenic factors were dose-dependently reduced by propranolol [4].

In an effort to apply animal model data to humans, a subsequent trial studied fifty-two preterm newborns with Stage 2 ROP who were randomized to receive oral propranolol in addition to standard treatment versus standard treatment alone [13]. They found that newborns treated with oral propranolol showed not only less progression to Stage 3 or Stage 3 plus but also that they required fewer laser treatments as well as less need for rescue treatment with intravitreal bevacizumab. These benefits, however, needed to be weighed against a number of serious adverse effects of systemic propranolol, such as hypotension and bradycardia, which were noted in 5 out of the 26 newborns treated with propranolol [13]. The use of oral propranolol was also studied by Makhoul et al in 2013 whose group determined that placebo infants required twice as many interventions as those treated with propranolol. However, due to the small number of participants, it was noted that the results were not statistically significant [14].

Given the concern for the potentially harmful systemic side effects of oral propranolol, the use of propranolol eye drops was first looked at in a pilot study by Dal Monti et al in 2013. They looked at topical applications of propranolol as related to prevention of retinal vascular proliferation in OIR mouse models [15]. In the first arm, the study demonstrated that topical propranolol did indeed reach the retina and resulted in drug concentrations that were effective. While these researchers admit that it might be difficult to extrapolate these results to humans, they were nonetheless excited to report that β-AR blockade could counteract oxygen induced retinopathy by preventing angiogenic responses to hypoxia. Topical propranolol could be a cheap, easy, and safe alternate delivery route to systemic propranolol [15]. Further trials are necessary to bring this data to the point of human application.

5. Vitamin A

In 2012, it was hypothesized that dark-adapted retinal sensitivity in preterm infants is improved by early high dose vitamin A [13]. This is explained by an increased availability of retinaldehyde for incorporation into rhodopsin in the developing retina. Mactier et al were the first to measure functional ocular stores of retinol in preterm infants, and found that early high-dose intramuscular vitamin A supplementation for infants at risk of retinopathy of prematurity improves retinal function at 36 weeks' post menstrual age [16]. However, the association between vitamin A and hypoxia-induced retinal neovascularization was not explored until Wang et al showed that systemic administration of retinoic acid in OIR mouse models can increase endogenous VEGF production. This, in turn, has beneficial effects on retinal vasculature and ultimately counteracts the first vaso-obliterative phase of ROP [17]. The reasons, as proposed by Wang and his colleagues, for strongly considering systemic vitamin A amongst the prevention strategies for ROP are compelling. Systemic application of retinoic acid is a more feasible mode of drug delivery in neonates than, for example, intravitreal administration. It also generates an endogenous supply of VEGF to the retina. Furthermore it should be noted that retinoic acid administration in extremely low birth weight infants has been shown to reduce the rate of bronchopulmonary dysplasia and associated pulmonary comorbidities. Finally, it is no small matter that the pharmacology, pharmacodynamics, and toxicology of retinoic acid in humans is well understood because it has been used safely and effectively in treating other conditions such as acute promyelocytic leukemia [17]. Clinical trials looking specifically at retinoic acid administration in neonates and the impact of progression of ROP promises to be an exciting area of research in the realm of ROP prevention.

6. Vitamin E

Since the 1940s, there have been a number of clinical trials of Vitamin E supplementation in premature infants to prevent ROP [10]. A Cochrane review of vitamin E studies concluded that supplemental vitamin E significantly reduced the risk of severe ROP in very low birth weight infants, however at the increased risk of sepsis [18]. One of these trials from the late 1980s found that the incidence of severe ROP was not significantly decreased; however they showed an increased incidence of sepsis and late-onset necrotizing enterocolitis (NEC) in Vitamin E-treated infants weighing less than or equal to 1500 gm at birth who received study medication for greater than or equal to 8 days [19]. An additional study by Phelps *et al.* in 1987 documented increased incidence of hemorrhagic complications of prematurity, especially in infants weighing less than 1000 g [20]. It appears that above studies have come to a unanimous conclusion that the benefits of using vitamin E as prophylaxis against ROP do not come close to outweighing the risks of sepsis, NEC, and hemorrhagic complications.

7. Serum IGF-1

Scientists have postulated that in addition to oxygen related risk factors, non-oxygen related growth factors affected by prematurity itself are also known to play an important role in pathogenesis of ROP. It has been shown that lack of IGF-1, such as in IGF-1 knock out mice, is associated with the lack of vascular growth that subsequently leads to hypoxia-driven proliferative ROP [21]. Hellstrom et al subsequently applied this data to humans and showed that persistently low serum IGF-1 did indeed correlate with increased incidence of ROP. These authors went so far as to state that IGF-1 is as strong a predictor for ROP as is low birth weight and post menstrual age at birth [22]. In 2006, they established an algorithm called WINROP (Weight, Insulin-like growth factor I, Neonatal, Retinopathy of Prematurity) in which, IGF-I values can be used to screen for infants who might be at risk of ROP [23].

Scientists have explored methods at exogenous IGF-1 delivery to preterm infants. Human milk increases serum IGF-1 more than formula feeding, however given feeding intolerance that many premature infants face, there are efforts to increase IGF-1 by parenteral administration [10]. Fresh frozen plasma has been shown to be a source of exogenous IGF-1. Dani et al, in an effort to determine whether FFP infusions can decrease the rate of ROP, found that 2 or more transfusions of FFP in the first week of life decreased the risk of developing any grade of ROP in preterm infants [24].

8. Omega-3 Supplements

Supplementing omega-3-PUFA may be of benefit in preventing retinopathy. In 2007 Connor et al used a mouse model to study the influence of omega-3- and omega-6-polyunsaturated fatty acids (PUFAs) on vascular loss and hypoxia-induced neovascularization as it pertained to oxygen induced retinopathy. They successfully showed that increasing omega-3-PUFA served to increase vessel regrowth after injury, thereby decreasing the avascular area of the retina. This reduced the hypoxic stimulus for neovascularization [25].

It had been previously noted that DHA, a major long chain poly unsaturated fatty acid (LCPUF), is a fundamental structural component of retinal cells and that DHA concentration affects the enzyme activity of membranes of retinal photoreceptors and their function. DHA was noted to be necessary for optimal retinal function [26]. A metaanalyses recently published aimed to evaluate whether supplementation of infant formula LCPUFA before the age of 1 improves infants' visual acuity. Researches did find a significant benefit of LCPUFA supplementation to visual acuity, as assessed by visual evoked potentials and behavioral methods [26].

The impact of fortification of infant formula with DHA or supplementation with omega-3 fatty acids to breast-feeding mothers on phase I or phase II ROP in low birth weight infants needs further study [18]. If additional research does support this hypothesis, then an approach similar to folic acid prenatal supplementation can be undertaken [27].

9. D-Pencillamine

A known chelator in medicine, D-pencillamine, which had been used in prevention of hyperbilirubinemia in premature infants, was also thought to possibly contribute to lower incidence of ROP. In 2001, as part of a larger review, two randomized trials on the effects of prophylactic D-pencillamine on ROP were identified. When combined, they showed a significantly lower incidence of acute ROP in the treated infants [28].

Subsequent to these findings, as part of a Cochrane review, a study was conducted looking at outcome of ROP in controlled trials where D-penicillamine was administered as compared with no treatment or placebo. A meta-analysis of 3 randomized trials meeting inclusion criteria revealed that there was no significant difference in the risk of any stage of ROP. Based on this data the authors of the review could not recommend the use of D-penicillamine for the prevention of ROP [29].

10. Inositol

Human milk has many antioxidant constituents including inositol, vitamin E, and beta-carotene that may protect against the development of ROP. An observational cohort study was designed to look at the effect of human milk feedings on the incidence of ROP in infants weighing less than 1500 g. It was determined that the incidence of ROP differed significantly by type of feeding *i.e.* human milk (41%) vs. formula (63.5%) [30].

This study paved the way for further research targeting specific nutrients such as inositol. In 2000, Friedman et al designed a prospective study looking at the relationship between inositol and ROP. They found that infants receiving high inositol formula and with higher serum inositol concentrations at birth and after 30 days had a statistically significant lower incidence of severe ROP than those receiving the lower inositol formula and with lower serum concentrations [31].

11. Conclusion

This brief review serves as a whirlwind look at preventative strategies for tackling ROP given what we already know about the pathogenesis of a potentially blinding disease. Certain strategies for prevention have been confirmed by numerous trials, namely the role of oxygen therapy as an independent risk factor for the development of ROP and the benefits of strict control of premature infant oxygen saturations in the NICU. There is valuable data that supports use of other approaches, such as beta adrenergic blockade and IGF-1 supplementation, for which clinical trials are still in the works to establish clear protocols for their clinical use. Supplementation with vitamin A, omega-3 fatty acids, and inositol are all exciting arenas for further trials as preliminary data shows promising results in ROP prevention. It has also been shown that the benefit of vitamin E is not worth the increased incidence of NEC and sepsis as potential side effects. Furthermore, while it was an interesting idea to use the chelator D-penicillamine as a preventative strategy for ROP, the results of multiple trials seemed to be equivocal. This brief review is not all-inclusive, as there are many more modes of prevention currently being studied. It is an exciting period in medicine as clinical trials continue to establish easier, safer, and more effective modes of prevention of ROP.

References

[1]   National Eye Institute: Facts about Retinopathy of Prematurity (ROP). https://www.nei.nih.gov/health/rop/rop

[2]   Fleck, B.W. and McIntosh, N. (2008) Pathogenesis of Retinopathy of Prematurity and Possible Preventive Strategies. *Early Human Development*, **84**, 83-88. http://dx.doi.org/10.1016/j.earlhumdev.2007.11.008

[3]   Penn, J.S., Madan, A., Caldwell, R.B., Bartoli, M., Caldwell, RW. and Hartnett, M.E. (2008) Vascular Endothelial Growth Factor in Eye Disease. *Progress in Retinal and Eye Research*, **27**, 331-371. http://dx.doi.org/10.1016/j.preteyeres.2008.05.001

[4]   Filippi, L., Cavallaro, G., Bagnoli, P., Dal Monte, M., Fiorini, P., Donzelli, G., Tinelli, F., Araimo, G., Cristofori, G., La Marca, G., Della Bona, M.L., La Torre, A., Fortunato, P., Furlanetto, S., Osnaghi, S. and Mosca, F. (2010) Study Protocol: Safety and Efficacy of Propranolol in Newborns with Retinopathy of Prematurity (PROP-ROP): ISRCTN18523491. *BMC Pediatrics*, **10**, 83. http://dx.doi.org/10.1186/1471-2431-10-83

[5]   Tin, W., Milligan, D.W., Pennefather, P. and Hey, E. (2001) Pulse Oximetry, Severe Retinopathy, and Outcome at One Year in Babies of Less than 28 Weeks Gestation. *Archives of Disease in Childhood—Fetal and Neonatal Edition*, **84**, F106-F110. http://dx.doi.org/10.1136/fn.84.2.F106

[6]   VanderVeen, D.K., Mansfield, T.A. and Eichenwald, E.C. (2006) Lower Oxygen Saturation Alarm Limits Decrease the Severity of Retinopathy of Prematurity. *Journal of AAPOS*, **10**, 445-448. http://dx.doi.org/10.1016/j.jaapos.2006.04.010

[7]   Chow, C., Wright, K.W. and Sola, A. (2003) Can Changes in Clinical Practice Decrease the Incidence of Severe Retinopathy of Prematurity in Very Low Birth Weight Infants? *Pediatrics*, **111**, 339-345. http://dx.doi.org/10.1542/peds.111.2.339

[8]   Wright, K.W., Sami, D., Thompson, L., Ramanathan, R. and Joseph, R. (2006) A Physiologic Reduced Oxygen Protocol Decreases the Incidence of Threshold Retinopathy of Prematurity. *Transactions of the American Ophthalmological Society*, **104**, 78-84.

[9]   Sink, D., Thomas, P., Bober, B. and Hagadom, J.I. (2012) Oxygen with Love (OWL) Improves Oxygen Saturation Target Achievement and Eye Outcomes in Preterm Newborn. http://www.docstoc.com/docs/73625317/OxygenwithLove_OWL_ImprovesOxygenSaturationTarget

[10]   Raghuveer, T.S. and Bloom, B.T. (2011) A Paradigm Shift in the Prevention of Retinopathy of Prematurity. *Neonatology*, **100**, 116-129. http://dx.doi.org/10.1159/000322848

[11]   The STOP-ROP Multicenter Study Group (2000) Supplemental Therapeutic Oxygen for Prethreshold Retinopathy of Prematurity (STOP-ROP): A Randomized, Controlled Trial. I: Primary Outcome. *Pediatrics*, **105**, 295-310.

[12]   Cavallaro, G., Filippi, L., Bagnoli, P., La Marca, G., Cristofori, G., Raffaeli, G., Padrini, L., Araimo, G., Fumagalli, M., Groppo, M., Dal Monte, M., Osnaghi, S., Fiorini, P. and Mosca, F. (2014) The Pathophysiology of Retinopathy of Prematurity: An Update of Previous and Recent Knowledge. *Acta Ophthalmologica*, **92**, 2-20.

[13]   Filippi, L., Cavallaro, G., Bagnoli, P., Dal Monte, M., Fiorini, P., Donzelli, G., Tinelli, F., Araimo, G., Cristofori, G., la Marca, G., Della Bona, M.L., La Torre, A., Fortunato, P., Furlanetto, S., Osnaghi, S. and Mosca, F. (2013) Oral Propranolol for Retinopathy of Prematurity: Risks, Safety Concerns, and Perspectives. *The Journal of Pediatrics*, **163**, 1570-1577. http://dx.doi.org/10.1016/j.jpeds.2013.07.049

[14]   Makhoul, I.R., Peleg, O., Miller, B., Bar-Oz, B., Kochavi, O., Mechoulam, H., Mezer, E., Ulanovsky, I., Smolkin, T., Yahalom, C., Khoury, A., Lorber, A., Nir, A. and Blazer, S. (2013) Oral Propranolol versus Placebo for Retinopathy of Prematurity: A Pilot, Randomised, Double-Blind Prospective Study. *Archives of Disease in Childhood*, **98**, 565-567. http://dx.doi.org/10.1136/archdischild-2013-303951

[15]   Dal Monte, M., Casini, G., la Marca, G., Isacchi, B., Filippi, L. and Bagnoli, P. (2013) Eye Drop Propranolol Administration Promotes the Recovery of Oxygen-Induced Retinopathy in Mice. *Experimental Eye Research*, **111**, 27-35. http://dx.doi.org/10.1016/j.exer.2013.03.013

[16]   Mactier, H., McCulloch, D., Hamilton, R., Galloway, P., Bradnam, M.S., Young, D., Lavy, T., Farrell, L. and Weaver, L.T. (2012) Vitamin A Supplementation Improves Retinal Function in Infants at Risk of Retinopathy of Prematurity. *The Journal of Pediatrics*, **160**, 954-959. http://dx.doi.org/10.1016/j.jpeds.2011.12.013

[17]   Wang, L., Shi, P., Xu, Z., Li, J., Xie, Y., Mitton, K., Drenser, K. and Yan, Q. (2014) Up-Regulation of VEGF by Retinoic Acid during Hyperoxia Prevents Retinal Neovascularization and Retinopathy. *Investigative Ophthalmology & Visual Science*, **55**, 4276-4287. http://dx.doi.org/10.1167/iovs.14-14170

[18]   Brion, L.P., Bell, E.F. and Raghuveer, T.S. (2003) Vitamin E Supplementation for Prevention of Morbidity and Mortality in Preterm Infants. *Cochrane Database of Systematic Reviews*, Article ID: CD003665. http://dx.doi.org/10.1002/14651858.cd003665

[19]   Johnson, L., Quinn, G.E., Abbasi, S., Otis, C., Goldstein, D., Sacks, L., Porat, R., Fong, E., Delivoria-Papadopoulos, M., Peckham, G., *et al.* (1989) Effect of Sustained Pharmacologic Vitamin E Levels on Incidence and Severity of Retinopathy of Prematurity: A Controlled Clinical Trial. *The Journal of Pediatrics*, **114**, 827-838. http://dx.doi.org/10.1016/S0022-3476(89)80149-0

[20]   Phelps, D.L., Rosenbaum, A.L., Isenber, S.J., Leake, R.D. and Dorey, F.J. (1987) Tocopherol Efficacy and Safety for Preventing Retinopathy of Prematurity: A Randomized, Controlled, Double-Masked Trial. *Pediatrics*, **79**, 489-500.

[21]   Smith, L.E.H. (2008) Through the Eyes of a Child: Understanding Retinopathy through ROP the Friedenwald Lecture. *Investigative Ophthalmology & Visual Science*, **49**, 5177-5182. http://dx.doi.org/10.1167/iovs.08-2584

[22]   Hellström, A., Engström, E., Hård, A.L., Albertsson-Wikland, K., Carlsson, B., Niklasson, A., Löfqvist, C., Svensson, E., Holm, S., Ewald, U., Holmström, G. and Smith, L.E. (2003) Postnatal Serum Insulin-Like Growth Factor I Deficiency Is Associated with Retinopathy of Prematurity and Other Complications of Premature Birth. *Pediatrics*, **112**, 1016-1020. http://dx.doi.org/10.1542/peds.112.5.1016

[23]   Löfqvist, C., Engström, E., Sigurdsson, J., Hard, A.L., Niklasson, A., Ewald, U., *et al.* (2006) Postnatal Head Growth Deficit among Premature Infants Parallels Retinopathy of Prematurity and Insulin-Like Growth Factor-I Deficit. *Pediatrics*, **117**, 1930-1938. http://dx.doi.org/10.1542/peds.2005-1926

[24]   Dani, C., Poggi, C., Bresci, C., Corsini, I., Frosini, S. and Pratesi, S. (2014) Early Fresh-Frozen Plasma Transfusion

Decreases the Risk of Retinopathy of Prematurity. *Transfusion*, **54**, 1002-1007.
http://dx.doi.org/10.1111/trf.12432

[25] Connor, K.M., SanGiovanni, J.P., Lofqvist, C., Aderman, C.M., Chen, J., Higuchi, A., *et al.* (2007) Increased Dietary Intake of ω-3-Polyunsaturated Fatty Acids Reduces Pathological Retinal Angiogenesis. *Nature Medicine*, **7**, 868-873. http://dx.doi.org/10.1038/nm1591

[26] Qawasmi, A., Landeros-Weisenberger, A. and Bloch, M.H. (2013) Meta-Analysis of LCPUFA Supplementation of Infant Formula and Visual Acuity. *Pediatrics*, **131**, e262-e272. http://dx.doi.org/10.1542/peds.2012-0517

[27] Mantagos, I.S., Vanderveen, D.K. and Smith, L.E. (2009) Emerging Treatments for Retinopathy of Prematurity. *Seminars in Ophthalmology*, **24**, 82-86. http://dx.doi.org/10.1080/08820530902800322

[28] Phelps, D.L., Lakatos, L. and Watts, J.L. (2001) D-Penicillamine for Preventing Retinopathy of Prematurity in Preterm Infants. *Cochrane Database of Systematic Reviews*, Article ID: CD001073. http://dx.doi.org/10.1002/14651858.cd001073

[29] Qureshi, M.J. and Kumar, M. (2013) D-Penicillamine for Preventing Retinopathy of Prematurity in Preterm Infants. *Cochrane Database of Systematic Reviews*, **9**, Article ID: CD001073. http://dx.doi.org/10.1002/14651858.cd001073.pub2

[30] Hylander, M.A., Strobino, D.M., Pezzullo, J.C. and Dhanireddy, R. (2001) Association of Human Milk Feedings with a Reduction in Retinopathy of Prematurity among Very Low Birth-Weight Infants. *Journal of Perinatology*, **21**, 356-362. http://dx.doi.org/10.1038/sj.jp.7210548

[31] Friedman, C.A., McVey, J., Borne, M.J., James, M., May, W.L., Temple, D.M., Robbins, K.K., Miller, C.J. and Rawson, J.E. (2000) Relationship between Serum Inositol Concentration and Development of Retinopathy of Prematurity: A Prospective Study. *Journal of Pediatric Ophthalmology & Strabismus*, **37**, 79-86.

28

Effectiveness of Music Therapy on Social Skill Growth in Educable Intellectual Disability Boys

Peyman Hashemian[1]*, Mansoureh Mohammadi[2]

[1]Psychiatry and Behavioral Sciences Research Center, Ibn-e-Sina Hospital, Faculty of Medicine, Mashhad University of Medical Sciences, Mashhad, Iran
[2]Islamic Azad University, Ghochan, Iran
Email: *hashemianp@mums.ac.ir

Abstract

Introduction: Social skills include the ability to establish interpersonal relationships with others in a way that is acceptable in terms of norms of society and it should be beneficial to society and have mutual interest. **Method:** Sample was taken from especial elementary school for educable intellectual disability children in Mashhad, Iran. The sample was boys between 9 - 11 years. After the initial selection of students, they were randomly assigned to two groups of twenty (experimental and control groups). 7 sessions of music therapy were performed for each one in the experimental group whereas no sessions were applied for anyone in the control group. Winelend Social Growth Scale was used to measure their social skill before and after intervention. **Result:** The mean difference in social skill between the two groups were statistically less than the 0.01 which is highly significant (P-value = 0.0005). This shows that art and music therapy are effective on the growth of social skills in educable intellectual disability children. **Conclusion:** This research shows that music therapy is effective for improvement of social skills in educable intellectual disability children.

Keywords

Social Skills, Music Therapy, Educable Intellectual Disability Children

1. Introduction

Intellectual disability children do not have enough social skill in finding friends, maintaining the friendship and

---

*Corresponding author.

proper relationship with others, managing any teamwork.

Social skill is to have good relationship with others and find friends and maintain the friendship and cooperate with each other and to be active in social activities. This characteristic is low in intellectual disability children.

Social skill is an important factor in avoidance of negative reaction [1] [2].

One of the important factors in formation of social skill is family function. Kumar *et al.* [3] in 2009 found that social growth in children with intellectual disability depends on the severity of intellectual disability. Dunn and colleagues [4] in 2004 found the positive effect of social problem solving in individuals with intellectual disability. Heward [5] in 2005 showed that children with intellectual disability need special support and remediation for social growth.

As music therapy provide a field for social activity, they are used in this study to evaluate whether social skill will improve in these intellectual disability students.

Mental disability children are usually unable to socially interact with friends and classmates; and their adjustment in social life is difficult.

Some studies revealed that music has positive impact on human behaviors and mood [6]-[8]. Therefore music has been used for treatment of medical and psychiatric disorders [8] [9]. Some of the most common psychiatric disorders that are treated with music therapy are pain, grief, anxiety, and relationship issues [10]-[12]. Music therapy can regulate the mood and decrease pain by releasing endorphins [13] [14]. Music can also improve function of brain in coping with stress and increases self-satisfaction and self-confidence [15].

Music brings a safe environment for proper social relationship and positive self-esteem and decreases social withdrawal, lack of interest, and aggression [16]-[20].

2. Method

This research has been conducted as case-control trial in children with intellectual disability in especial elementary school in Mashhad, Iran in 2013. All children were boys between 9 to 11 years of age who were diagnosed as having mild intellectual disability. 40 children in two groups of 20 were selected randomly. Children in experimental group had taken 7 sessions of music and art therapy whereas control group did not take any sessions of any kind. Both groups were compared by Winelend Social Growth Scale. SPSS software version 20 was used for statistical analysis. Data were analyzed by descriptive test, Leven's test, t-test and one-way ANCOVA for comparison of social growth with art and music therapy.

3. Results

The statistical analysis shows the average age in experimental group was 9.9 versus 9.8 in control group. In experimental group, mean score of pre-test was 74.73 and 79.79 in post-test whereas in control group pre-test score was 76.76 and post-test score was 79.36.

Distribution of social growth in the two groups was normal (Z = 0.63, P-value = 0.82).

Leven's test was used to evaluate homogeneity of social growth scale in educable mental retarded children (Leven's index = 90, P-value = 0.35).

Independent t-test shows no significant difference in pre-test score of the two groups (t = 0.23, P-value = 0.32).

Table 1 shows highly significant difference in social growth between the two groups in post-test (P-value = 0.0005).

4. Discussion

As known, intellectual disability is characterized by developmental delay in many area of growth such as social, individual, academic achievement and so on. One of the most important difficulties in intellectual disability children is low ability of social interaction that maybe due to poor interaction.

Table 1. The result of ANCOVA between experimental and control groups in social growth.

Source	F	2 Partial η	P-value
Group	152.31	0.83	0.0005

This study compares social skill changes in the two groups of educable intellectual disability male students where only one group goes through music therapy sessions. This study was performed only on male subjects.

The result of this study shows normal distribution of social growth in the two groups. Age and social skill scores in pre-test of the two groups were not significantly different. The result after intervention in the experimental group shows that music therapy made a highly significant change in their social skills. So it is compatible with the results achieved in previous studies on the effect of music therapy in improving psychological function and resolve of some psychiatric disorders including anxiety and improve stress management [7] [10] [11] [16]-[20]. The effect music therapy on social growth may be due to mood regulation [6]-[8] or by improving function of brain in coping with stress, self-satisfaction and self-confidence increases [13]-[15]. As music induces safe environment for good social relationship, it may cause positive self-esteem and increases social approach and interests [16]-[19]. Music therapy may decreases aggression as Habibipour *et al.*, Smeijsters *et al* and Hashemian *et al.* showed that music can be effective for control of aggression [16] [17] [20].

5. Limitation and Suggestion

This study shows that music therapy was effective in social skill improvement. This may be a trigger for initiation of social relationship and it is probably due to mood improvement. Further researches are suggested to evaluate the effect of art and music therapy on mood state.

Similar research is recommended on female individuals.

6. Conclusion

This study shows that music therapy can increase social skill in children with intellectual disability. This fact can be used to solve their social problems. So art and music therapy is recommended as one of the treatments for social skill improvement in these children.

References

[1]   Cartledge, G. and Milburn, J.A.F. (1996) Cultural Diversity and Social Skills Instruction: Understanding Ethnic and Gender Differences. 1st Edition, Research Press, Champaign.

[2]   Cartledge, G. and Kourea, L. (2008) Culturally Responsive Classrooms for Culturally Diverse Students with and at Risk for Disabilities. *Journal of Exceptional Children*, **74**, 351-371.

[3]   Kumar, I., Singh, A.R. and Akhtar, S. (2009) Social Development of Children with Mental Retardation. *Industrial Psychiatry Journal*, **18**, 56-59. http://dx.doi.org/10.4103/0972-6748.57862

[4]   Dunn, C. and Crites, S.A. (2004) Teaching Social Problem Solving to Individuals with Mental Retardation. *Education and Training in Developmental Disabilities*, **39**, 301-309.

[5]   Heward, W.L. (2003) Ten Faulty Notions about Teaching and Learning That Hinder the Effectiveness of Special Education. *The Journal of Special Education*, **36**, 186-205. http://dx.doi.org/10.1177/002246690303600401

[6]   Robb, S.L., Burns, D.S., Stegenga, K.A., Haut, P.R., Monahan, P.O., Meza, J., *et al.* (2014) Randomized Clinical Trial of Therapeutic Music Video Intervention for Resilience Outcomes in Adolescents/Young Adults Undergoing Hematopoietic Stem Cell Transplant: A Report from the Children's Oncology Group. *Cancer*, **120**, 909-917. http://dx.doi.org/10.1002/cncr.28355

[7]   Fritz, T.H., Halfpaap, J., Grahl, S., Kirkland, A. and Villringer, A. (2013) Musical Feedback during Exercise Machine Workout Enhances Mood. *Frontiers in Psychology*, **4**, 921. http://dx.doi.org/10.3389/fpsyg.2013.00921

[8]   Ghetti, C.M. (2013) Effect of Music Therapy with Emotional-Approach Coping on Preprocedural Anxiety in Cardiac Catheterization: A Randomized Controlled Trial. *Journal of Music Therapy*, **50**, 93-122. http://dx.doi.org/10.1093/jmt/50.2.93

[9]   Fritz, T.H., Hardikar, S., Demoucron, M., Niessen, M., Demey, M., Giot, O., *et al.* (2013) Musical Agency Reduces Perceived Exertion during Strenuous Physical Performance. *Proceedings of the National Academy of Sciences of the United States of America*, **110**, 17784-17789. http://dx.doi.org/10.1073/pnas.1217252110

[10] Sili, A., Fida, R., Proietti, D., Vellone, E. and Alvaro, R. (2013) Decreasing Preoperative Anxiety by Music: Experimental Study in a Vascular Surgery Unit. *Assistenza Infermieristica e Ricerca: AIR*, **32**, 13-19.

[11] Nightingale, C.L., Rodriguez, C. and Carnaby, G. (2013) The Impact of Music Interventions on Anxiety for Adult Cancer Patients: A Meta-Analysis and Systematic Review. *Integrative Cancer Therapies*, **12**, 393-403. http://dx.doi.org/10.1177/1534735413485817

[12] Blain-Moraes, S., Chesser, S., Kingsnorth, S., McKeever, P. and Biddiss, E. (2013) Biomusic: A Novel Technology for Revealing the Personhood of People with Profound Multiple Disabilities. *Augmentative and Alternative Communication*, **29**, 159-173. http://dx.doi.org/10.3109/07434618.2012.760648

[13] Vollert, J.O., Stork, T., Rose, M. and Mockel, M. (2003) Music as Adjuvant Therapy for Coronary Heart Disease. Therapeutic Music Lowers Anxiety, Stress and Beta-Endorphin Concentrations in Patients from a Coronary Sport Group. *Deutsche Medizinische Wochenschrift*, **128**, 2712-2716.

[14] Boso, M., Politi, P., Barale, F. and Enzo, E. (2006) Neurophysiology and Neurobiology of the Musical Experience. *Functional Neurology*, **21**, 187-191.

[15] McKinney, C.H., Tims, F.C., Kumar, A.M. and Kumar, M. (1997) The Effect of Selected Classical Music and Spontaneous Imagery on Plasma Beta-Endorphin. *Journal of Behavioral Medicine*, **20**, 85-99. http://dx.doi.org/10.1023/A:1025543330939

[16] Habibipour, M., Habibipour, H., Habibipour, M. and Rejaee, A. (2008) Effect of Iranian Nonverbal Soft Music on the Reduction of Aggression among Boy Students of Mashhad Guidance School. *Quarterly Educational Psychology*, **3**, 45-55.

[17] Smeijsters, H. and Cleven, G. (2006) The Treatment of Aggression Using Arts Therapies in Forensic Psychiatry: Results of a Qualitative Inquiry. *The Arts in Psychotherapy*, **33**, 37-58. http://dx.doi.org/10.1016/j.aip.2005.07.001

[18] Saarikallio, S. and Erkkilä, J. (2007) The Role of Music in Adolescents' Mood Regulation. *Psychology of Music*, **35**, 88-109. http://dx.doi.org/10.1177/0305735607068889

[19] Labbe, E., Schmidt, N., Babin, J. and Pharr, M. (2007) Coping with Stress: The Effectiveness of Different Types of Music. *Applied Psychophysiology and Biofeedback*, **3**, 163-168. http://dx.doi.org/10.1007/s10484-007-9043-9

[20] Hashemian, P., Mashoogh, N. and Jarahi, L. (2015) Effectiveness of Music Therapy on Aggressive Behavior of Visually Impaired Adolescents. *Journal of Behavioral and Brain Science*, **5**, 96-100. http://dx.doi.org/10.4236/jbbs.2015.53009

29

Outcomes of Severely Malnourished Children Aged 6 - 59 Months on Outpatient Management Program in Kitui County Hospital, Kenya

Dorothy Mbaya[1,2*], **Lucy Kivuti Bitok**[2], **Anna K. Karani**[2], **Boniface Osano**[3], **Michael Habtu**[4]

[1]Chuka District Hospital, Chuka, Kenya
[2]School of Nursing Sciences, College of Health Sciences, University of Nairobi, Nairobi, Kenya
[3]Department of Pediatrics and Child Health, School of Medicine, College of Health Sciences, University of Nairobi, Nairobi, Kenya
[4]Institute of Tropical Medicine and Infectious Diseases, Jomo Kenyatta University of Agriculture and Technology, Nairobi, Kenya
Email: *dmicheni10@gmail.com

Abstract

Background: Severe acute malnutrition is a widely prevalent problem in developing countries and a major cause of morbidity and mortality. Traditionally, children with severe acute malnutrition were rehabilitated within inpatient services. Advent of ready to use therapeutic food made it possible to treat majority of these children in their homes. However, there is limited data about the outcomes of the program. Objectives: To determine the outcomes (recovery, default, mean weight gain and non-response rates) of severely malnourished children aged 6 - 59 months enrolled in outpatient therapeutic program at Kitui County Hospital. Methodology: A prospective longitudinal study design was carried out for one month. Hundred and four (104) children with SAM were recruited in the study. Anthropometric measurements, physical examination and appetite test of the children were conducted on a weekly basis for 28 days. Descriptive analysis was conducted using means, frequency and proportions. Paired *t* test was computed for mean weight gain and mid-upper arm circumference between admission and subsequent visits. Results: The findings of the study revealed that the recovery rate was 73.3%, weight gain rate of 5.1 g/kg/day, defaulter rate was 2.9% and non-response rate was 13.9% (WHZ = −3SD). Mean weight increased from 6.8 kg on the 1st visit to 7.5 kg in the 4th visit (P = 0.000) and the meanmid-upper arm circumferenceincreased from 11.1 cm at admission to 11.9 cm at 4th visit (P = 0.000). Conclusion: The recovery and weight gain rates were below the global acceptable SPHERE of minimum standards

---

*Corresponding author.

(recovery rate > 75% and weight gain rate > 8 g/kg/day). The defaulter rate was within the acceptable international standards (<15%).

Keywords

Default, Outcomes, Recovery Rate, Severe Acute Malnutrition, Weight Gain

---

1. Introduction

Severe acute malnutrition (SAM) is defined by an extremely low weight for height, by visible severe wasting (marasmus), and/or by the presence of nutritional oedema (kwashiorkor). SAM or wasting is measured by one or more of the following criteria: Weight-for-height (WFH) ≤ -3 Z-scores; Weight-for-height less than 70% of the median; Mid-upper arm circumference (MUAC) less than 115 mm and Presence of bilateral pitting oedema [1].

Worldwide nearly 24 million children (younger than 5 years) experience SAM and 19 million severely wasted children are living in developing countries. It is common in sub-Saharan Africa, with approximately 3% of children less than five years affected at any one time. It is associated with several hundred thousand child deaths each year [2] [3]. An estimated 53% of the preventable causes of death in children less than five years are attributed to malnutrition [4]. It also has negative implications for morbidity, long-term growth, cognitive and behavioural development, and work capacity among survivors [5].

The outpatient therapeutic program (OTP) offers services to severely malnourished children age 6 - 59 months. Until recently, the management of SAM has been limited to hospital cares with limited coverage [6]. OTP brings the service of management of SAM closer to the community by making services available at decentralized health facilities (primary health care units) in different resource limited countries [7]. It is operational at health centers and health posts and offers the lifesaving treatments with ready-to-use therapeutic foods (RUTF), usually Plumpy'Nut. In addition to Plumpy'Nut, severely malnourished children are provided with routine medications such as de-wormers, antibiotics, vitamin A, folic acid and measles vaccine. Only children who have appetite with Plumpy'Nut and those who don't have medical complications are eligible to the OTP [8].

Practitioners and World Health Organization (WHO) experts endorse community-based management for uncomplicated SAM while still advising that children who are severely malnourished and have medical complications, such as severe oedema, should be treated in an appropriate health facility [9]. However, two trial studies comparing children treated in outpatient care after one week of stabilization in inpatient setting against full inpatient care have shown outcome discrepancies. The first trial in Malawi reported better results in outpatients than in inpatients (recovery: 72% vs 49%) probably related to more infections in inpatient care and mortality rate was 5.4% in inpatient and 3.0% for home-based therapy [10]. The second trial in Bangladesh reported the reverse (recovery: 67% vs 86%) but no food supplement was provided to outpatients and mortality rate was 3.5% in inpatient, 5% in day care and 3.5% at home (after one week of day care) [11].

Although the prevalence of malnutrition in Kenya especially Eastern province including Kitui County is still high, the outcome data on outpatient therapeutic program of severe acute malnourished children is still unclear. This study, therefore, sought to establish the outcomes of outpatient therapeutic program among children aged 6 - 59 months with SAM in Kitui County Hospital.

2. Materials and Methods

2.1. Study Setting

The study was carried out in Kitui County Hospital. It has a catchment population of 75,000 and serves as the main referral hospital in the Southern part of Kitui County. It has a bed capacity of 200 beds and 44 cots and an outpatient department with an OTP. Patients enrolled to OTP are detected from maternal and child health (MCH) clinics after routine screening, those referred from in-patient of the hospital or referred by community health workers (CHWs).

2.2. Study Design

A short prospective longitudinal study was conducted among children aged 6 - 59 months with SAM enrolled under OTP. Each child was followed for 4 weeks on a weekly basis.

2.3. Study Population and Sampling Technique

Children aged 6 - 59 months enrolled in OTP were recruited into the study. Children with poor appetite, edema and medical complications were excluded. SAM was determined by WHO reference classification W/H < −3 Z-score, MUAC < 11.5 cm, a good appetite, no medical complications and no severe edema (do not have moderate or severe edema).There were 104 children consecutively recruited to the study as they came to OTP. The sample size was calculated using Israel [12] formula $\left[n = N/1 + N(e)^2 \right]$; where n = the sample size, N = the population, e = margin of error (5%).

2.4. Data Collection Tools and Data Quality Control

The anthropometric measurements (weight, height/Length and left mid upper arm circumference) were obtained using a follow up checklist in a private room within the OTP clinic. In addition, physical examination and appetite test were conducted. The anthropometric measurements were conducted at the onset then weekly for 4 weeks.

Research assistants were trained on data collection tools and procedures of the study before the actual study commenced. Quality assurance was maintained through monitoring of data collection activities on daily and weekly basis by the principal investigator. The weighing machines were calibrated for validity and standardization of reporting was ensured.

2.5. Outcome Measures

The main outcomes in the study were recovered (cured), defaulted, failure to respond and mean weight gain.

Recovered was defined when children attained target W/H -2 Z-score, MUAC > 11.5 cm and no edema for two consecutive visits and has attained discharge criteria.

Defaulter referred to a child that was absent for two consecutive weeks and confirmed that the patient is not dead by home visit.

Non-respondent is a patient that has not reached discharge criteria after staying under OTP intervention for 28 days.

Mean weight gain is the difference between two weights taken on admission and on 4th visit divided by the number of intervening days; and then by the mid-point of the two weights. The units of mean weight gain were grams per kilogram per day.

2.6. Data Management and Analysis

After data collection, cleaning and validation was done and then entered into a Statistical Package format (using SPSS version 20.0) ready for analysis. Descriptive analysis using means, frequency and proportions was computed. Paired t test ($P < 0.05$) was computed for continuous variables (mean weight gain and MUAC) between admission and subsequent visits.

2.7. Ethical Considerations

Study approval was sought from the Ethics and Research Committees of the Kenyatta National Hospital/University of Nairobi (KNH/UON) and administrative permission from the Kitui County Hospital. Voluntary informedwritten consent was obtained from all mothers/guardians of the child. Confidentiality was maintained while handling participants' information.

3. Results

3.1. Characteristics of the Children

We recruited 104 children aged 6 - 56 months, 44 (42.3%) were males and 60 (57.7%) were female children. As shown in **Table 1**, the highest age group were those aged 6 - 12 months 36 (34.6%) followed by 13 - 18 months 29 (27.9%).The mean age of the children was18 months. About a quarter 28 (26.9%) of the children were first born.

3.2. Outcomes of the Outpatient Therapeutic Program

Of the 104 children enrolled into the study 3 (2.9%) defaulted. Children with WHZ −2SD and above were classified as recovered while below −2SD of WHZ were considered as not recovered. Out of the 101 children who were followed for four visits 74 (73.3%) recovered and 27 (26.7%) didn't recover. Fourteen children (13.9%) failed to respond (WHZ = −3SD) and only 7 (6.9%) had attained full nutritional recovery (WHZ = −1SD). More than half 55 (54.5%) of the children had WHZ of −2SD by fourth visit. The overall mean weight gain was 5.12 grams. About half of the children 49 (48.5%) and 47 (46.5%) had gained mean weight of 5 to 10 g/kg/day and <5 g/kg/day respectively. However, there were only 5 (5.0%) who gained mean weight of >10 g/kg/day (**Table 2**).

Table 1. Characteristics of the children.

Variables	n = 104	%
Age in months		
6 - 12 months	36	34.6
13 - 18 months	29	27.9
19 - 24 months	23	22.1
25 - 56 months	16	15.4
Sex		
Male	44	42.3
Female	60	57.7
Birth order		
First	28	26.9
Second	22	21.2
Third	21	20.2
Fourth	14	13.5
Fifth and above	19	18.3

Table 2. Outcomes of the outpatient therapeutic program.

Variables	n = 104	%
Default		
Yes	3	2.9
No	101	97.1
Recovery		
Yes	74	73.3
No	27	26.7
Overall mean weight gain in grams (5.12 ± 2.5)		
Mean weight gain		
>10 g/kg/day	5	5.0
5 to 10 g/kg/day	49	48.5
<5 g/kg/day	47	46.5
WHZ on 4th visit		
−1SD	7	6.9
<−1SD and >−2SD	11	10.8
−2SD	56	55.4
<−2SD and >−3SD	13	12.9
−3SD	14	13.9

3.3. Trend and Comparison of Mean Weight and MUAC

Figure 1 shows the mean trend of weight and MUAC among children enrolled in the outpatient management program for 4 weeks duration. The figure shows that the mean weight and MUAC increased over the four weeks of follow up till the 4th visit.

Paired samples t test was computed to determine the mean differences of weight and MUAC between the visits (**Table 3**). There was significant differences between the mean weights of 1st visit and 2nd visit (P = 0.000), 1st visit and 3rd visit (P = 0.000) as well as 1st visit and 4th visit (P = 0.000). Likewise, the mean MUAC was significantly higher between 1st visit and 3rd visit (P = 0.000) as well as between 1st visit and 4th visit (P = 0.000). However, the mean MUAC between 1st visit and 2nd visit was not significant (P = 0.143).

4. Discussion

The recovery rate in this study (73.3%) was lower than the international standards which set the lower threshold at 75%. The rate is lower than findings from studies carried out in Southern Ethiopia which shows 87% [13] and in Southern Malawi where the recovery rate was 89% [14]. However, it was higher than the study done in Nairobi which reported 58% [15] and in Tigray Northern Ethiopia (61.78%) [16]. These discrepancies could be as a result of differences in adherence to optimal management of children under OTP across regions, low frequency of feeding per day and sharing of the Plumpy'Nut with other members of the household which is a likely predictor of poor recovery of children treated at home. It was reported that sharing of RUTF with other family members, mostly children, was justified by social norms favoring sharing of food, a shortage of food in the household, the good taste of RUTF and its perceived good treatment properties [17].

In addition, genetic variations among SAM children may play a role in the recovery rate. Results from several ethnic groups (Bagandan, Peruvian, Chilean, South African Coloured) show that previously malnourished children do not attain, at least for several years, the weight, height, and bone age as children of the same ethnic background but of a higher social class [18] [19]. Considering that children from a higher social class may be nutritionally above average.

The overall defaulter rate (2.9%) was well within the minimum international standard (<15%). This figure is lower as compared to similar studies conducted on RUTF based therapeutic feeding programs in Maradi-Niger [20], Darfur-Sudan [21], Bedawacho-Ethiopia and Arbegoba-Ethiopia [22] [23]. This may signify that the

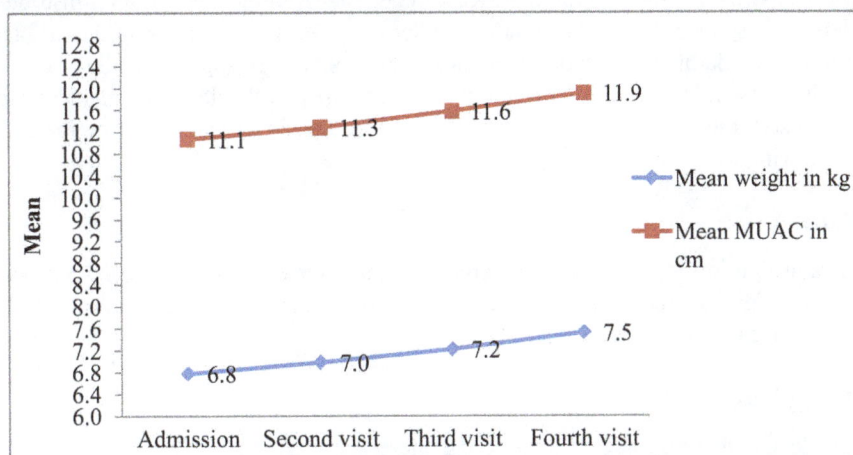

Figure 1. Trend of mean weight and MUAC between admission and consecutive visits.

Table 3. Comparison of mean weight and MUAC between first and consecutive visits.

Variables	Paired *t* test between 1st and 2nd visit	Mean difference (95% CI)	Paired *t* test between 1st and 3rd visit	Mean difference (95% CI)	Paired *t* test between 1st and 4th visit	Mean difference (95% CI)
Mean weight in kg	0.000	0.20 (0.16 - 0.25)	0.000	0.43 (0.38 - 0.40)	0.000	0.70 (0.65 - 0.80)
Mean MUAC in cm	0.143	0.21 (−0.07 - 0.50)	0.000	0.51 (0.30 - 0.72)	0.000	0.80 (0.54 - 1.12)

mothers/guardians in the study area are aware about the consequences of defaulting from the program. It could also be attributed to shortage of food among the community/households which may compel them to attend the outpatient program for Plumpy'Nut/RUTF.

The mean weight gain of 5.12 g/kg/day in this study was substantially less than the predicted rate based on the international standards which recommends weight gain of greater than or equal to 8 g/kg/day. Yet it was higher compared to a similar study conducted in Nairobi which was 3.79/kg/day [15] and was comparable to a study conducted in Tigray Northern Ethiopia (5.24 g/kg/day) [16]. However, it was lower than in studies carried out by Chane *et al.* [24] (10.1 g/kg/day), by Hossain *et al.* [25] (10 g/kg/day) and by Gebremichael *et al.* [26] in Ayder referral in Ethiopia (10.7 g/kg/day). These discrepancies could have been due to differences in causes of malnutrition across various settings. In addition, the weights may not be taken on all visits and yet the RUTF should be given according to the body weight.

Even though the mean weight gain ($P < 0.000$) and mean MUAC ($P < 0.000$) were significantly different on admission and at 4th visit, only (6.0%) had attained nutritional recovery rate (defined as a WHZ equal to or greater than $-1SD$). About half (48.5%) of the children had moderate to good mean weight gain (5 to 10 g/kg/day), 46.5% had poor mean weight gain (<5 g/kg/day) and only 5.0% had good mean weight gain (>10 g/kg/day). However, the findings are higher compared to study done in India by Patel *et al.* [27] during home based rehabilitation that reported only (11.5%) children achieved weight gain of more than 5 gm/kg/day, while (89.5%) children had weight gain of less than 5 gm/kg/day.

5. Conclusion

The recovery and weight gain rates in this study were below the acceptable standards of Global SPHERE. However, the defaulter rate was within the acceptable international standards.The findings highlight the need to enhance implementation of essential nutrition action approach during management of severe malnutrition in outpatient program.

Acknowledgements

The funding is from the Linked-Strengthening Maternal, Newborn and Child Health Research Training in Kenya. The grant is linked to Partnership for Innovative Medical Education in Kenya (PRIME-K). The project described was supported by Award Number 5R24TW008907 from the US National Institutes of Health. The content is solely the responsibility of the authors and does not necessarily represent the official views of the US National Institutes of Health. The authors would also like to sincerely appreciate all the study participants for their time and willingness to participate. The authors also give special thanks to the medical superintendent, data collectors and all staff members of Kitui County Hospital for their cooperation during the collection of data for this study and allowing us to conduct this research.

Limitation

During malnutrition low hemoglobin and serum albumin concentrations are common but due to financial constraints the study did not make provision for taking blood samples for biochemical information, therefore only anthropometric measurement were used.

Competing Interests

The authors declare that they have no competing interests.

References

[1]   Isanaka, S., Villamor, E., Shepherd, S. and Grais, R.F. (2009) Assessing the Impact of the Introduction of the World Health Organization Growth Standards and Weight-for-Height Z-Score Criterion on the Response to Treatment of Severe Acute Malnutrition in Children: Secondary Data Analysis. Malnutrition in Children. *Paediatrics*, **123**, e54-e59. http://dx.doi.org/10.1542/peds.2008-1375

[2]   Collins, S., Sadler, K., Dent, N., Khara, T., Guerrero, S., Myatt, M., Saboya, M. and Walsh, A. (2006) Key Issues in the Success of Community-Based Management of Severe Malnutrition. *Food and Nutrition Bulletin*, **27**, S49-S82. http://dx.doi.org/10.1177/15648265060273S304

[3]   Briend, A. and Collins, S. (2010) Therapeutic Nutrition for Children with Severe Acute Malnutrition Summary of African Experience. *Indian Pediatrics*, **47**, 655-659. http://dx.doi.org/10.1007/s13312-010-0094-2

[4]   Black, R.E., Morris, S.S. and Bryce, J. (2003) Where and Why 10 Million Children Are Dying Every Year? *Lancet Child Survival Series* 1, **361**, 2226-2234.

[5]   Alderman, H. (2006) Long Term Consequences of Early Childhood Malnutrition. *Oxford Economic Papers*, **58**, 450-474. http://dx.doi.org/10.1093/oep/gpl008

[6]   Del, R. and Joy, M. (2008) Madagascar's Pilot Program for Community Management of Acute Malnutrition: Evaluation Highlights. *Basic Support for Institutionalizing Child Survival (BASICS) for USAID* 2008, Arlington.

[7]   Lapidus, N., Luquero, F.J., Gaboulaud, V., Shepherd, S. and Grais, R.F. (2009) Prognostic Accuracy of WHO Growth Standards to Predict Mortality in a Large-Scale Nutritional Program in Niger. *PLOS Medicine,* **6**, e1000039. http://dx.doi.org/10.1371/journal.pmed.1000039

[8]   Econinck, H., Swindale, A., Grant, F. and Navarro-Colorado, C. (2008) Review of Community-Based Management of Acute Malnutrition (CMAM) in the Postemergency Context: Synthesis of Lessons on Integration of CMAM into National Health Systems. The Cases of Ethiopia, Malawi and Niger. FANTA Project, Academy for Educational Development, Washington DC.

[9]   WHO (2013) Guideline Update: Technical Aspects of the Management of Severe Acute Malnutrition in Infants and Children. World Health Organization, Geneva.

[10] Ciliberto, M.A., Sandige, H., Ndekha, M.J., Ashorn, P., Briend, A., Ciliberto, H.M. and Manary, M.J. (2005) Comparison of Home-Based Therapy with Ready-to-Use Therapeutic Food with Standard Therapy in the Treatment of Malnourished Malawian Children: A Controlled, Clinical Effectiveness Trial. *American Journal of Clinical Nutrition*, **81**, 864-870.

[11] Khanum, S., Ashworth, A. and Huttly, S.R. (1994) Controlled Trial of Three Approaches to the Treatment of Severe Malnutrition. *The Lancet*, **344**, 1728-1732. http://dx.doi.org/10.1016/S0140-6736(94)92885-1

[12] Israel, G.D. (1992) Sampling: The Evidence of Extension Program Impact. Program Evaluation and Organizational Development, IFAS, University of Florida; PEOD-5. http://edis.ifas.ufl.edu/pdffiles/PD/PD00500.pdf3/6/2011

[13] Teferi, E., Lera, M., Sita, S., Bogale, Z., Datiko, D.G. and Yassin, M.A. (2010) Treatment Outcome of Children with Severe Acute Malnutrition Admitted to Therapeutic Feeding Centers in Southern Region of Ethiopia. *Ethiopian Journal of Health Development*, **24**, 234-238.

[14] Dent, N. (2009) Outpatient Management of Acute Malnutrition in a Kenyan Urban Slum Context: Caseloads and Challenges. *Malawi Medical Journal*, **21**, 123-159.

[15] Nalwa, G.M. (2012) Outcomes of Severely Malnourished Children Aged 6 to 60 Months on Outpatient Management in Nairobi.

[16] Yebyo, H.G., Kendall, C., Nigusse, D. and Lemma, W. (2013) Outpatient Therapeutic Feeding Program Outcomes and Determinants in Treatment of Severe Acute Malnutrition in Tigray, Northernethiopia: A Retrospective Cohort Study. *PLoS ONE*, **8**, e65840.

[17] Tadesse, E., Berhane, Y., Hjern, A., Olsson, P. and Ekström, E. (2015) Perceptions of Usage and Unintended Consequences of Provision of Ready-to-Use Therapeutic Food for Management of Severe Acute Child Malnutrition. A Qualitative Study in Southern Ethiopia. *Health Policy and Planning*, **2015**, 1-8.

[18] Messina, M.J. (1999) Legumes and Soybeans: Overview of Their Nutritional Profiles and Health Effects. *American Journal of Clinical Nutrition*, **70**, 439S-450S.

[19] Perdigón, G., Nader de Macías, M.E., Álvarez, S., Oliver, G. and Pescede Ruiz Holgado, A. (1986) Effect of Perorally Administered Lactobacilli on Macrophage Activation in Mice. *Infection and Immunity*, **53**, 104-410.

[20] Defourny, I., Drouhin, E., Terzian, M., Tatay, M., Sekkenes, J., *et al.* (2006) Scaling up the Treatment of Acute Childhood Malnutrition in Niger. *Field Exchange*, **28**, 2-4.

[21] Taylor, A. (2002) Outpatient Therapeutic Programme (OTP): An Evaluation of a New SC UK Venture in North Darfur, Sudan. Taken from Field Exchange Issue 16, 2002.

[22] Chaiken, S., Deconinck, H. and Degefie, T. (2006) The Promise of a Community-Based Approach to Managing Severe Malnutrition: A Case Study from Ethiopia. *Food and Nutrition Bulletin*, **27**, 95-104. http://dx.doi.org/10.1177/156482650602700201

[23] Collins, S. (2002) Outpatient Care for Severely Malnourished Children in Emergency Relief Programs: A Retrospective Cohort Study. *The Lancet*, **360**, 1824-1830. http://dx.doi.org/10.1016/S0140-6736(02)11770-3

[24] Chane, T., Oljira, L., Atomesa, G.E. and Agedew, E. (2014) Treatment Outcome and Associated Factors among Under-Five Children with Severe Acute Malnutrition Admitted to Therapeutic Feeding Unit in Woldia Hospital, North Ethiopia. *Journal of Nutrition & Food Sciences*, **4**, 329. http://dx.doi.org/10.4172/2155-9600.1000329

[25] Hossain, M.I., Dodd, N.S., Ahmed, T., *et al.* (2009) Experience in Managing Severe Malnutrition in a Government Tertiary Treatment Facility in Bangladesh. *Journal of Health, Population and Nutrition*, **27**, 72-80. http://dx.doi.org/10.3329/jhpn.v27i1.3319

[26] Gebremichael, M., Bezabih, A.M. and Tsadik, M. (2014) Treatment Outcomes and Associated Risk Factors of Severely Malnourished under Five Children Admitted to Therapeutic Feeding Centers of Mekelle City, Northern Ethiopia. *Open Access Library Journal*, **1**, e446. http://dx.doi.org/10.4236/oalib.1100446

[27] Patel, D., Gupta, P., Shah, D. and Sethi, K. (2010) Home-Based Rehabilitation of Severely Malnourished Children in Resource Poor Setting. *Indian Paediatrics*, **47**, 694-710. http://dx.doi.org/10.1007/s13312-010-0102-6

Hereditary Vesicoureteral Reflux: A Study of 66 Families

Zsuzsa I. Bartik[1], Agneta Nordenskjöld[2], Sofia Sjöström[1], Rune Sixt[1], Ulla Sillén[1]

[1]The Pediatric Uro-Nephrologic Centre, The Queen Silvia Children's Hospital, Sahlgrenska Academy, University of Gothenburg, Gothenburg, Sweden
[2]Department of Women and Children Health, Karolinska Institutet and Center of Molecular Medicine, Karolinska University Hospital, Stockholm, Sweden
Email: zsuzsa.bartik@vgregion.se

Abstract

Purpose: We studied the inheritance pattern, clinical features and outcome in children with vesicoureteral reflux (VUR). Characteristics of known familial VUR cases were also compared with those of sporadic VUR. Material and Methods: 726 patients were treated for VUR between 1990-2004. The families were contacted by letter inquiring if other members of the family were affected. The phenotype of all cases (familial and non-familial) was characterized in terms of presenting symptoms, reflux grade, recurrent urinary tract infections, kidney damage, and the natural course of reflux. Results: The response rate was 79%. A total of 99 individuals (22%) reported relatives with VUR. Since some of the 99 index cases belonged to the same family, the total number of families was ultimately 66. The distribution of relatives with VUR was: 38 siblings, 20 parents (15 mothers), 19 cousins, 15 aunts/uncles and 12 grandparents. The phenotype of VUR did not differ between familial and non-familial cases. However, VUR among relatives was of milder grade than index and sporadic cases. Conclusions: The proportion of hereditary reflux in our material was lower than in other studies (22%). We found a strong overrepresentation of maternal transmission of reflux. Severity of the disease did not differ between familial and non-familial VUR.

Keywords

Vesicoureteral Reflux, Heredity, Phenotype

1. Introduction

Vesicoureteral reflux (VUR) is a common abnormality affecting 1% - 2% of the pediatric population [1]. The association between VUR and urinary tract infection (UTI) is well known, with risk for scarring of the renal pa-renchyma. Several studies have shown familial clustering of VUR, implying that genetic factors play an impor-tant role in its pathogenesis. For example, siblings of children with VUR are at higher risk of reflux than the general population, with reported prevalences between 27% and 51% [2]-[4]. Among multiple gestation births the concordance is higher in monozygotic twins than in dizygotic ones (80% vs. 35%) [5]. Moreover, the risk for offspring of parents with previously diagnosed VUR of having VUR themselves is reported to be 66% [6].

Although subjects with VUR may present with similar initial symptoms, some cases have a benign natural course with no recurrent UTIs, no progressive renal damage and a high rate of spontaneous resolution of the reflux. Others, on the other hand, have recurrent UTIs, deterioration of renal status and persistent reflux [7]. These two phenotypes may have different etiological and genetic backgrounds. Therefore, it is of great interest to establish whether this previously described inherited (familial) form of VUR represents the same disease as the sporadic cases (when only one individual in the family has VUR) or whether it has a more aggressive course. In order to answer this question we assessed clinical features including severity of reflux, frequency of recurrent infections, renal damage, overall kidney function, and natural course in familial VUR compared with sporadic reflux cases. The aim of this study was to increase the understanding of the etiology of VUR. This knowledge can be further used to predict prognosis and individually tailor appropriate treatment.

2. Material and Methods

Figure 1 illustrates the data selection process for the study. Seven hundred and twenty-six children with VUR

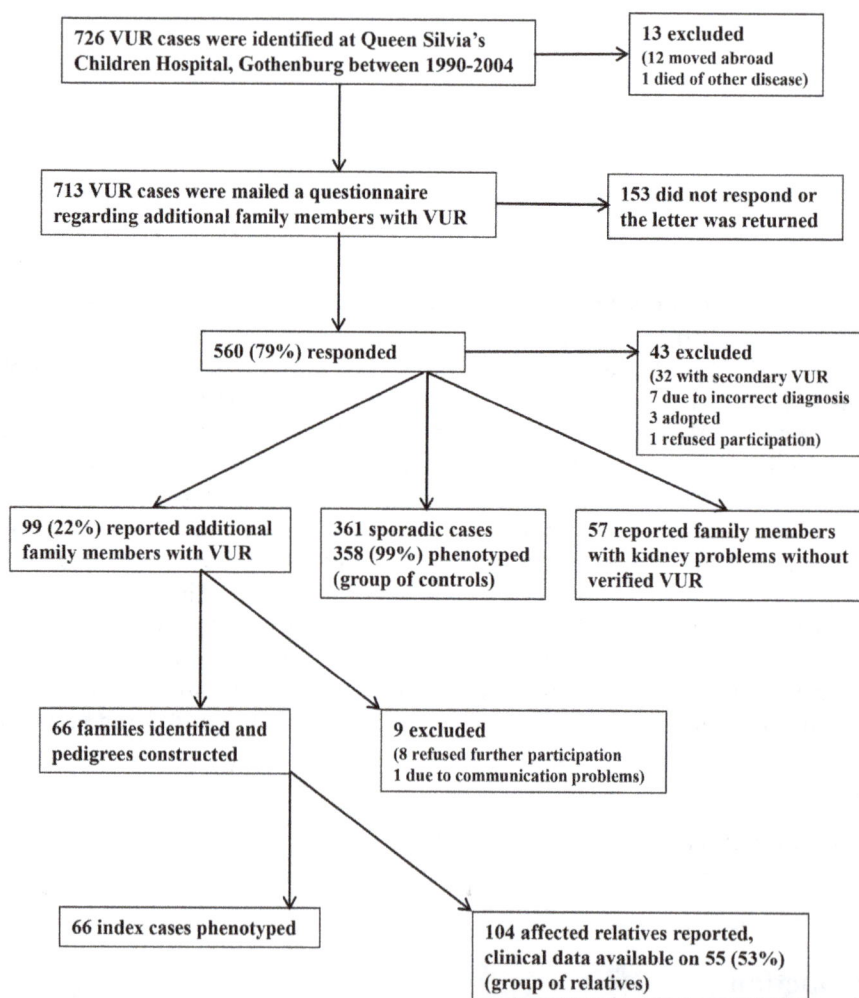

Figure 1. Flow chart showing the collection of cases. VUR = Vesicoureteral reflux.

treated at Queen Silvia's Children Hospital (a tertiary referral center) in Gothenburg, Sweden between 1990 and 2004 were identified through medical records. Letters were sent to all but 13 index cases, inquiring as to whether there were other members of the family or close relatives with VUR. The 99 cases that reported more than one individual with VUR were interviewed by telephone. During this conversation we inquired as to which members of the family had diagnosed VUR or had symptoms indicating such a problem, *i.e.* recurrent UTIs, bladder function symptoms or kidney problems. We also asked about possible consanguinity in the family. In this study, familial VUR cases were defined as patients with one or more first, second or third degree relatives with VUR. These affected relatives were analyzed as a separate group and compared with index and non-familial cases. Patients with VUR secondary to urethral valves, myelomeningocele or high anal atresia with neurogenic bladder were excluded from the study.

For inclusion of family members in the group of relatives with VUR, a previously performed voiding cystourethrography (VCU) showing reflux was mandatory, except for older relatives diagnosed in an era when VCU was not in general use. A history of recurrent febrile UTIs during childhood with or without renal damage suggesting high probability for VUR was accepted in these cases. Relatives with radiologically confirmed diagnosis were marked as certain VUR cases in the pedigrees (n = 55), while cases with a strong history but with no radiological investigations available were labelled probable affected cases (n = 49) (**Figure 2**). Fifty-seven index patients who reported other members of the family with vague history of diffuse urinary tract problems, such as cystitis during adulthood, were excluded.

Owing to the fact that some individuals with VUR in our material belonged to the same family, the total number of families with hereditary reflux was ultimately 66. These 66 families were invited to participate in our study, and informed consent from patients and family members was obtained to examine medical records regarding their VUR and kidney status. The families were also asked to provide blood samples for a genetic study [8].

To clarify the relationship and analyse the pattern of inheritance, pedigrees were constructed for each family. VUR in all affected individuals was characterised regarding presenting symptoms, grade of reflux, recurrent UTIs, kidney damage, natural course of the reflux, surgical treatment and additional anomalies. Data was also collected from medical records on subjects who did not report any relatives with VUR (controls), a total of 361 individuals. In these patients we recorded presenting symptoms, grade of reflux at presentation, recurrent UTIs (yes or no) and renal damage.

When recording the recurrent UTIs, only the febrile infections (>38.5°C) with positive urinary culture (at least 100,000 cfu/ml) were counted in the hereditary groups. In the group of controls such data about symptoms and urinary culture were not always available.

In the characterisation of the subjects, grade of reflux was registered from VCU investigations according to the international grading system, both at presentation and at the latest follow-up before eventual surgical treatment [9]. In case of bilateral VUR, the patient was classified by the more severe side. Resolution of VUR was defined as grade II or less. DMSA and MAG-3 scintigraphy results were used for evaluation of renal damage, including split function, parenchymal abnormalities and size of kidneys. Focal damage was defined as one or more areas with reduced uptake or indentation of the renal outline. Generalised damage was classified as a small kidney with reduced tracer uptake or diffuse parenchymal anomaly. Reference values for split function were between 45% and 55%. Usually more than one scintigraphy was performed during the follow-up time. In this study we present the results from the latest available investigations regarding renal abnormality.

Glomerular filtration rate (GFR) was assessed using 51Cr-EDTA. In the cases where no direct GFR measurement was available, indirect GFR estimation was performed according to the formula of Schwartz [10] from serum creatinine and the height (cm) of the patient. The reference value used for normal GFR was 110 mmol/l/ 1.73 m^2 after two years of age according to Bröchner-Mortensen [11] and GFR < 80% (<2SD) of expected GFR was considered subnormal. Before two years of age, steady state of GFR is not achieved, and for this age group we operationally used the equation developed by Winberg for estimation of expected clearance [12]. Deterioration of renal status at follow up was defined as loss of ≥7% of split function seen on scintigram or decrease of GFR with ≥12%.

Statistical methods. In the statistical analysis of VUR phenotype in the group of relatives, only the 55 cases (of 104) were included, *i.e.* those who had performed VCU, whereas in the index and control groups VCU was performed in all cases and thus included. For categorical variables n (%) is presented, and for continuous variables Median (Min-Max). For comparisons between groups the chi-square test was used for non-ordered categorical variables, while Kruskal-Wallis test was used for continuous variables. For pairwise comparison be-

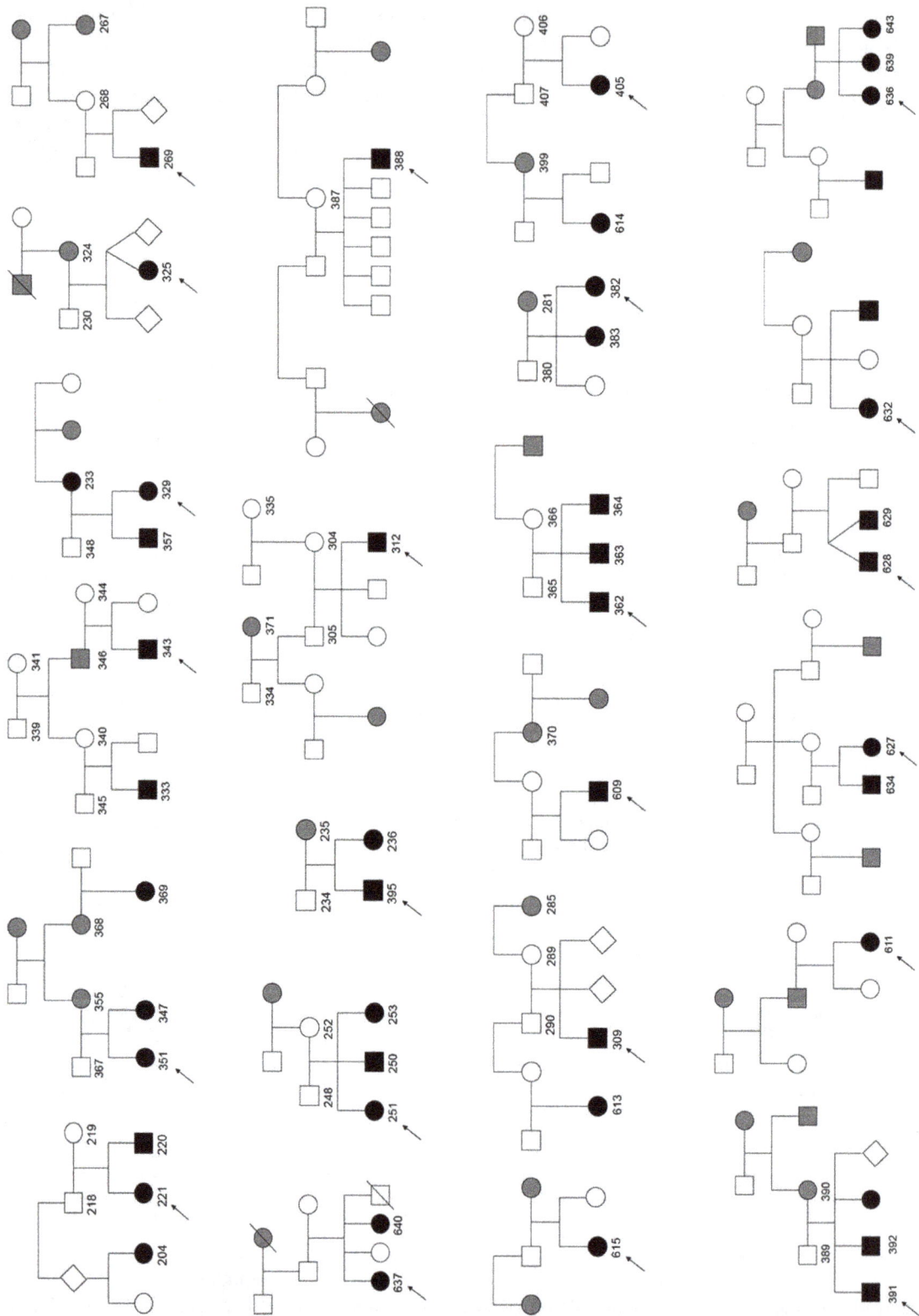

Figure 2. Pedigrees describing the families with three or more vesicoureteral reflux cases. *Squares* males, *circles* females, *rhombuses* sex unknown, *black symbols* diagnosis confirmed by voiding cystouretherography, *gray symbols* strong history of VUR but no radiological investigations available, *crossed over symbols* deceased, *arrow* index cases.

tween groups, Fisher's exact test was used for dichotomous variables, Mantel-Haenszel chi-square test was used for ordered categorical variables, chi-square test was used for non-ordered categorical variables and Mann-Whitney U-test for continuous variables. All tests were 2-tailed and conducted at the 5% significance level.

Approval from the Regional Ethical Review Board in Gothenburg was obtained

3. Results

3.1. Familial Aggregation

The response rate of the VUR patients to the questionnaire regarding relatives with VUR was 79% (560 of 713 subjects). Of 560 individuals with VUR, 99 reported additional family members, 361 reported no relatives with VUR and 57 reported diffuse urinary tract problems in family members but without diagnosed reflux. Since it was uncertain whether or not individuals in this latter group had hereditary reflux, they were excluded. Thus, 22% (99/460) had relatives with reflux.

Some of these 99 index cases belonged to the same family and therefore the total number of families with hereditary reflux was ultimately 66. The distribution of relatives with a history of VUR including both confirmed and probable affected cases was: 38 siblings, 20 parents (15 of whom were mothers), 19 cousins and second cousins, 15 aunts/uncles and 12 grandparents (**Table 1**). The proportion of girls among siblings and cousins was 22/38 (58%) and 10/17 (59%) respectively, which does not differ from the proportion in the entire material (58%).

The numbers of affected members in the families are shown in **Table 2**. 25/66 (38%) families had three or more affected members, whereas 41 only had two. In this latter group with 2 affected individuals, 21 of 41 were sibs. In total, VUR was inherited from the mother's family in 25 cases while paternal inheritance was seen in 15 cases. In four cases the families of both parents were affected and in one case sufficient data was missing. Pedigrees are shown for subjects with three or more affected family members (**Figure 2**).

3.2. Phenotype of Familial and Non-Familial VUR

For analysis the material was divided into index patients (n = 66), relatives with confirmed VUR (n = 55) and controls (n = 358). The results are presented in **Table 3**. There was overrepresentation of females in all three groups, with no significant difference between the groups. The presenting symptom was pyelonephritis in the majority of cases. However, VUR in relatives had been detected to a significantly higher extent by pre- or postnatal screening than in index cases and controls. Fourteen of 52 (27%) relatives were diagnosed by screening in comparison with only 2 of 65 (3%) index patients and 25 of 342 (7%) controls (p < 0.0001). Nine of the 14 screened

Table 1. Sixty-six families with hereditary VUR; relationship between 66 index cases and 104 affected relatives.

Affected relatives	Number (%)
Siblings	38 (37)
Parents	20 (19)
Grandparents	12 (12)
Aunts/uncles	15 (14)
Cousins/second cousins	19 (18)
Total number (%)	104 (100)

Table 2. Sixty-six families with hereditary VUR; number of affected subjects per family and maternal/parental transmission.

No. of VUR patients/family	No. of families	Maternal transmission	Paternal transmission	Unknown transmission
2 affected/family	41	12	7	1 unknown side, 21 only sibs
3 affected/family	18	7	8	3 both sides
4 affected/family	4	4		
5 affected/family				
6 affected/family	3	2		1 both sides
Total number	66	25	15	26

Table 3. Dermographic data, VUR grades, renal abnormalities and function split by hereditary (index and relatives) and non-hereditary (controls) VUR.

Variable	Index	Relatives	Controls	Test between groups		
				p-value		
	n = 66	n = 55	n = 358	Index vs relatives	Index vs controls	Relatives vs controls
Sex						
Female	38 (58%)	37 (67%)	201 (56%)			
Male	28 (42%)	18 (33%)	157 (44%)	0.365	0.925	0.152
Presenting symptom VUR						
Pyelonephritis	61 (94%)	36 (69%)	308 (90%)			
Pre- and postnatal screening	2 (3%)	14 (27%)	25 (7%)			
Other symptoms	2 (3%)	2 (4%)	9 (3%)	0.001	0.449	<0.0001
Age at presentation (months)	8 (0.1 - 84)	7.0 (0.1 - 98)	8 (0 - 141)	0.674	0.637	0.893
Grade of reflux						
I	2 (3%)	4 (8%)	9 (3%)			
II	7 (11%)	11 (23%)	42 (12%)			
III	21 (32%)	22 (45%)	123 (34%)			
IV	24 (36%)	8 (16%)	140 (39%)			
V	12 (18%)	4 (8%)	44 (12%)	0.002	0.436	0.0003
Grade of reflux at follow up						
0 - II	18 (32%)	18 (47%)				
III - V	38 (68%)	18 (53%)		0.136		
Recurrent UTIs						
No	27 (44%)	20 (47%)	168 (50%)			
Yes	35 (56%)	23 (53%)	171 (50%)	0.919	0.465	0.831
Renal abnormality						
No	18 (28%)	13 (36%)	90 (26%)			
Yes	46 (72%)	23 (64%)	255 (74%)	0.543	0.840	0.276
Total renal function						
Normal	50 (82%)	34 (79%)	226 (87%)			
Subnormal	11 (18%)	9 (21%)	33 (13%)	0.900	0.378	0.235

relatives were examined due to reflux in sibling. Age at presentation was median 8 months (range: 0 - 141), with no difference between the groups.

3.3. VUR Grade

The grade of reflux at presentation was significantly lower among the relatives than the index patients (p = 0.002) and the same was seen for relatives vs. controls (p = 0.0003) (**Table 3**, **Figure 3**). The grades of reflux in both the index and control groups showed the same distribution. Bilateral reflux was more common than unilateral reflux, with no differences between the groups. The rate of resolution of VUR was only analyzed in the hereditary groups. The reflux resolved spontaneously in 18 of 56 (32%) in the index group and 18 of 36 (50%) in the group with relatives but the difference did not reach significance. The follow-up time was median 32 months (range: 5 - 117) counting the last VCU prior to eventual surgical treatment. However, persistent VUR was corrected surgically significantly more often in index cases than in relatives (p = 0.034).

3.4. Urinary Tract Infection

The number of individuals with recurrent UTIs was high, with no difference between the groups (56%, 53% and

50% in index, relatives and controls, respectively) (**Table 3**).

3.5. Renal Status

The number of children with renal damage was similarly high in all three groups. Forty-six of 64 (72%) in the index group, 23 of 36 (64%) in the group with relatives and 255 of 345 (74%) in the control group showed renal abnormalities (**Table 3**). Focal damage was seen in 22 of 64 (34%) index patients, 5 of 36 (14%) relatives and 101 of 345 (29%) controls, whereas generalized damage was present in 23 of 64 (36%) in the index group, 18 of 36 (50%) in the group with relatives and 143 of 345 (42%) of controls (p = 0.284) (**Figure 4**). Most of the renal damage was unilateral, with no differences between the groups. After median 62 months (range: 4 - 233) of follow-up, very few individuals showed deterioration in renal status (4 of 44 (9%) and 4 of 25 (16%) in the index and relative groups, respectively).

GFR did not differ between the groups (median 92%, 93% and 98% of normal, for the index, relatives and controls respectively). Furthermore, the number of individuals with subnormal GFR was also similar in index (11 of 61 (18%)), relative (9 of 43, (21%)) and control (33 of 253 (13%)) (**Table 3**).

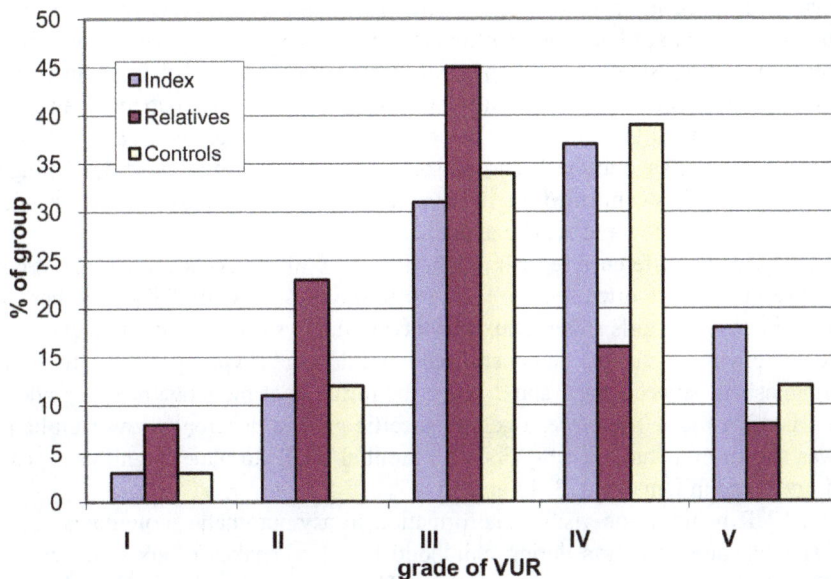

Figure 3. Grade of VUR according to study group, hereditary (index patients and relatives) and non-hereditary (controls).

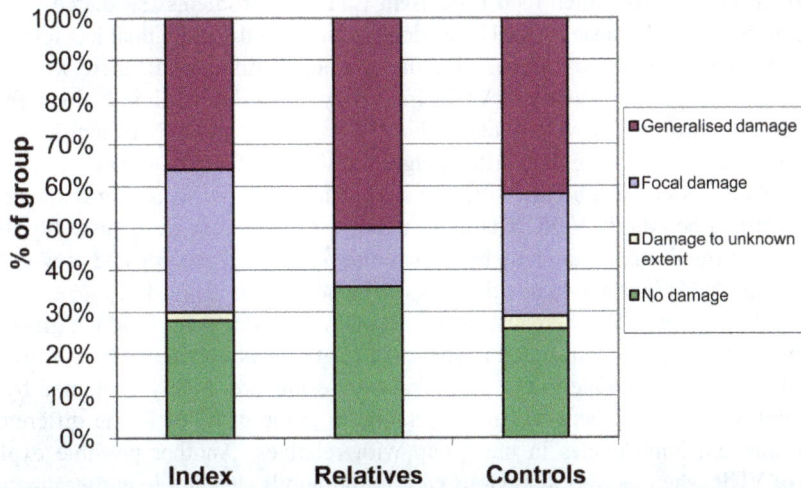

Figure 4. Prevalence of renal abnormality according to study group, hereditary (index patients and relatives) and non-hereditary (controls).

3.6. Additional Anomalies of the Urinary Tract (UT) and Other Organs

In 50 of 66 (76%) index cases and 44 of 55 (80%) relatives, VUR was the only abnormality of the UT. The most common associated UT anomaly was duplex kidney, which was seen in 18% and 13% of cases in the index and relative groups, respectively. In 13 of 66 families (20%) VUR could be a part of the CAKUT syndrome (congenital anomalies of the kidney and urinary tract) as duplex kidney or congenital generalised renal damage was seen in more than one family member. The majority of individuals in the two hereditary groups showed no anomalies in other organs (11/66 (17%) and 3/55 (6%) for index and relatives).

4. Discussion

Vesicoureteral reflux is a congenital defect of the urinary tract with a high risk of inheritance if a parent or sibling is affected. However, of the 560 individuals who responded to our questionnaire, 99 had other relatives with VUR while 361 had none. There was strong overrepresentation of maternal transmission of VUR. In 20 families, VUR was inherited from a parent, and in 15 of these 20 cases the inheritance was maternal. In addition, when all affected family members (except siblings) are taken into account, maternal inheritance was seen in 25 families and paternal inheritance in 15 cases. This overrepresentation of maternal inheritance has been noted in other studies but has not been attributed any particular significance [13]-[15]. One should be aware of selection bias when interpreting these results. One possible explanation in our study is that the questionnaire and the telephone interview were answered to a higher extent by the mothers of the index patients than the fathers, thereby reflecting the health problems of the maternal relatives to a higher degree. Scott *et al.* [15] put forward a similar explanation, rather than linkage to the X-chromosome, as suggested in a report describing a large family [16]. To date, no genetic study has confirmed the involvement of the X-chromosome in transmission of VUR. The maternal transmission of VUR could also be explained by imprinting mechanism.

The above discussed difference regarding inheritance of VUR versus gender can of course be associated with the fact that reflux is more often seen in females, in the present study 58%. Another interesting difference regarding VUR in boys and girls is the reflux phenotype. In boys reflux is often diagnosed early during infancy, is high-grade and often with congenital generalised renal damage (hypo/dysplasia). In girls, on the other hand, the peak for diagnosis is between age 1 and 2 years, the reflux is of moderate or low grade and when renal damage is present it is often focal. Therefore, a gender-specific genetic difference may well be possible, which actually recently was shown in a study of sib-pairs with familial VUR: in males significant peaks were found on chromosome 1 and 5 and in females on 3, 13 and 15 [17].

However, VUR being a non-visible malformation in asymptomatic individuals and with a possible natural course of spontaneous resolution during childhood [18] [19] makes reflux a difficult abnormality to study in terms of heredity from one generation to another. Moreover, the fact that VCU is the only existing investigation for confirming the diagnosis leads to uncertainty in older generations, for whom this examination was not in common use. These relatives often report recurrent UTIs and problems associated with renal damage but there are no VCU films, either because no VCU was done or because the individual has forgotten.

When comparing the two study groups, familial and non-familial VUR, there were no significant differences in sex, presenting symptoms, severity of VUR, frequency of breakthrough infections, renal damage or total renal function. However, differences were noted within the hereditary group between the index group and the group with relatives. The relatives were more often diagnosed through screening than index patients (27% vs 3%). The 14 screened relatives were all siblings. Still, our study showed a low screening frequency as compared with other studies regarding hereditary VUR. The explanation for this difference is probably the method of confirming VUR diagnosis in relatives: in our study by questionnaire, hospital records and previous VCU films, whereas in most other studies VCU investigations of siblings were performed [3] [4] [20] [21].

Differences in grade of VUR were also noted between the index group and the group with relatives, with significantly lower grades in the latter group. The same relation has previously been shown in screened siblings of children with reflux [2] [4]. One might think that our results are mainly explained by low-grade reflux in the screened siblings. However, there was no difference in grade of VUR in the different relationships: siblings, parents, cousins and aunts/uncles in the group with relatives. Another possible explanation is an increased knowledge of VUR when there is a previous case in the family, leading to earlier diagnosis even without active screening.

Overall, the prevalence of renal damage was high in the total material (74%), with no difference between the hereditary and the non-hereditary groups. In other materials comparing index patients with their refluxing siblings the prevalence of renal damage was 30% [20]. The explanation for the difference is suggested to be the fact that fewer children with low-grade reflux are diagnosed and treated in Scandinavia. In fact, the frequency of renal damage found here is very similar to that found in a recent Swedish reflux trial [22]. Cascio *et al.* reported an increased number of cases with normal kidneys in the relatives as compared with both index and controls [23]. A simmilar relationship was detected in the present study but the difference was not significant. In addition a lower frequency of mild renal damage (focal) was reported by Menezes *et al.* in relatives without UTI as compared with both index patients and relatives with a history of UTI [20]. A similar tendency with lower number of relatives with focal damage was also seen in the present study.

Thus, the lower frequency of focal damage in relation to generalized damage in the relative group, as mentioned above, could theoretically be explained by lower frequency of recurrent febrile UTIs causing fewer new scars, which was reported in the study by Menezes *et al.* [20]. Even if we found in the present study that the VUR in the relative group was milder with regard to grade of VUR we saw no difference in incidence of infections between the groups. This could of course be explained by the low number of patients and difficulties in finding reliable data about UTI in older relatives.

Methodological limitations of our study was the lack of VCU in almost half of the relatives with VUR, owing to the fact that this radiological examination was not performed prior to the 1960s. In addition, relatives of patients with VUR were not routinely screened in Sweden, which could be responile for the lower prevalence of familial VUR in our material. Relatives with VUR could be underreported in both the herditary and control groups. The missed cases probably presented with less symptoms, given the availability of the Swedish health care. We agree that VCU is the gold standard method to detect VUR. However, it is a higly invasive investigation, which limits its use in asymptomatic relatives.

5. Conclusion

In conclusion, we found a possible increased inheritance of VUR via the mother, a result that is worthy of further examination both regarding inheritance and genetics. No difference was found between the phenotype of familial and non-familial reflux, whereas there was a difference between the index and relative groups, such as lower grade of reflux in the latter group.

References

[1]   Amar, A.D. (1972) Familial Vesicoureteral Reflux. *The Journal of Urology*, **108**, 969-971.

[2]   Jerkins, G.R. and Noe, H.N. (1982) Familial Vesicoureteral Reflux: A Prospective Study. *The Journal of Urology*, **128**, 774-778.

[3]   Parekh, D.J., Pope, J.C.T., Adams, M.C. and Brock 3rd., J.W. (2002) Outcome of Sibling Vesicoureteral Reflux. *The Journal of Urology*, **167**, 283-284. http://dx.doi.org/10.1016/S0022-5347(05)65450-X

[4]   Wan, J., Greenfield, S.P., Ng, M., Zerin, M., Ritchey, M.L. and Bloom, D. (1996) Sibling Reflux: A Dual Center Retrospective Study. *The Journal of Urology*, **156**, 677-679. http://dx.doi.org/10.1016/S0022-5347(01)65782-3

[5]   Kaefer, M., Curran, M., Treves, S.T., Bauer, S., Hendren, W.H., Peters, C.A., Atala, A., Diamond, D. and Retik, A. (2000) Sibling Vesicoureteral Reflux in Multiple Gestation Births. *Pediatrics*, **105**, 800-804. http://dx.doi.org/10.1542/peds.105.4.800

[6]   Noe, H.N., Wyatt, R.J., Peeden Jr., J.N. and Rivas, M.L. (1992) The transmission of Vesicoureteral Reflux from Parent to Child. *The Journal of Urology*, **148**, 1869-1871.

[7]   Sjostrom, S., Sillen, U., Jodal, U., Sameby, L., Sixt, R. and Stokland, E. (2010) Predictive Factors for Resolution of Congenital High Grade Vesicoureteral Reflux in Infants: Results of Univariate and Multivariate Analyses. *The Journal of Urology*, **183**, 1177-1184. http://dx.doi.org/10.1016/j.juro.2009.11.055

[8]   Zu, S., Bartik, Z., Zhao, S., Sillen, U. and Nordenskjold, A. (2009) Mutations in the ROBO2 and SLIT2 Genes Are Rare Causes of Familial Vesico-Ureteral Reflux. *Pediatric Nephrology*, **24**, 1501-1508. http://dx.doi.org/10.1007/s00467-009-1179-9

[9]   Lebowitz, R.L., Olbing, H., Parkkulainen, K.V., Smellie, J.M. and Tamminen-Mobius, T.E. (1985) International System of Radiographic Grading of Vesicoureteric Reflux. International Reflux Study in Children. *Pediatric Radiology*, **15**, 105-109. http://dx.doi.org/10.1007/BF02388714

[10] Schwartz, G.J., Brion, L.P. and Spitzer, A. (1987) The Use of pLasma Creatinine Concentration for Estimating

Glomerular Filtration Rate in Infants, Children, and Adolescents. *Pediatric Clinics of North America*, **34**, 571-590.

[11] Brochner-Mortensen, J., Haahr, J. and Christoffersen, J. (1974) A Simple Method for Accurate Assessment of the Glomerular Filtration Rate in Children. *Scandinavian Journal of Clinical and Laboratory Investigation*, **33**, 140-143. http://dx.doi.org/10.3109/00365517409082481

[12] Winberg, J. (1959) The 24-Hour True Endogenous Creatinine Clearance in Infants and Children without Renal Disease. *Acta Paediatrica*, **48**, 443-452.

[13] Conte, M.L., Bertoli-Avella, A.M., de Graaf, B.M., Punzo, F., Lama, G., La Manna, A., Grassia, C., Rambaldi, P.F., Oostra, B.A. and Perrotta, S. (2008) A Genome Search for Primary Vesicoureteral Reflux Shows Further Evidence for Genetic Heterogeneity. *Pediatric Nephrology*, **23**, 587-595. http://dx.doi.org/10.1007/s00467-007-0675-z

[14] Feather, S.A., Malcolm, S., Woolf, A.S., Wright, V., Blaydon, D., Reid, C.J., Flinter, F.A., Proesmans, W., Devriendt, K., Carter, J., Warwicker, P., Goodship, T.H. and Goodship, J.A. (2000) Primary, Nonsyndromic Vesicoureteric Reflux and Its Nephropathy Is Genetically Heterogeneous, with a Locus on Chromosome 1. *American Journal of Human Genetics*, **66**, 1420-1425. http://dx.doi.org/10.1086/302864

[15] Scott, J.E., Swallow, V., Coulthard, M.G., Lambert, H.J. and Lee, R.E. (1997) Screening of Newborn Babies for Familial Ureteric Reflux. *Lancet*, **350**, 396-400. http://dx.doi.org/10.1016/S0140-6736(97)01515-8

[16] Naseri, M., Ghiggeri, G.M., Caridi, G. and Abbaszadegan, M.R. (2010) Five Cases of Severe Vesico-Ureteric Reflux in a Family with an X-Linked Compatible Trait. *Pediatric Nephrology*, **25**, 349-352. http://dx.doi.org/10.1007/s00467-009-1293-8

[17] Marchini, G.S., Onal, B., Guo, C.Y., Rowe, C.K., Kunkel, L., Bauer, S.B., Retik, A.B. and Nguyen, H.T. (2012) Genome Gender Diversity in Affected Sib-Pairs with Familial Vesico-Ureteric Reflux Identified by Single Nucleotide Polymorphism Linkage Analysis. *BJU International*, **109**, 1709-1714. http://dx.doi.org/10.1111/j.1464-410X.2011.10634.x

[18] Esbjorner, E., Hansson, S. and Jakobsson, B. (2004) Management of Children with Dilating Vesico-Ureteric Reflux in Sweden. *Acta Paediatrica*, **93**, 37-42. http://dx.doi.org/10.1111/j.1651-2227.2004.tb00671.x

[19] Sjostrom, S., Sillen, U., Bachelard, M., Hansson, S. and Stokland, E. (2004) Spontaneous Resolution of High Grade Infantile Vesicoureteral Reflux. *The Journal of Urology*, **172**, 694-699. http://dx.doi.org/10.1097/01.ju.0000130747.89561.cf

[20] Menezes, M. and Puri, P. (2009) Familial Vesicoureteral Reflux—Is Screening Beneficial? *The Journal of Urology*, **182**, 1673-1677. http://dx.doi.org/10.1016/j.juro.2009.02.087

[21] Noe, H.N. (1992) The Long-Term Results of Prospective Sibling Reflux Screening. *The Journal of Urology*, **148**, 1739-1742.

[22] Brandstrom, P., Esbjorner, E., Herthelius, M., Holmdahl, G., Lackgren, G., Neveus, T., Sillen, U., Sixt, R., Sjoberg, I., Stokland, E., Jodal, U. and Hansson, S. (2010) The Swedish Reflux Trial in Children: I. Study Design and Study Population Characteristics. *The Journal of Urology*, **184**, 274-279. http://dx.doi.org/10.1016/j.juro.2010.01.055

[23] Cascio, S., Yoneda, A., Chertin, B., Colhoun, E. and Puri, P. (2003) Renal Parenchymal Damage in Sibling Vesicoureteric Reflux. *Acta Paediatrica*, **92**, 17-20. http://dx.doi.org/10.1111/j.1651-2227.2003.tb00462.x

31

Performance of Children and Adolescents from a School of the City of Sogamoso on a Decision-Making Test

Patricia Bernal*, Johanna Montaña, Rocio Acosta, Yonathan Rojas

Universidad de San Buenaventura, Bogotá, Colombia
Email: *arlethpatriciab@gmail.com

Abstract

The aim of this study was to describe the performance on a decision-making task of children and adolescents (aged 7 - 17 years) from a school in the city of Sogamoso. This non-experimental descriptive, cross-sectional study was conducted by means of a non probability sampling of type cases. The sample consisted of 325 subjects, to whom the Hungry Donkey Task in its version adapted for Colombia was applied. Through descriptive statistics, the test performance trend was established, finding that participants aged 7 to 11 years had better performance than adolescents 12 to 14 years old, which partially supports the hypothesis of decision-making development in J shape. Subjects aged 15 to 17 years had the most disadvantageous performance, which may indicate immaturity and slow development of prefrontal areas and the influence of the trend towards risk-taking, characteristic of this age range.

Keywords

Decision-Making, Children and Adolescents, Somatic Marker, Hungry Donkey Task

1. Introduction

Decision-making is defined as the ability to select the course of action from a set of behavioral alternatives oriented to favorable or unfavorable options involving cognitive aspects, reward and punishment contingencies and emotional signals associated with each of the possible responses [1].

Decision-making requires the processing of emotions, according to the somatic marker model (MS) proposed by Damasio [2], where emotions and cognition are integrated to make decisions based on the future potential

---

*Corresponding author.

consequences of behavior, rather than on the immediate ones [3]-[9].

The MS model involves a processing system for primary emotions that depend on the limbic system (innate and prearranged reactions to an environmental stimulus) and another one for secondary emotions that require prefrontal and somato-sensory cortices [10]-[12]. Primary emotions are innate, while secondary ones are developed throughout life, although these have a major development peak during adolescence [3].

During adolescence, new synapses are established in the prefrontal area [13] and myelination progresses in the frontal cortex and in the paths that link it to other brain areas such as some limbic structures (amygdala, hippocampus and caudate nucleus), with an impact on the development of decision-making capacity, by improving the inhibitory control, organizing emotional inputs and determining the behavioral response [13]-[16] However, this is a process which is accompanied by periods of limbic over-activation generating imbalance between the adolescent's emotional experience and their ability to regulate their motivation and arousal [17]. Should it persist, will be related to increased risk behaviors [18], but should it mature, will lead to a reduction in the mesolimbic excitability and strengthening of cortical control with adoption of more adaptive behaviors [12].

The first studies carried out to assess decision-making in children and adolescents used two adapted versions of the Iowa Gambling Task (IGT): The Children's Gambling Task, adapted by Kerr and Zelazo in 2004 [19], and later The Hungry Donkey Task (HDT) adapted by Crone and Van der Molen in 2004 [20]. Regarding the HDT, it has been found that children between 7 - 12 years old, as well as patients with damage to the ventro-medial prefrontal cortex (VMPFC), choose options that result in higher immediate profits despite large future losses, because they base their performance on the number of items they win, no matter how many items they lose [21] [22]. Additionally, it has been found that with age, the strategy changes towards finding a more proportional gain [23], and children from 7 to12 years old, who seem to have a myopia about the future, increase their sensitivity to future consequences when the potential punishment is high [20].

It has further been found that the development of decision-making in subjects from 7 to 17 years old shows a trajectory in the form of a J, where the youngest showed a less unfavorable performance than early adolescents, who from the age of 14 begin to present a more advantageous performance, as prefrontal cortex development progresses, being better able to inhibit their initial impulsive responses [24]. According to these authors, the poor performance of early adolescents is not indicative of pathology, but of immaturity of the frontal areas, which will continue to mature throughout adolescence until achieving better control of their executive functions.

The aim of the study is to describe the performance of Colombian children and adolescents on the Hungry Donkey Task, according to three age ranges (7 - 11, 12 - 14 and 15 - 17 years), at a school in the city Sogamoso. This in order to understand the mechanisms that guide adequate or inadequate decision-making in different age groups, with particular emphasis on brain maturation as a fundamental aspect in the final configuration of an individual that fits the demands of the environment, making decisions based on future consequences.

2. Method

This is a non-experimental descriptive cross-sectional study, which it was made during 2014. A non-probability sampling was done for convenience, and included all children and adolescents of both genders aged 7 - 17 years, from a school of the medium stratum of city of Sogamoso, Colombia with semi-customized education, without learning or behavioral disorders and without neurological or psychiatric impairments. Through a non-probability sampling of type cases, participants were chosen with a similar profile, upon reviewing their medical history (reported by parents).

Exclusion criteria: Presence of history of behavioral or learning disorders, brain damage or neurological or psychiatric impairments whose implications persist today.

The informed consent was completed by 358 children (129 males and 196 females), with a homogeneous level of participation from grades 3° to 11°, except for grade 5° which had a better participation (4.3%), since not all students were at school that day. 25 data were eliminated for not having finished the task and 7 exclusions were made in accordance with established criteria. Finally, the sample consisted of 325 children and adolescents (see **Table 1**).

2.1. Instruments

"*The Hungry Donkey Task*" by Crone and Van der Molen [23] is a Colombian adaptation of the test. The task is presented through a software that displays 4 doors and the goal is to collect as many apples as possible. The four options (P1, P2, P3 and P4) systematically differ in the amount of gains, losses and frequency thereof. Participants must choose one of the four gates throughout 100 trials. The sum of gains doors 1 and 2 corresponds to 400 and the total losses of 500 blocks; while the doors 3 and 4, the gain is 200 apples and 100 apples losses. In the **Table 2** the description of income probabilities of each door is exposed.

Additional, we used a Personal Data Questionnaire and Medical History, which included personal information, prenatal, perinatal and postnatal history, developmental background, treatments undertaken, diagnoses received and family history.

2.2. Procedure

Parents were asked to give their informed consent and complete the *Personal Data Questionnaire and Medical History*. The Hungry Donkey Task was applied to children whose parents authorized their participation and did not meet any exclusion criteria.

All the principles governing scientific research in the field of psychology regarding informed consent, use of data and instruments with theoretical, practical and research support, were fulfilled (Chapter VII Articles 50, 52 and 55; Chapter VI Article 48 - Law 1090 of 2006: Deontological and Bioethical Code of the Psychologist in Colombia). Also, children and adolescents were asked to give their assent to participate (Article 37 of Act 1098 of 2006 - Code for Children and Adolescents of the Republic of Colombia).

3. Results

Statistical analysis was performed from SPSS-21 and measures of central tendency and dispersion measures of

Table 1. Frequencies of the sample by age and grade of education.

Age	Frequency	%	Grade	Frequency	%
7	2	0.6	3	38	11.7
8	39	12.0	4	32	9.8
9	28	8.6	5	14	4.3
10	15	4.6	6	53	16.3
11	56	17.2	7	44	13.5
12	40	12.3	8	41	12.6
13	38	11.7	9	37	11.4
14	38	11.7	10	35	10.8
15	39	12.0	11	31	9.5
16	29	8.9			
17	1	0.3			

Table 2. Characteristics of the gates.

Gate	Programming	Gain	Lost	Interpretation
P1	50 times	4	0	High magnitude of gain, high frequency and magnitude of loss
	10 times	4	8	
	30 times	4	10	
	10 times	4	12	
P2	90 times	4	0	Low loss frequency, high magnitude of loss and gain
	10 times	4	50	
P3	50 times	2	0	Loss high frequency and low magnitude of loss and gain
	10 times	2	1	
	30 times	2	2	
	10 times	2	3	
P4	90 times	2	0	Lower loss frequency and low magnitude of loss and gain
	10 times	2	10	

all test scores sheds were established. Data were grouped according to three age ranges (7 - 11, 12 - 14 and 15 - 17 years old).

The following are the results of the study describing the overall performance, the characteristics of the learning process throughout the test, the preference for reward or punishment options, and the reaction time for choosing advantageous and disadvantageous alternatives.

3.1. Overall Performance

To calculate the overall performance, the formula (P3 + P4) − (P1 + P2) was used, corresponding to the sum of the number of times advantageous gates are chosen (P3 and P4) minus the sum of the number of times disadvantageous gates are selected (P1 and P2) in a total of 100 trials. The calculation produces a positive or negative number (above or below zero). For this test it is assumed that a positive result indicates the choice of more advantageous options (P3 and P4), compared to the disadvantageous ones (P1 and P2).

Table 3 shows that the three groups had an average performance below zero, and that the youngest age group obtained the least disadvantageous performance. Although all three groups had an average yield below zero, it is noteworthy that it was the younger age group who had the least disadvantageous performance; however, it should be noted that the variability of the results in all age groups, proved to be extended as shown by the dispersion indices.

Regarding the overall performance trend, **Figure 1** shows that in the group of 7 to 11 years old, the frequency of data in relation to the mean was relatively homogeneous, whereas for subjects aged 12 to 14 years, it shows a higher distribution of the data to the right of the mean, that is, towards a more positive performance. Regarding the latter group (aged 15 to 17 years), a greater data distribution was found towards a negative result, that is, to the left of the mean.

3.2. Learning Process

To analyze the learning process achieved by the subjects during the course of the task, the average of the partial performance on the test was calculated using the same formula mentioned for overall performance, but this time

Table 3. Overall performance by age group.

Age Group	N	Mean	SD	Mínimum	Maximum
7 - 11	140	−2.9	21.1	−66	62
12 - 14	116	−6.2	23.5	−72	48
15 - 17	69	−8.3	21.2	−74	40

SD: Standard Deviation.

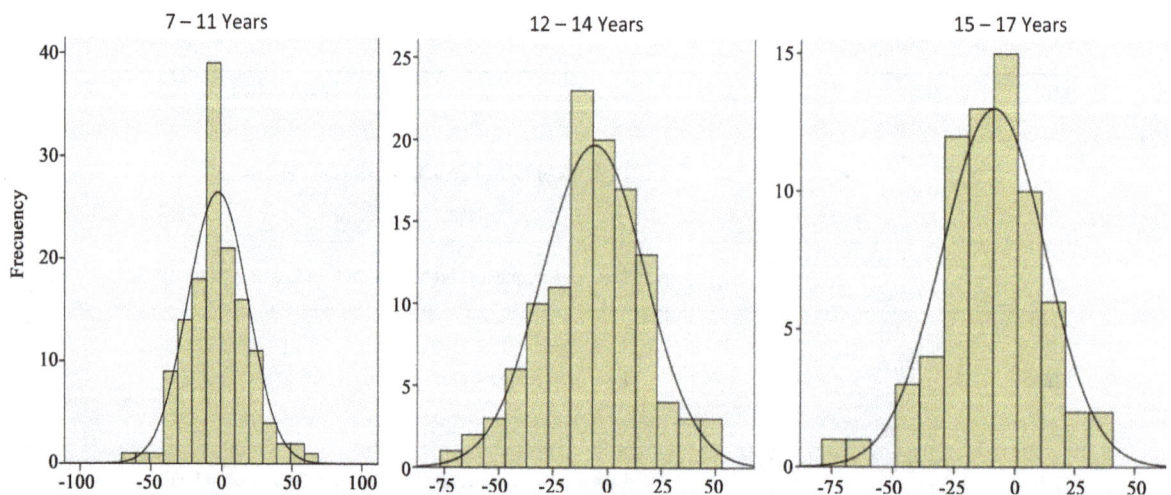

Figure 1. Overall performance trend by age group.

every 20 trials. **Figure 2** shows the average score obtained by each group on partial performances (R1 to R5). According to the observed, it can be deduced that there were not random performances, but that the three groups generated a learning process through the trials, resulting in an upward curve. It should be noted that the first group was the one that presented the most positive performance at the end of the test (mean = 1.16), followed by the group aged 12 to 14 years (mean = 1.1). In the case of older individuals (15 - 17 years), the averages of partial performances, although showing an upward trend, they presented a decline around the middle of the test and later regained control toward less disadvantageous choices.

3.3. Preference for Reward or Punishment Options

In general terms, children showed a greater preference for P2, which between the two unfavorable options, is the one that provides less frequent punishment. Among the advantageous options (P3 and P4), a slightly higher preference for the last gate was evidenced, which of the four options, is the one presenting the lowest frequency and magnitude of loss (see **Figure 3**).

3.4. Response Time

Children generally had very fast execution times, although there was a more impulsive trend in those who had a negative performance (see **Table 4**).

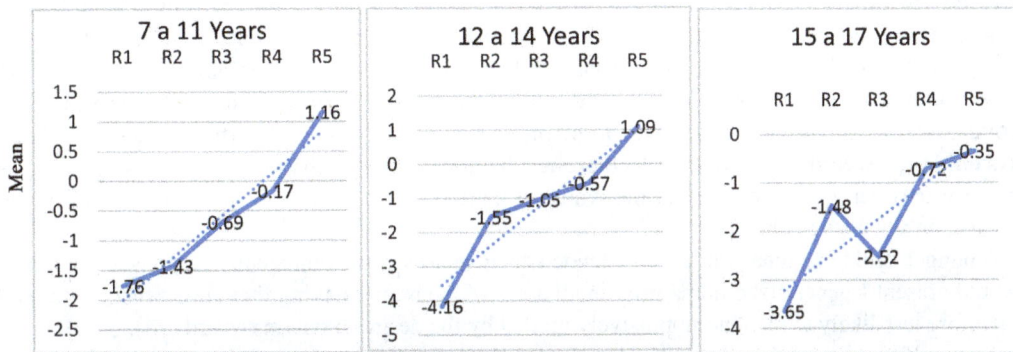

R1: trials 1-20, R2: trials 21-40, R3: trials 41-60, R4: trials 61-80, R5: trials 81-100

Figure 2. Learning curves by age group.

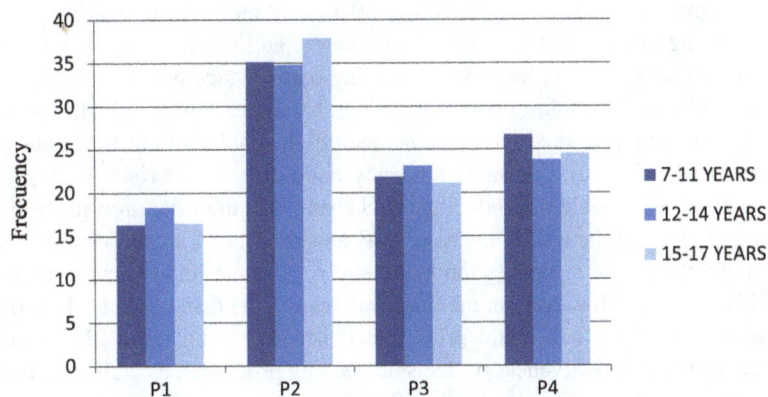

Figure 3. Response options to gate in each age group.

Table 4. Response time as performance in seconds.

Performance	N	Mean	SD	Mínimum	Maximum
Positive	139	1.3	0.72	−0.07	5.09
Negative	186	1.2	0.74	−0.58	4.37

SD: Standard Deviation.

As for the total execution time on the test, there was no evidence of relevant differences between the time spent by subjects with a positive performance and that of participants who had a negative one (2.27 and 2.23 minutes respectively).

4. Discussion

The interpretation of results was carried out on the basis of the somatic marker theory, which argues that the consequences of recent choices influence future decisions. As for overall performance, the theory has reported a linear increase from childhood to adolescence, in the performance of tasks with the IGT paradigm [22] [23] [25] [26]. On the contrary, the results of this study showed that younger individuals (7 - 11 years old) presented the most advantageous performance of the three groups, followed by the 12 - 14 years old group; and finally, with the lowest performance exhibited, by older teens (15 - 17 years).

These findings are consistent with the studies by Smith *et al.* [24], regarding the development trajectory of the decision-making process in the form of a J, which means that younger participants (8 - 11 years old) have a better performance than early adolescents (12 - 14 years old). However, a gradual improvement in performance was not found from this age (contrary to the assertions made by these authors), possibly due to a greater tendency in older adolescents (15 to 17 years old), to take risks and get away from the norm. It is noteworthy though, that the latter age group did not have a representative sample size to support these claims.

The performance showed by the group of 12 - 14 years old could be explained by the over-activation of limbic and subcortical structures such as the amygdala, hippocampus, caudate nucleus [15] and the nucleus accumbens [18] that occurs at the beginning of adolescence, and by hormonal factors of puberty in early adolescents [17], which would be more clearly demonstrated in tasks involving reinforcement such as the IGT. At the same time, it could be due to the relative immaturity of the prefrontal cortex, especially the ventromedial prefrontal cortex, whose development has proven to be much slower than some subcortical structures related to the reward system [14]. According to Oliva [12], these results may be due to the fact that at this age there is a greater imbalance between the cognitive and motivational circuits, which can lead to difficulties in imposing inhibitory control on impulsive behavior.

Younger children, meanwhile, who tended to give less disadvantageous responses than early adolescents, would present a generalized immaturity in all areas of the brain, making them less sensitive to reinforcement and therefore less likely to respond impulsively guided by the desire to obtain reward [24].

In the third group (15 - 17 years old), an upgrade in decision-making skills measured by the Hungry Donkey Task was not found, possibly because young people in middle and late adolescence, despite their advances in cognitive and executive functioning [27], tend to keep a preference for the search for new sensations and continue engaging in many risk behaviors, obviously affecting their decision-making process [28].

As for the learning process in the sample under study, an upward curve was found in the three groups. It is observed that subjects aged 7 - 11 years show a rising performance pattern relatively steady throughout the test, a result that coincides with that described by Crone and Van der Molen [23]. In the learning curve of the second group (12 - 14 years old), a marked increase was seen in the choice of advantageous options from the first to the second interval (trials 21 - 40); this same tendency is described by Crone *et al.* [20], who argue that children around the age of 14 are capable of producing rapid changes in their decision-making strategies.

Toward the last block of the test, in the same way as Crone and Van der Molen [23] have reported, the pattern of favorable and unfavorable responses tended to show a modest improvement, with a greater tendency toward choosing positive options. However, an increase was seen in the dispersion of data toward the final trials (higher standard deviation in R5) which could prove the existence of individual differences in the consolidation of learning, in the degree of effectiveness of decision-making processes, as well as in particular characteristics such as persistence and emotional and behavioral self-control.

In particular, the performance of the group aged 15 to 17 years presents a break halfway through the test, which may respond to a risk-taking behavior. Regarding this tendency, Hooper *et al.* [22] indicate that in this age group decision-making is not completely effective and even subjects aged just over 17 years fail to match the performance of adults, suggesting that the VMPFC and its connections continue maturing after this age.

The above has implications regarding the vulnerability of adolescents (15 - 17 years old) in risk-taking, since they require external control for their sensation-seeking tendencies [29]. Thus, real life for teens is strongly influenced by social determinants and feelings [17].

With regard to the preference of reward or punishment options, the greatest frequency of choice was found on P2. However, considering the upward learning curves for the three groups, it can be inferred that the choice of P2 was mostly present in the first test intervals, and that in the last trials the trend shifted towards a greater choice of P4.

It is observed that all groups showed high avoidance to P1, followed by P3, options having high frequency of punishment. It might be that, as predicted by prospect theory (Kahneman & Tversky, 1979 cited by Bechara, 2007 [30]), at the beginning, children and adolescents are oriented towards finding reinforcement (P1), but quickly realize the high frequency and magnitude of loss brought about by this first option and therefore opt for P2, which provides the same amount of reinforcement than P1, but with a lower frequency of punishment. As explained by this theory, when it comes to a choice between a sure loss (P1) and a possible loss (P2), although the possible loss may be of great magnitude, neurologically intact subjects prefer the less probable loss (P2).

In connection therewith, Crone et al., and Kerr and Zelazo [19] state that children will tend to prefer options with infrequent punishment, compared to options with frequent punishment, suggesting that the choice will initially be determined by a low probability of punishment even if this is high in magnitude. The shift toward an option as P4, also with low frequency of punishment but with a lower amount of gain and loss than P2, can be explained not only by a learning process within the test, but by the development of the ability to change an association previously learned and to anticipate future consequences, particularly in children aged 12 years and older [26]. This corroborates what Matthias-Brand, Recknor, Grabenhorst and Bechara [31] have stated, in terms that on the IGT, the first trials are conducted under ambiguity, and the latter trials under risk.

In the case of the youngest (aged 7 - 11 years), performance is driven by a low frequency of punishment rather than their ability to anticipate future consequences or damages ("future myopia"). This ability, according to Crone et al. [20], develops with age, especially in conditions of occasional punishment where it is necessary to implement it in order to anticipate, whereas when punishment is frequent the likelihood of future losses seems obvious.

Therefore, changes in the development of decision-making are not associated with hypersensitivity to reinforcement or insensitivity to punishment, but rather with the fact that as children grow older, they seem to learn to anticipate future consequences based on their lived experiences. That is how, throughout childhood, the development of somatic markers is sensitive to the frequency with which punishments are experienced [20].

It should be noted that the fact that the younger children had achieved a better performance than the older ones, does not mean that the latter do not have the capacity to make decisions advantageously. It rather means that there are additional variables characteristic of the psychological and neuropsychological development of teenagers, such as the search for identity and independence by distancing themselves from the norm and seeking risks [32], as well as a slow development of the prefrontal cortex and the immaturity of frontostriatal circuits, which would determine a greater inhibition of such behaviors [16]. This could suggest that teenagers under 15 would benefit considerably from training in self-control and decision-making, which may mitigate the tendency to taking risks shown by adolescents aged 15 to 18 years.

Regarding response time, it was found that subjects who had a positive performance had invested a little more time in the development of the task than those who had a negative performance. It has been found that subjects who have a more disadvantageous performance on the test show faster responses to unfavorable options, compared with those who show a better performance. This may reflect a degree of impulsiveness in disadvantageous performers [24].

However, although it is expected that with age the response time will decrease according to a linear improvement in other cognitive processes such as processing speed and working memory [24], a relationship between performance in IGT (nonlinear development) and response time has not been found, nor was it observed in this study.

To conclude, it can be said that age differences observed in the performance on the Donkey Hungry Task and described by different authors about IGT, are consistent with the differences observed in real life in terms of decision-making, often preceded by affective and emotional factors (over cognitive ones). From the above, it follows that an improvement in the decision-making process would be supported by the maturity of affective aspects, rather than cognitive aspects [25]. Likewise, the role of a slow and progressive course in the development of cortical and subcortical structures and their connections during childhood and adolescence [33] is highlighted.

As a proposal for future research in this area, it could be suggested carrying out a study with subjects aged 17 - 19 years, since according to the theory is from 17 years of age onward when the most significant improvements in the process of decision-making can begin to be appreciated. Therefore, it is likely that a research conducted with a large and representative sample of subjects within this age range, does show an improved performance in late adolescence that the present study could not determine, bearing in mind that the sample of subjects aged 17 years was minimal (one participant). A longitudinal study that considers gender, cultural and demographic variables, as well as correlations with cold executive functions, would be perhaps the closest alternative to reach an understanding of an increasingly complex and particularly changing process such as decision-making.

Another proposal would be to assess clinical backgrounds in a more precise way, such as neurological and neuropsychological implications of perinatal hypoxia in decision-making since this condition is related to possible impairment in subcortical structures.

As for the test, it would be interesting to inquire whether changes occur in trends and scores observed in this study, by introducing a larger number of trials (200 for example). As it could be seen, towards the end of the 100 trials, an improvement in performance of almost all subjects was evident leading to hypothesize that by including more trials the average scores would be more positive and beneficial.

Finally, it can be said that this study did constitute a contribution to the challenge of Neuropsychology in Colombia, by collaborating in the generation of information to enable obtaining the validity and reliability of neuropsychological instruments for this population. As limitations only one subject was assessed 17 years, so it can not be concluded towards the older age range, also it could have been considered a sample of subjects from 17 to 19 years to see the performance at the end of the test adolescence.

References

[1]   Verdejo-García, A., Benbrook, A., Funderburk, F., David, P., Cadet, J. and Bolla, K. (2007) The Differential Relationship between Cocaine Use and Marijuana Use on Decision-Making Performance over Repeat Testing with the Iowa Gambling Task. *Drug and Alcohol Dependence*, **90**, 2-11. http://dx.doi.org/10.1016/j.drugalcdep.2007.02.004

[2]   Damasio, A. (1994) Descartes' Error: Emotions, Reason, and the Human Brain. Avon Books, New York.

[3]   Bechara, A., Damasio, H. and Damasio, A. (2000) Emotion, Decision Making and the Orbitofrontal Cortex. *Cerebral Cortex*, **10**, 295-307. http://dx.doi.org/10.1093/cercor/10.3.295

[4]   García, M. (2012) Las funciones ejecutivas cálidas y el Rendimiento académico. Tesis Doctoral Universidad Complutense de Madrid.

[5]   Contreras, D., Catena, A., Cándido, A., Perales, J. and Maldonado, A. (2007) Funciones de la Corteza Prefrontal Ventromedial en la Toma de Decisiones Emocionales. *International Journal of Clinical and Health Psychology*, **8**, 285-313.

[6]   Gordillo, F., Arana, J., Salvador, J. and Mestas, L. (2011) Emoción y Toma de Decisiones: Teoría y Aplicación de la Iowa GamblingTask. *Revista Electrónica de Psicología Iztacala*, **14**, 333-353.

[7]   Levav, M. (2005) Neuropsicología de la emoción. Particularidades en la infancia. *Revista Argentina de Neuropsicología*, **5**, 15-24.

[8]   Verdejo, A. and García, M. (2006) Funciones Ejecutivas y Toma de Decisiones en Drogodependientes: Rendimiento Neuropsicológico y Funcionamiento Cerebral. Editorial de la Universidad de Granada.

[9]   Martínez-Selva, J., Sánchez, J. Bechara, A. and Román, F. (2006) Mecanismos cerebrales de la toma de decisiones. *Revista de Neurología*, **42**, 411-418.

[10]   Acuña, I. Castillo, D. Bechara, A. and Godoy, J. (2013) Toma de decisiones en adolescentes: Rendimiento bajo diferentes condiciones de información e intoxicación alcohólica. *International Journal of Psychology and Psychological Therapy*, **13**, 195-214.

[11]   Daza, M. and Arcas, P. (2002) Una apuesta teórica: Damasio y El error de Descartes.

[12]   Oliva, A. (2007) Desarrollo cerebral y asunción de riesgos durante la adolescencia. *Apuntes de Psicología*, **25**, 239-254. http://www.apuntesdepsicologia.es/index.php/revista/article/view/77/79

[13]   Spear, L. (2007) The Developing Brain and Adolescent-Typical Behavior Patterns: An Evolutionary Approach. In: Walker, E., Bossert, J. and Romer, D., Eds., *Adolescent Psychopathology and the Developing Brain: Integrating Brain and Prevention Science*, Oxford University Press, Oxford, 11-32.

[14]   Ernst, M. and Spear, L. (2009) Reward Systems. In: de Haan, M. and Gunnar, M.R., Eds., *Handbook of Developmental Social Neuroscience*, Guilford Press, New York, 324-341.

[15]   Goldberg, E. (2001) The Executive Brain: Frontal Lobes and the Civilized Mind. Oxford University Press, New York.

[16]   Moreno, A. (2012) Alteraciones Neuroanatómicas en los núcleos caudado y accumbens como marcador neurobiológico de mala respuesta al metilfenidato en el TDAH Infantil. Tesis Doctoral, Universidad Autónoma de Barcelona, Bellaterra.

[17]   Steinberg, L. (2005) Cognitive and Affective Development in Adolescence. *Trends in Cognitive Sciences*, **9**, 69-74. http://dx.doi.org/10.1016/j.tics.2004.12.005

[18]   Verdejo, A., Orozco, C., Meersmans, M., Aguilar, F. and Pérez, M. (2004) Impacto de la gravedad del consumo de drogas sobre distintos componentes de la función ejecutiva. *Revista de Neurología*, **38**, 1109-1116.

[19]   Kerr, A. and Zelazo, P. (2004) Development of "Hot" Executive Function: The Children's Gambling Task. *Brain & Cognition*, **55**, 148-157. http://dx.doi.org/10.1016/S0278-2626(03)00275-6

[20]   Crone, E., Bunge, S., Latenstein, H. and Van der Molen, M. (2005) Characterization of Children's Decision Making Sensitivity to Punishment Frequency, Not Task Complexity. *Child Neuropsychology*, **11**, 245-263. http://dx.doi.org/10.1080/092970490911261

[21]   Crone, E., Vendel, I. and Van der Molen, M. (2003) Decision-Making in Disinhibited Adolescents and Adults: Insensitivity to Future Consequences or Driven by Immediate Reward? *Personality and Individual Differences*, **35**, 1625-1641. http://dx.doi.org/10.1016/S0191-8869(02)00386-0

[22]   Hooper, C., Conklin, M. and Yarger, R. (2004) Adolescents' Performance on the Iowa Gambling Task: Implications for the Development of Decision Making and Ventromedial Prefrontal Cortex. *Developmental Psychology*, **40**, 1148-1158. http://dx.doi.org/10.1037/0012-1649.40.6.1148

[23]   Crone, E. and Van der Molen, M. (2004) Developmental Changes in Real Life Decision Making: Performance on a Gambling Task Previously Shown to Depend on the Ventromedial Prefrontal Cortex. *Developmental Neuropsychology*, **25**, 251-279. http://dx.doi.org/10.1207/s15326942dn2503_2

[24]   Smith, D., Xiao, L. and Bechara, A. (2012) Decision Making in Children and Adolescents: Impaired Iowa Gambling Task Performance in Early Adolescence. *Developmental Psychology*, **48**, 1180-1187. http://dx.doi.org/10.1037/a0026342

[25]   Cauffman, E., Shulman, E., Steinberg, L., Claus, E., Banich, M. and Graham, S. (2010) Age Differences in Affective Decision Making as Indexed by Performance on the Iowa Gambling Task. *Developmental Psychology*, **46**, 193-207. http://dx.doi.org/10.1037/a0016128

[26]   Overman, W., Frassrand, K., Ansel, S., Trawalter, S., Bies, B. and Redmond, A. (2004) Performance on the IOWA Card Task by Adolescents and Adults. *Neuropsychologia*, **42**, 1838-1851. http://dx.doi.org/10.1016/j.neuropsychologia.2004.03.014

[27]   Best, J., Miller, P. and Jones, L. (2009) Executive Functions after Age 5: Changes and Correlates. *Developmental Review*, **29**, 180-200. http://dx.doi.org/10.1016/j.dr.2009.05.002

[28]   Reyna, V. and Farley, F. (2006) Risk and Rationality in Adolescent Decisión Making: Implications for Theory Practice, and Public Policy. *Psychological Science in the Public Interest*, **7**, 1-44. http://dx.doi.org/10.1111/j.1529-1006.2006.00026.x

[29]   Galvan, A., Hare, T., Parra, C., Penn, J., Voss, K. and Glover, G. (2006) Earlier Development of the Accumbens Relative to Orbitofrontal Cortex Might Underlie Risk-Taking Behavior in Adolescents. *Journal of Neuroscience*, **26**, 6885-6892. http://dx.doi.org/10.1523/JNEUROSCI.1062-06.2006

[30]   Bechara, A. (2007) Iowa Gambling Task Professional Manual. Psychological Assessment Resources, Lutz.

[31]   Matthias-Brand, E., Recknor, F., Grabenhorst, A. and Bechara, A. (2007) Decisions under Ambiguity and Decisions under Risk: Correlations with Executive Functions and Comparisons of Two Different Gambling Tasks with Implicit and Explicit Rules. *Journal of Clinical and Experimental Neuropsychology*, **29**, 86-99. http://dx.doi.org/10.1080/13803390500507196

[32]   Oliva, A. and Antolin, L. (2010) Cambios en el cerebro adolescente y conductas agresivas y de asunción de riesgos. *Estudios de Psicología*, **31**, 53-66. http://dx.doi.org/10.1174/021093910790744563

[33]   Welsh, M. (2002) Developmental and Clinical Variations in Executive Functions. In: Molfese, D.L. and Molfese, V.J., Eds., *Developmental Variations in Learning: Applications to Social, Executive Function, Language, and Reading Skills*, Erlbaum, Mahwah, 139-185.

32

Syrup versus Drops of Iron III Hydroxide Polymaltose in the Treatment of Iron Deficiency Anemia of Infancy

Ayala Yahav[1], Chaim Kaplinsky[2], Miguel M. Glatstein[3]*, Yaakov Shachter[1], Aryeh Simmonds[1], Yakov Shiff[1], Dennis Scolnik[4], Nechama Sharon[1,5]

[1]Department of Pediatrics, Laniado Hospital, Netanya, Israel
[2]Department of Pediatric Hemato-Oncology, Sheba Hospital, Tel Hashomer, Israel
[3]Divisions of Pediatric Emergency Medicine and Clinical Pharmacology and Toxicology, Dana-Dwek Children Hospital, Tel Aviv Sourasky Medical Center, Affiliated to the Sackler Faculty of Medicine, Tel Aviv, Israel
[4]Divisions of Pediatric Emergency Medicine and Clinical Pharmacology and Toxicology, Department of Pediatrics, The Hospital for Sick Children, University of Toronto, Toronto, Canada
[5]Pediatric Hemato-Oncology, Laniado Hospital, Netanya, Israel
Email: *Nopasara73@hotmail.com

Academic Editor: Carl E. Hunt, George Washington University School of Medicine and Health Sciences, USA

Abstract

Background: Iron deficiency anemia in infants is the most common micronutrient deficiency worldwide. The main cause is low iron intake in the presence of accelerated physiologic growth rate. Objective: The current study aimed at prospectively comparing the efficacy of iron III hydroxide polymaltose syrup (IPS) versus iron III hydroxide polymaltose drops (IPD) in treating iron deficiency among infants attending the hematology outpatient clinic. Our hypothesis was that IPS would be less effective possibly related to the difficulty of giving the medication. Methods: Participants diagnosed with iron deficiency anemia between 11-24 months were randomly assigned to receive either IPS or IPD for 3 months. The main outcome parameter was hemoglobin blood level, while the secondary outcome parameters were: 1) iron; 2) ferritin; 3) transferrin (*i.e.* total iron binding capacity); 4) mean corpuscular volume; and 5) red blood cell distribution width. Results: Out of the 104 recruited infants, 55 (52%) completed the study: 29 in the IPS group and 26 in the IPD group. There was no significant difference in the main outcome parameter at either 1 or 3 months of treatment: mean hemoglobin was 10.5 versus 10.7 g/dL within a 1 month treatment, P = 0.4; mean hemoglobin was 11.0 versus 11.1 g/dL within a 3 months of

Syrup versus Drops of Iron III Hydroxide Polymaltose in the Treatment of Iron...

217

treatment, P = 0.59. Likewise, no significant differences were found with respect to the occurrence of side effects. Conclusion: Oral IPD and IPS are equally effective in treating iron deficiency anemia in infants aged 11 - 24 months.

Keywords

Iron Deficiency Anemia (IDA), Treatment, Iron III Hydroxide Polymaltose, Formulation

1. Background

Iron deficiency anemia (IDA) is currently the most common micronutrient deficiency, affecting more than 2 billion people worldwide [1]. Although most common in developing countries, it is also a major health problem in developed countries [2] and in Israel [3]. IDA, usually due to low intake in the presence of an accelerated growth rate, is a risk factor for developmental delay and disturbed cognitive function in infants. These adverse effects may be irreversible and may lead to behavioral problems in childhood and adolescence [4] [5]. Supplemental iron administration improves behavioral and cognitive development [6], stressing the public health importance of preventing iron deficiency.

The World Health Organization defines IDA in infants and toddlers aged 6 - 60 months living at sea level as a hemoglobin level ≤11 g/dL, or hematocrit ≤ 33% [7]. For infants, the amount of iron necessary to supply growth requirements is 1 mg/day. A joint UNICEF/USAID consultation has recommended that the most practical iron supplement for infants and young children is either an aqueous solution of a soluble ferrous salt such as ferrous sulfate, or a ferric complex, such as iron polymaltose complex [1] [8]. The gold standard for response to treatment is defined as an increase of 1 g/dL in hemoglobin level after one month of treatment [9]. Iron salts with divalent iron have been associated with more gastrointestinal adverse effects such as nausea, vomiting, and disturbances in stool consistency, although they are more readily absorbed [9] [10]. Iron III hydroxide polymaltose complex is available both as drops and syrup. The drops are more concentrated and therefore require a smaller volume/dose, which is especially useful in the first year of life. However, it should be noted that the use of higher concentration drops can be associated with more damaging therapeutic mishaps [11]. The current study aimed at prospectively comparing the efficacy of iron III hydroxide polymaltose syrup (IPS) versus iron III hydroxide polymaltose drops (IPD) in treating iron deficiency among infants attending the hematologic outpatient clinic of a large tertiary-care paediatric hospital. Additionally the two preparations were compared for patient compliance and outcome.

2. Methods

Participants were infants between the ages of 11 - 24 months, referred to the pediatric hematology clinic at Laniado Hospital by local pediatricians and family physicians IDA. The main outcome measures were change in blood levels of hemoglobin, iron, transferrin, MCV, and RDW.

1. Inclusion criteria:

Otherwise healthy term infants with birth weights > 2500 g and without any symptoms of gastrointestinal pathology.

2. Exclusion criteria:

1) Any systemic medical condition; 2) inborn errors of metabolism; 3) birth defects; 4) hemoglobinopathy; 5) medication consumption on a regular basis; and 6) family history of a significant systemic or chronic condition.

The study was approved by the Helsinki Committee of Laniado Hospital and written consent was obtained from the parent or guardian of each participant.

IDA was defined as hemoglobin ≤ 10.5 g/dL with biochemical evidence of iron deficiency as reflected by low ferritin and transferrin saturation levels [6]. Participants were treated with 3 mg/kg of elemental iron twice daily for three months using either IPD ("Tiptipot Ferripel-3" Oral Drops, CTS, Israel) or IPS ("Ferripel-3 Syrup", CTS, Israel). Randomization was achieved by assigning consecutive patients alternately to each group. Participants were scheduled for two additional clinic visits at one and three months after starting treatment ("Visit 2" and "Visit 3", respectively). At each of these three visits blood was drawn for hemoglobin, iron, ferritin, total iron binding capacity (TIBC), mean corpuscular volume (MCV), and red blood cell distribution width (RDW).

All patients were also followed by a study nurse weekly for the first month, using a structured telephone interview, to assess compliance and to collect data regarding adverse effects such constipation.

3. Statistical Analysis

The study was designed to identify a 25% - 50% response with a strength of 80% and significance of 0.05 (P-value), taking into account a dropout rate of 20%. For continuous variables, the means of the two groups were compared using the Student's t-test. For discrete variables, chi-square test was used. Statistical significance was set at $P \leq 0.05$.

3. Results

Of the 104 infants recruited 55 (52%) took the assigned treatment for the full three months of the study: 26 in the IPD group and 29 in the IPS group. The remaining 49 children were excluded only because they failed to complete the full three month treatment (mainly because they refused to complete the study period or failed to show-up for follow-up visits or blood tests), and not because of any side-effects reported. No significant differences were found between the IPS and IPD groups in any of the demographic characteristics such as gender, gestational age, birth weight and duration of breast feeding (**Table 1**).

Gastrointestinal side effects, such as vomiting, diarrhea, or constipation, were noted in two patients in the IPD group and 5 in the IPS group.

Laboratory values from the three visits are detailed in **Table 2**. No significant differences were noted between the two groups in serum iron, serum transferrin, MCV and RDW.

4. Discussion

A joint UNICEF/USAID consultation recommended an aqueous solution of a soluble ferrous salt such as ferrous sulfate, or a ferric complex such iron polymaltose, for iron supplementation in infants and young children with IDA [12]. They have equivalent bioavailability in infants [13] [14]. Ours is the first study to compare trivalent iron as syrup versus drops in the treatment of IDA in infants and we found the two preparations equally effective.

There is limited data comparing the efficacy of different preparations of oral iron in the management of iron deficiency [6]-[15]. One recent study by Jaber *et al.* compared divalent to trivalent iron-containing preparations in the prevention of IDA among 4 - 12 month old infants, and showed no significant superiority for either form in the prevention of IDA, though demonstrating that iron gluconate was less tolerable [16]. Jaber *et al.* demonstrated that bivalent iron is more effective than trivalent iron, however latter is more tolerable than bivalent iron since it has less reported side effects resulting in reduced compliance. For this reason the net efficacy of both preparations is very similar [5].

Despite a weekly telephone follow-up during the first month and a low incidence of side effects in both of our study groups, there was a significant drop-out rate, resulting in about half of the participants completing all visits. The poor compliance may reflect parents' lack of perceived importance of iron supplementation and is probably unrelated to the ease of dosing.

Until recently, the Israeli Ministry of Health recommended that all infants aged 4 - 12 months receive daily

Table 1. Demographic characteristics of study patients.

Variable	IPD* (n = 48)	IPS** (n = 56)	P-Value
Gender (%)			
Male	24 (50)	23 (41)	0.36
Female	24 (50)	33 (59)	
Gestational age (weeks)	39.5	39.2	0.56
Birth weight (kg)	3.15	3.17	0.79
Breast feeding (months)	7	7.3	0.77

IPD* = Iron III Hydroxide polymaltose drops;
IPS** = Iron III Hydroxide polymaltose syrup.

Table 2. Iron status of participating infants. IPD: Iron III Hydroxide polymaltose drops; IPS: Iron III Hydroxide polymaltose syrup. 32/48 and 43/56 patients were followed up in the IPD and IPS groups, respectively, P = 0.251. **Patients in the IPD and IPS groups, respectively.

Variables	IPD 32/48 completed the study (Mean + SD)	IPS 43/56 completed study (Mean + SD)	P-Value
Breast feeding [months]	7.0 + 5.8	7.3 + 7.0	0.779
Birth term [weeks]	39.5 + 1.7	39.3 + 2.3	0.561
Birth weight [kg]	3.1 + 0.5	3.2 + 0.6	0.791
Age of first eating meat [months]	6.5 + 1.6	7.2 + 3.0	0.115
Age of first eating vegetables [months]	6.2 + 1.2	6.4 + 2. 1	0.704
Age of first eating fruit [months]	6.2 + 1.1	6.2 + 2.2	0.532
Hemoglobin—Visit 1 [gm/dl]	9.8 + 0.6	9.8 + 0.7	0.872
Hemoglobin—Visit 2 [gm/dl]*	10.5 + 0.7	10.7 + 08	0.401
Hemoglobin—Visit 3 [gm/dl] (26 - 29)**	11.0 + 0.8	11.2 + 0.8	0.591
Iron—Visit 1 (38 and 47)**	41 + 32	41 + 32	0.909
Iron—Visit 2 (24 and 34)**	51 + 26	49.6 + 26	0.786
Iron—Visit 3 (17 and 20)**	64.60 + 32	47 + 19	0.264
TIBC—Visit 2 (32 and 37)**	267 + 59	282 + 39	0.197
TIBC—Visit 3 (23 and 30)**	269 + 35	282 + 42	0.214
MCV—Visit 2 (45 and 52)**	70 + 7	70 + 7	0.950
MCV—Visit 3 (29 and 40)**	69 + 7	71 + 6	0.110
RDW—Visit 2 (46 and 51)**	16 + 2	17 + 3	0.271
RDW—Visit 3 (46 and 51)**	17 + 2	16 + 2	0.058

supplemental iron (7.5 mg/day up to six months and 15 mg/day up to one year) for primary prevention of iron deficiency. Due to the high prevalence of IDA, the Ministry of Health recently issued new guidelines extending the duration of preventative treatment to 18 months. Primary preventive therapy consists of nutritional recommendations [17], and secondary prevention includes screening for hemoglobin level at one year.

5. Conclusion

In conclusion, the current study shows that IDA may be treated effectively with trivalent iron in both drop and syrup forms.

References

[1]   Bopche, A.V., Dwiverdi, R., Mishra, R., *et al.* (2009) Ferrous Sulfate versus Iron Polymaltose Complex for Treatment of Iron Deficiency Anemia in Children. *Indian Pediatrics*, **46**, 883-885.

[2]   DeMaeyer, E. and Adiels-Tegman, M. (1985) The Prevalence of Anaemia in the World. *World Health Statistics Quarterly*, **38**, 302-316.

[3]   Meyerovitch, J., Sherf, M., Antebi, F., Barhoum-Noufi, M., Horev, Z., Jaber, L., Weiss, D. and Koren, A. (2006) The Incidence of Anemia in an Israeli Population: A Population Analysis for Anemia in 34,512 Israeli Infants Aged 9 to 18 Months. *Pediatrics*, **118**, e1055-e1060. http://dx.doi.org/10.1542/peds.2006-0024

[4]   Lozoff, B., De Andraca, I., Castillo, M., *et al.* (2003) Behavioral and Developmental Effects of Preventing Iron Deficiency Anemia in Healthy Full Term Infants. *Pediatrics*, **112**, 846-854.

[5]   Jaber, L., Tamary, H., *et al.* (2010) Iron Polymatose versus Ferrous Gluconate in the Prevention of Iron Deficiency

Anemia of Infancy. *Journal of Pediatric Hematology/Oncology*, **32**, 585-588.
http://dx.doi.org/10.1097/MPH.0b013e3181ec0f2c

[6] Wright, C.M., Kelly, J., Trail, A., Parkinson, K.N. and Summerfield, G. (2004) The Diagnosis of Borderline Iron Deficiency: Results of a Therapeutic Trial. *Archives of Disease in Childhood*, **89**, 1028-1031.
http://dx.doi.org/10.1136/adc.2003.047407

[7] Lozoff, B., Jimenez, E. and Wolf, A.W. (1991) Long Term Development Outcome of Infants with Iron Deficiency. *The New England Journal of Medicine*, **325**, 687-694. http://dx.doi.org/10.1056/NEJM199109053251004

[8] Pizarro, F., Yip, R., Dallman, P.R., *et al.* (1991) Iron Status with Different Infant Feeding Regimens: Relevance to Screening and Prevention of Deficiency. *Journal of Pediatrics*, **118**, 687-692.
http://dx.doi.org/10.1016/S0022-3476(05)80027-7

[9] Glazer, Y. and Bilenko, N. (2010) Effect of Iron Deficiency and Iron Deficiency Anemia in the First Two Years of Life on Cognitive and Mental Development during Childhood. *Harefuah*, **149**, 309-314, 335.

[10] Mujica-Coopman, M.F., Borja, A., Pizarro, F. and Olivares, M. (2015) Effect of Daily Supplementation with Iron and Zinc on Iron Status of Childbearing Age Women. *Biological Trace Element Research*.

[11] Devaki, P.B., Chandra, R.K. and Geisser, P. (2008) Effects of Oral Supplementation with Iron (III) Hydroxide Polymaltose Complex on the Hematological Profile of Adolescents with Varying Iron Status. *Arzneimittel-Forschung*, **58**, 389-397.

[12] Nestel, P. and Alnwick, D. (1996) Iron-Micronutrient Supplements for Young Children. Summary and Conclusions of a Consultation Held at UNICEF, Copenhagen, 19-20 August 1996.

[13] Borbolla, J.R., Cicero, R.E., Dibildox, M.M., Sotres, D.R. and Gutierrez, R.G. (2000) IPC *vs.* Iron Sulphate in the Treatment of Iron Deficiency in Infants. *Rev Mex Padiatr*, **67**, 63-67.

[14] Jacobs, P. (1984) Oral Iron Therapy in Human Subjects: Comparative Absorption between Ferrous Salts and Iron Polymaltose. *Journal of Medicine*, **3**, 387-377.

[15] Ortiz, R., Toblli, J.E., Romero, J.D., Monterrosa, B., Frer, C., Macagno, E. and Breymann, C. (2011) Efficacy and Safety of Oral Iron (III) Polymaltose Complex versus Ferrous Sulfate in Pregnant Women with Iron-Deficiency Anemia: A Multicenter, Randomized, Controlled Study. *Journal of Maternal-Fetal and Neonatal Medicine*, **24**, 1347-1352.

[16] Geltman, P.L., Meyers, A.F., Mehta, S.D., Brugnara, C., Villon, I., Wu, Y.A. and Bauchner, H. (2004) Daily Multivitamins with Iron to Prevent Anemia in High-Risk Infants: A Randomized Clinical Trial. *Pediatrics*, **114**, 86-93.
http://dx.doi.org/10.1542/peds.114.1.86

[17] Walter, T., Dallman, P.R., Pizarro, F., *et al.* (1993) Effectiveness of Iron Fortified Infant Cereal in Prevention of Iron Deficiency Anemia. *Pediatrics*, **91**, 976-982.

Specific Injuries Management in the Postoperative of Congenital Heart Diseases (II): Univentricular Hearts

A. Sánchez Andrés[1], C. González Miño[2], E. Valdés Diéguez[3], L. Boni[3], J. I. Carrasco Moreno[1]

[1]Pediatric Cardiology Unit, Hospital Universitario y Politécnico La Fe, Valencia, Spain
[2]Pediatric Intensive Care Unit, Hospital General de Castellón, Castellon, Spain
[3]Pediatric Surgery Unit, Hospital Universitario y Politécnico La Fe, Valencia, Spain
Email: tonisanchan@hotmail.com

Abstract

It is very important to understand that the univentricular heart surgery is just palliative, not being in anyway a definitive or curative surgery, but nowadays it's the best initial treatment of this complex heart disease. The fundamental philosophy of treatment of every univentricular heart is to ensure the flow system and/or restrict the lung flow. Thus, initially a patient with univentricular heart who is undergoing surgery may need to ensure systemic flow (reconstruction of the aortic arch type Norwood), to restrict the lung flow (pulmonary banding) or to provide enough pulmonary flow (pulmonary-systemic fistulae). However, some heart diseases with univentricular physiology remain "balanced" autonomously, until the "second" stage of palliation is performed (cavo-pulmonary anastomosis type Glenn), but others require performance of pulmonary banding, if there's no native lung protection and/or repair of the systemic circuit in a first stage, to reach next palliation steps in the best possible conditions.

Keywords

Univentricular heart, Postoperative, Congenital heart disease, Norwood, Glenn, Fontan

1. Introduction

Biventricular circulatory system consists of a double circuit (pulmonar and systemic) connected in series through blood flows driven by two distinct, well developed ventricular chambers which have enough contractile power to act as pumps. From an anatomical segmental view, the heart must then be essentially a biventricular atrioventricular connection with two atrioventricular orifices: normal, permeable and competent.

Certain complex cardiac malformations are characterized by only a functionally useful ventricular chamber to keep the requirement to simultaneously hold the circulation in both circuits (pulmonary and systemic) when they are connected in parallel as occurs after birth. For identification, colloquially the name "univentricular heart" or "single ventricle" is used, even if it's actually possible to verify in many cases the presence of two ventricles regardless of the absolute size of each. The vast majority of these hearts have a univentricular atrioventricular connection, and the classic example is the tricuspid atresia. It is noted, that there are certain malformations with two well developed ventricles in which a biventricular surgical correction is impossible, so in these cases it is necessary to resort to univentricularization.

The postnatal circulation of cardiac malformations with univentricular context involves two fundamental problems: volume overload of the single ventricle and systemic desaturation; this is because both circuits, pulmonary and systemic flow are receiving the blood flow simultaneously in parallel. From the perspective of hemodynamics, the result of the surgery is a univentricular circulatory model number, even if the transaction has a marked palliative.

The application of mitigation techniques in such patients, atrioseptostomy Rashkind, surgical atrioseptectomy (Blalock-Hanlon), and those aimed to regulate the pulmonary blood flow (aortopulmonary anastomosis and pulmonary artery banding), projected a ray of hope on these malformations (there are cases of prolonged survival with these techniques). Throughout these years there have been other variants of surgical intervention called "repair" that, when applied appropriately respond to this group of patients with previous or palliative surgery have helped reduce mortality significantly, these are veno-atrium-pulmonary shunt techniques.

The main objective of this article is to provide a list of the most common surgical procedures performed trough the stages of palliation for univentrcular hearts, along with the possible complications to be expected in the postoperative period. Some recommendations as to their diagnoses and management are also discussed.

2. Perioperative Management of Univentricular Hearts

Univentricular heart diseases have different physiology depending on stage of palliation in which they are (**Table 1** and **Table 2**). Following the procedures that are performed, either systemic-pulmonary shunt or pulmonary artery banding, the relationship between pulmonary and systemic blood flow (Qp:Qs) depends on the systemicvascular resistance, the size of the pulmonary artery shunt and to a lesser degree, of pulmonary vascular resistance. The

Table 1. Univentricular heart surgery.

▫ **Stage 1 (Norwood):** Neoaorta formation and pulmonary flow through systemic pulmonary fistula (Blalock-Taussig) or from the right ventricle through the pulmonary trunk (Sano)

- Low cardiac output.
- High Qp:Qs.
- Low Qp:Qs.
- Residual aortic arch stenosis.
- AV valve dysfunction.

▫ **Stage 2 (Glenn):** Bidirectional cavo-pulmonary anastomosys:

- Cyanosis.
- Arterial hypertension.
- Pleural effusion.
- Superior vena cava syndrome.

▫ **Stage 3 (Fontan):** Bicavo (superior and inferior)—Pulmonary anastomosys:

- Third space fluid loss.
- Cyanosis.
- Low cardiac output.
- Arrhythmias.

Table 2. Palliative procedures.

▫ **Systemic to Pulmonary Shunts (Blalock-Taussig, Modified Blalock-Taussig, Central Fistulae)**
• Excessive pulmonary flow.
• Arterial Hypotension.
• Thrombosis.
▫ **Pulmonary Artery Banding**
• Cyanosis.
• Excessive pulmonary flow.

arterial saturation is definitely half between systemic and pulmonary venous saturations, weighted by the Qp:Qs, therefore, any circumstance that produces a decrease in venous admixture, pulmonary venous saturation or Qp:Qs, can produce increases in the degree of cyanosis. The problems in the immediate postoperative period usually lead mainly to a ***decrease in oxygen delivery to tissues due to low cardiac output and/or excessive level of cyanosis***, so it is of vital importance to determine if the problem is related to low heart output, an unequal distribution of the cardiac output (increases or decreases in Qp:Qs) or problems in pulmonary venous saturation. Poor systemic perfusion or high difference in arterio-venous mixing suggests a problem related to low output or increased Qp:Qs. In contrast, the hemodynamic maintenance cyanosis suggests a primary lung problem or decrease in Qp:Qs.

One of the most important principles to consider during the postoperative management of heart disease with univentricular physiology is that ***increases in systemic vascular resistance can increase blood pressure***, Qp:Qs and arterial saturation at the expense of systemic perfusion. Therefore, adequate blood pressure should not be taken itself as a sign of adequate systemic perfusion. Many of the current studies suggest that high blood pressure is actually associated with low tissue oxygen delivery. Hence, the use of afterload reducing agents such as milrinone, nitroprusside or phenoxybenzamine in order to improve systemic perfusion is becoming widespread. Blood pressure can be maintained within acceptable ranges by improving cardiac output with the use of low doses of epinephrine or norepinephrine.

Another goal in the management of these patients is to ***maximize cardiac output*** to ensure adequate tissue oxygenation and to assess those adjustments that can be made by manipulating the ratio Qp:Qs. Again, this principle supports the use of afterload reducing agents that can increase cardiac output and counteract pulmonary circulatory overload. Therapeutic strategies aimed at increasing pulmonary vascular resistance have their limitations in practice, overall because the mayor component of pulmonary resistance takes place where shunt or banding have been made.

The **first stage of palliative surgery or Norwood procedure** is one of the leading major efforts to palliate the hypoplastic left heart syndrome (HLHS), but operative mortality remains worrisome. Several factors associated with poor prognosis have been described, such as preoperative hemodynamic instability, the diminutive size of the ascending aorta, the commitment of the ventricular function, significant tricuspid regurgitation, prematurity and low birth weight. Instead, it is a good prognostic factor type of diagnosis, being more favorable, for example, those diseases that do not correspond to HLHS. For this reason, some groups considered a contraindication to perform this operation, at least at this early stage, prematurity, weight below 2.5 kg, significant ventricular dysfunction, significant tricuspid regurgitation, the presence of anomalous pulmonary venous drainage total obstruction and the presence of other severe associated malformations. These conditions can contraindicate surgery up to 25% of patients with this diagnosis [1] [2].

Currently, most diagnoses are made in the antenatal period, what constitutes a significant contribution in the management strategy of these children. HLHS antenatal diagnosis can be made from the eighteenth week of pregnancy, allowing to properly plan patient's birth and timely implement measures to stabilize the patient hemodynamics, including early onset of prostaglandins or early and scheduled completion of the Rashkind maneuver if there were any restriction at the level of the fossa ovalis. Note that this disease can go unnoticed initially and the patient may present with cardiogenic shock after a few days of life, the result of spontaneous closure of the ductus.

Many groups continue to perform what is known as "classic Norwood", because the reconstruction of the ascending aorta and arch with homograft offers better results in terms of lower incidence of recoarctation and less distortion of the pulmonary valve in comparison with other techniques. However, these differences are not so clear so it is permissible to choose the technique with which the surgical team feels most comfortable. Other groups have designed variants tailored for each individual case, but that conceptually belong to the same intervention and therefore have been arbitrarily called "modified Norwood". Patients who develop postoperative gradient at the aortic arch usually correspond to "classical" repairs, because of redundancy of the patch, which can generate an invagination thereof. The use of "cardiac arrest" is an interesting technical contribution in recent years, aimed at reducing the cerebral ischemia time. Its routine implementation in the Norwood operation can help to preserve brain function in the medium and long term.

The reported perioperative mortality figures have historically been around 20% - 30%. The best series have managed to lose 10% but others reach more than 50%. Bartram et al performed a detailed analysis of the post Norwood causes of death, being coronary irrigation problems and those derived from the most common shunt the main causes. The initial mortality of this series is comparable to international studies, however, it has the important limitation of being a small series. It is not a minor event that these patients remain with abnormal physiology, with pulmonary flow dependent on a systemic-pulmonary shunt, so the intra and postoperative management is a real challenge.

Several methods have been gradually incorporated to optimize postoperative management, such as adding carbon dioxide or nitrogen to air mixture, continuous measurement of mixed venous saturation and, recently, the use of phenoxybenzamin (POB) with promising results. The principle of the use of phenoxybenzamin is the increase in systemic cardiac output by maximal dilatation of the systemic circulation. This effect results in a more stable parallel circulation through prevention of fluctuations in systemic vascular resistance in the early postoperative period. However, there is a technical amendment introduced lately, which seems to contribute significantly in reducing mortality and facilitate the handling in the intensive care unit, because the balance between pulmonary and systemic circulation ceases to be critical. This modification is to replace the Blalock-Taussig shunt (**Figure 1**) with one that connects the ventricle and the pulmonary artery (**Figure 2**), so as to obtain only systolic flow, rather than systolic and dyastolic as in the first situation. While there are some problems in relation to this option, popularized by Sano et al, it seems to be one of the most important contributions of recent times and it seems reasonable to consider its use selectively. The risk of death continues in the medium term, especially before the Glenn operation. There is unpublished evidence that the Sano modification could also help to reduce this attrition before the second stage [3] [4].

The **second and the third stage in palliation of univentricular hearts** are unique from the standpoint of pulmonary blood flow becoming dependent on non-pulsatile venous flow. The ***bidirectional cavopulmonary shunt, the classic Glenn anastomosis*** (**Figure 3**), by virtue of increasing the effective pulmonary flow improves the systemic arterial oxygen saturation, volume unloads the ventricle, and also alters the ventricular geometry, whether the ventricle is of right or left ventricular morphology [5]. One of the mechanisms by which the bidirectional cavopulmonary connection improves the systemic arterial oxygen saturation is to increase the so-called effective pulmonary blood flow [6].

A particular aspect in bidirectional cavo-pulmonary anastomosis is that the pulmonary flow is dependent heavily on the strength of two distinct vascular beds. Both circulations, the brain and lung, have opposite responses to changes in the levels of carbon dioxide (CO_2), acid-base balance and oxygen. This can cause particular difficulties in the treatment of elevated pulmonary vascular resistance or low arterial oxygen saturation. Hyperventilation and alkalosis, for example, have limited utility in this aspect, as though they are effective pulmonary vasodilators, the hyperventilation and alkalosis produce cerebral vasoconstriction. Because pulmonary blood flow is dependent on venous return through the superior vena cava (largely composed of cerebral blood flow), maneuvers that cause decreased cerebral blood flow, may decrease the pulmonary blood flow and increase the degree of hypoxemia. Hyperventilation after the completion of a Glenn produces in fact a decrease in cerebral blood flow and thus a decrease in arterial oxygen saturation [7]. Other techniques commonly used to decrease pulmonary vascular resistance as the deep sedative drug can also cause a decrease in cerebral blood flow. Inhaled NO [8], which acts selectively on the pulmonary vessels has proven to be an effective measure in reducing the transpulmonary pressure gradient in patients undergoing such surgery Glenn and thus work in combination with moderate hypoventilation in case of high pulmonary vascular resistance and cyanosis. When the degree of cyanosis is not excessive, expectant attitude with adequate hemodynamic support and maintenance of hemoglobin levels within normal limits, may be sufficient. This is because the saturation tends to improve gradually in the first days after surgery and again at the

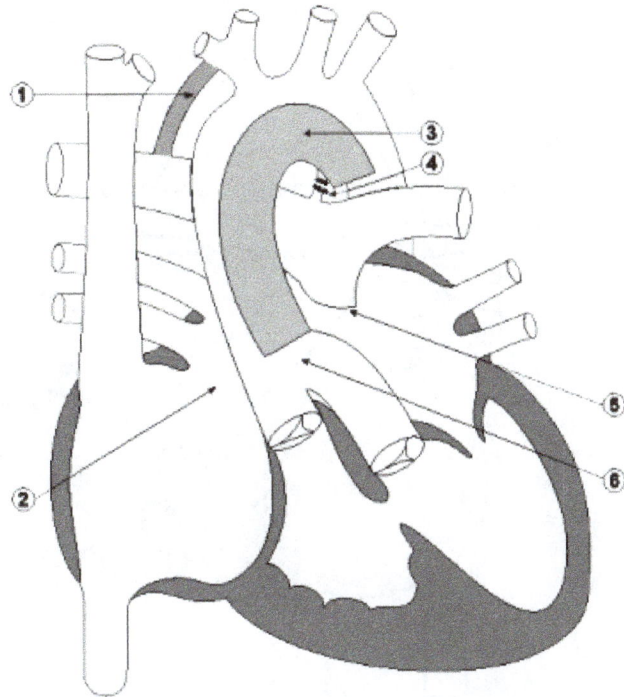

Figure 1. Norwood repair of the aortic arch with systemic-pulmonary shunt (modified Blalock-Taussig). 1. BT shunt. 2. Atrioseptectomy. 3. Norwood arch repair. 4. Clips on ductus. 5. Pulmonary trunk section. 6. Neo-aorta (Native pulmonary trunk with small native aorta).

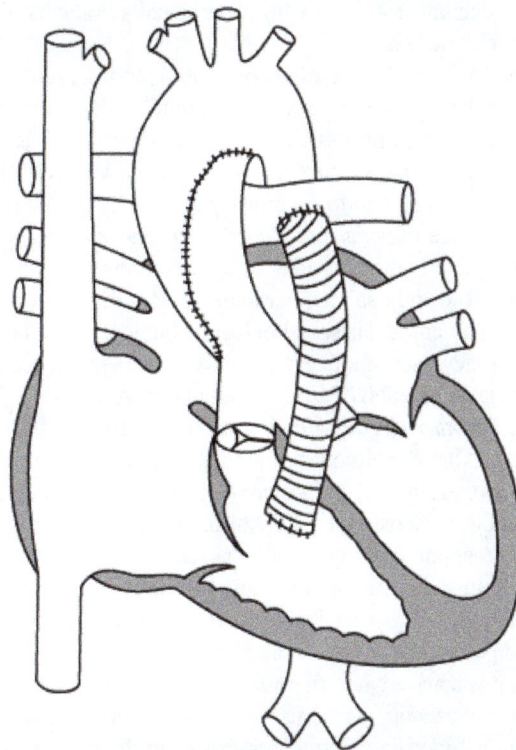

Figure 2. Norwood repair of the Aortic arch with right ventricle to pulmonary bifurcation conduit (Sano's conduit).

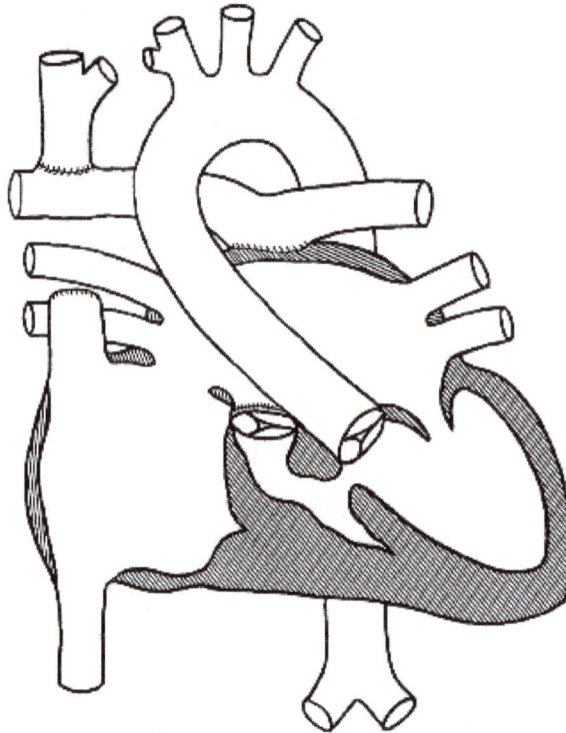

Figure 3. Superior cavo-pulmonary connection (Bidireccional Glenn).

time of extubation, provided that there are no problems in the lung or airways. Persistent cyanosis, can produce a series of problems such as decompression of veno-venous collaterals that divert the flow of the superior vena cava away from the pulmonary circulation.

Systemic hypertension is a common phenomenon after such interventions Glenn. This could occur in response to increased cerebral venous pressure or an improvement in the cost of a ventricle that is volume unloaded. Treatment with vasodilators is often necessary and blood pressure tends to decrease to normal range in the first days after surgery, a proportion of patients requiring treatment with ACE inhibitors for long periods of time [9].

The presence of residual shunts and aorto-pulmonary collaterals can be problematic in the post-Glenn. They have been associated with the presence of persistent pleural effusions, elevated venous pressures and low cardiac output. It is very important to recognize that ventricular structure suffers so many changes with this type of intervention, mainly because it reduces left to right shunts, particularly with the bidirectional Glenn. When systemic flow is dependent on the flow through a ventricular septal defect or bulbo-ventricular foramen, sharp decreases in ventricular dimensions may precipitate the onset of subaortic stenosis. The emergence of an ejection murmur in a patient with susceptible anatomy after the completion of a bidirectional Glenn should lead to screening for this injury [10].

The physiology of the *Fontan circulation* is a mixture between the bidirectional Glenn and normal cardiovascular physiology. As in Glenn, pulmonary blood flow is dependent on the systemic venous pressure, and all pulmonary flow is effective. However, pulmonary and systemic circulations are well differentiated, as in the normal heart. If circulation is composed of a Fontan fenestration in the atrial septum [11] [12], there may be varying degrees of left-right shunt causing a mild systemic desaturation. In this unique circulation, the two principal determinants of long-term outcome are low pulmonary vascular resistance (PVR) and adequate single-ventricle myocardial function. Drugs that lower PVR and/or improve myocardial performance could optimize circulatory efficiency and potentially improve outcomes [13] [14].

Major issues for intensivists arise when there is elevation of pulmonary arterial pressure, as this can occur either because the pulmonary vascular resistance is elevated, mechanical obstruction in the pulmonary artery or when there is myocardial dysfunction causing an increase in the pressure on pulmonary veins to left atrium level [14]. Numerous studies have shown that high pressures in the pulmonary artery (> 10 - 15 mmHg) are associated with poor prognosis in patients undergoing Fontan surgery, mainly because it is very difficult to maintain central venous pressures in these values without producing output of the third space fluid. When this loss of fluids progresses, patients develop pleural effusions, ascites and peripheral edema. It becomes necessary then to increase the pressure of the respirator to maintain adequate functional residual capacity and an adequate tidal volume against a distended abdomen, a heavy chest and small effective pleural lung distension. The increases in airway pressures, particularly in the absence of pulmonary parenchymal disease, increase pulmonary vascular resistance, and therefore even higher venous pressures are needed to maintain cardiac output. Also, when intraabdominal pressure increases, renal perfusion pressure decreases, specially when there is low cardiac output or blood pressure is at the lower limit, what is common in these circumstances. In general, the fenestration in the Fontan surgery can reduce the risk of some of these complications by providing a source of systemic flow which is not dependent on passage through the pulmonary circulation, but can also cause a decrease in pulmonary arterial pressure sufficient to reduce the loss of third space fluid [15].

When a patient with Fontan circulation physiology is in a state of low cardiac output, it is essential to identify and treat the underlying cause. It is very common for patients during the Fontan postoperative period, to require large amounts of volume on the first day after surgery.

The persistence of low central pressures strongly suggests the need of volume. The obstruction of the pulmonary artery should be considered as the cause of low cardiac output when left atrial pressure is low and central venous pressure is high. If the central venous pressure was not monitored, the heavy losses of third space fluid with low or normal pressures in the left atrium should increase the degree of suspicion. Even in the presence of fenestration, its ability to maintain cardiac output against an anatomical or physiological obstruction to pulmonary blood flow is significantly limited compared to the situation that occurs after the Glenn. Therefore, a limited pulmonary blood flow leads to a situation of low cardiac output and when there is fenestration significant cyanosis. Cyanosis may also be observed when there are intrapulmonary arteriovenous malformations (such as after the Glenn) or due to ventilation-perfusion imbalance that occurs in these situations of low cardiac output [16].

If the high pulmonary vascular resistance is responsible for the elevation of central venous pressure it is indicated to start with conventional treatments as supplemental oxygen, hyperventilation and alkalosis. As in patients with bidirectional Glenn, the use of high positive pressure during ventilation to achieve these ends may be counterproductive. To avoid high pressure ventilation may increase the minute volume and cardiac output and high frequency ventilation may decrease the PaCO2 at low airway pressures [13]. Intravenous vasodilators such as prostacyclin or prostaglandin E, should be used with caution, because of the risk of systemic vasodilatation with limited cardiac output. Inhaled NO has been referred to in several studies as an effective drug to lower the transpulmonary pressure gradient [8].

The presence of a low cardiac output with high central venous pressure in left atria, indicates dysfunction in patients with Fontan circulation. Myocardial dysfunction may occur during ischemia-reperfusion period, when aortic clamping and cardioplegia used to create the connection. You may also be related to poor preoperative myocardial function. The only effective therapy for low cardiac output due to ventricular dysfunction Fontan intervention is to improve cardiac output by inotropic agents and reduce the pressure in the left atrium. The use of inotropic agents such as phosphodiesterase inhibitors, dobutamine or low doses of epinephrine (less than 0.05 microgrs/kg/minute) may be helpful. If systemic blood pressure could tolerate it, an aggressive reduction of afterload with vasodilating agents (ONi in short term and sildenafil in long term [14]) may also reduce left atrial pressure in a meaningful way. If there is good reason to believe that the ventricular dysfunction is reversible, mechanical circulatory support (ECMO) could also be an effective therapy [15]. Because in those with persistent Fontan aorto-pulmonary collaterals may be associated with hemodynamic status similar to those with left ventricular dysfunction, aggressive evaluation and embolization of these collateral could be useful in these situations [17].

3. Conclusions

"Univentricular heart" denotes a wide variety of rare and complex congenital cardiac malformations whereby both atria predominantly egress into a functional single ventricle. Although most patients will be managed by a staged surgical approach in view of an ultimate Fontan procedure, a minority will not undergo Fontan palliation either because they maintain reasonably balanced systemic and pulmonary circulations or as a result of unfavorable hemodynamics.

Following major improvements of the surgical technique, modified Fontan operations represent a well accepted treatment for separation of pulmonary and systemic circulation in children with functionally univentricular hearts. Optimisation of flow dynamics was achieved by introduction of total cavopulmonary anastomosis, which can be performed either as a lateral tunnel (**Figure 4**) or as an extracardiac conduit procedure (**Figure 5**). Staging the Fontan procedure by a bidirectional cavopulmonary anastomosis with early relief

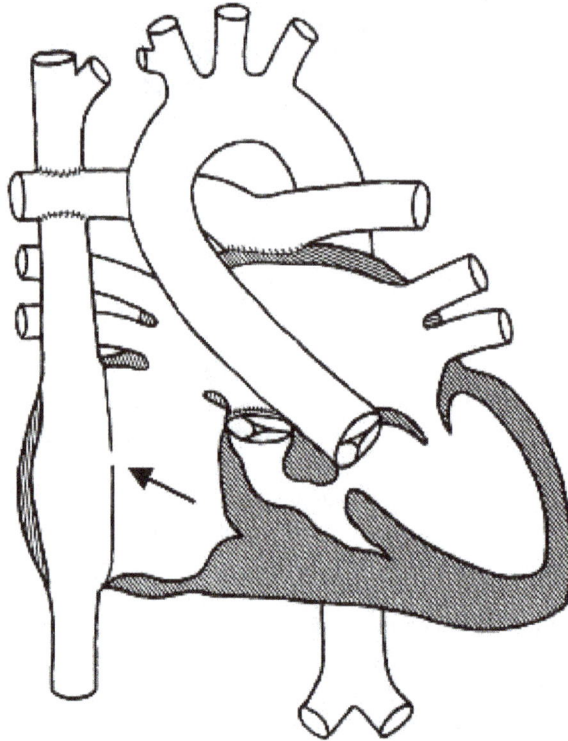

Figure 4. Superior and inferior cavo-pulmonary connection with lateral tunnel (Intracardiac Fontan).

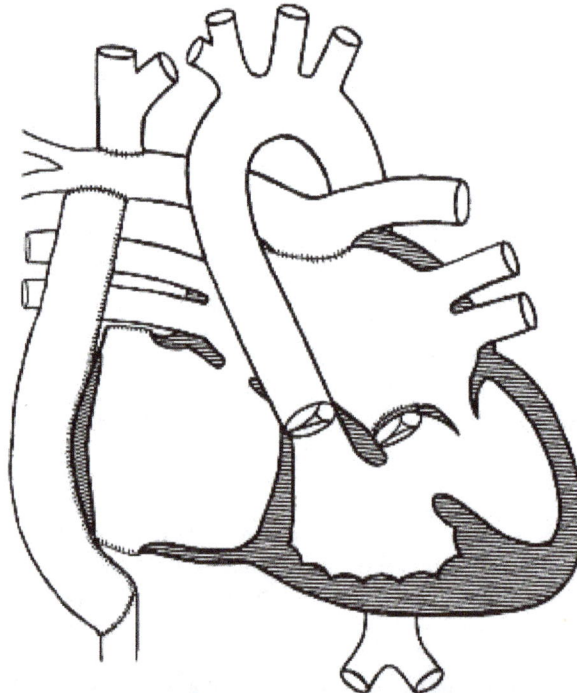

Figure 5. Superior and inferior cavo-pulmonary connection with extracardiac conduit (Extracardiac Fontan).

of volume load on the single ventricle and later completion of the Fontan circulation reduced the perioperative risk. Despite reduced operative mortality there remains a worrying decrement during long term follow up due to sequelae and complications of the univentricular circulation [18].

References

[1]   Khairi, P., Poirier, N. and Mercier, L.-A. (2007) Congenital Heart Desease for the Adult Cardiologist. Univentricular Heart. *Circulation*, **115**, 800-812.

[2]   De Oliveira, N.C., Ashburn, D.A., Khalid, F., *et al.* (2004) Prevention of Early Sudden Circulatory Collapse after the Norwood Operation. *Circulation*, **110**, II133-II138. http://dx.doi.org/10.1161/01.CIR.0000138399.30587.8e

[3]   Hoffman, G.M., Tweddell, J.S., Ghanayem, N.S., *et al.* (2004) Alteration of the Critical Arteriovenous Oxygen Saturation Relationship by Sustained Afterload Reduction after the Norwood Procedure. *Journal of Thoracic and Cardiovascular Surgery*, **127**, 738-745. http://dx.doi.org/10.1016/S0022-5223(03)01315-1

[4]   Chang, A.C., Hanley, F.L., Wernovsky, G., *et al.* (1993) Early Bidireccional Cavopulmonary Shunt in Young Infants. Postoperative Course and Early Results. *Circulation*, **88**, II149-II158.

[5]   Berdat, P.A., Belli, E., Lacour-Gayet, F., Planché, C. and Serraf, A. (2005) Additional Pulmonary Blood Flow Has No Adverse Effect on Outcome after Bidirectional Cavopulmonary Anastomosis. *The Annals of Thoracic Surgery*, **79**, 29-37. http://dx.doi.org/10.1016/j.athoracsur.2004.06.002

[6]   Freedom, R.M., Nykanen, D. and Benson Lee, N. (1998) The Physiology of the Bidirectional Cavopulmonary Connection. *The Annals of Thoracic Surgery*, **66**, 664-667. http://dx.doi.org/10.1016/S0003-4975(98)00618-3

[7]   Bradley, S.M., Simsic, J.M. and Mulvihill, D.M. (1998) Hyperventilation Impairs Oxygenation after Bidirectional Superior Cavopulmonary Connection. *Circulation*, **98**, II372-II376.

[8]   Gamillscheg, A., Zobel, G., Urlesberger, B., *et al.* (1997) Inhaled Nitric Oxide in Patients with Critical Pulmonary Perfusion after Fontan-Type Procedures and Bydireccional Glenn Anastomosis. *Journal of Thoracic and Cardiovascular Surgery*, **113**, 435-442. http://dx.doi.org/10.1016/S0022-5223(97)70355-6

[9]   Lee, T.M., Aiyagari, R., Hirsch, J.C., Ohye, R.G., Bove, E.L. and Devaney, E.J. (2012) Risk Factor Analysis for Second-Stage Palliation of Single Ventricle Anatomy. *The Annals of Thoracic Surgery*, **93**, 614-619. http://dx.doi.org/10.1016/j.athoracsur.2011.10.012

[10]   Alsoufi, B., *et al.* (2012) Current Outcomes of the Glenn Bidirectional Cavopulmonary Connection for Single Ventricle Palliation. *European Journal Cardio-Thoracic Surgery*, **72**, 42-49. http://dx.doi.org/10.1093/ejcts/ezr280

[11]   Bridges, N.D., Lock, J.E. and Castaneda, A.R. (1990) Baffle Fenestration with Subsequent Transcatheter Closure. Modification of the Fontan Operatión for Patients at Increased Risk. *Circulation*, **82**, 1681-1689. http://dx.doi.org/10.1161/01.CIR.82.5.1681

[12]   Lemler, M.F., Scott, W.A., Leonard, S.R., *et al.* (2002) Fenestration Improves Clinical Outcome of the Fontan Procedure. *Circulation*, **105**, 207-212. http://dx.doi.org/10.1161/hc0202.102237

[13]   Shekerdemian, L.S., Bush, A., Shore, D.F., *et al.* (1997) Cardiopulmonary Interaction after Fontan Operations: Augmentation of Cardiac Output Using Negative Pressure Ventilation. *Circulation*, **96**, 3934-3942. http://dx.doi.org/10.1161/01.CIR.96.11.3934

[14]   Tunks, R.D., *et al.* (2014) Sildenafil Exposure and Hemodynamic Effect after Fontan Surgery. *Pediatric Critical Care Medicine*, **15**, 28-34. http://dx.doi.org/10.1097/PCC.0000000000000007

[15]   Kaulitz, R. and Hofbeck, M. (2005) Current Treatment and Prognosis in Children with Functionally Univentricular Hearts. *Archives of Disease in Childhood*, **90**, 757-762. http://dx.doi.org/10.1136/adc.2003.034090

[16]   Spicer, R.L., Uzark, K.C., Moore, J.W., *et al.* (1996) Aortopulmonary Collateral Vessels and Prolonged Pleural Effusions after Modified Fontan Procedures. *American Heart Journal*, **131**, 1164-1168. http://dx.doi.org/10.1016/S0002-8703(96)90092-7

[17]   Triedman, J.K., Bridges, N.D., Mayer, J.E.J., *et al.* (1993) Prevalence and Risk Factors for Aortopulmonary Collateral Vessels after Fontan and Bidireccional Glenn Procedures. *Journal of the American College of Cardiology*, **22**, 207-215.

[18]   Lastinger, L. and Zaidi, A.N. (2013) The Adult With a Fontan: A Panacea without a Cure? *Circulation Journal*, **77**, 2672-2681. http://dx.doi.org/10.1253/circj.CJ-13-1105

Changes in Congenital Anomaly Incidence in West Coast and Pacific States (USA) after Arrival of Fukushima Fallout

Joseph Mangano*, Janette D. Sherman

Radiation and Public Health Project, New York, USA
Email: *odiejoe@aol.com

Abstract

Radioactive fallout after the March 2011 Fukushima nuclear meltdown entered the U.S. environment within days; levels of radioactivity were particularly elevated in the five western states bordering on the Pacific Ocean. The particular sensitivity of the fetus to radiation exposure, and the ability of radioisotopes to attach to cells, tissues, and DNA raise the question of whether fetuses/newborns with birth defects with the greater exposures suffered elevated harm during the period after the meltdown. We compare rates of five congenital anomalies for 2010 and 2011 births from April-November. The increase of 13.00% in the five western states is significantly greater than the 3.77% decrease for all other U.S. states combined (CI 0.030 - 0.205, p < 0.008). Consistent patterns of elevated increases are observed in the west (20 of 21 comparisons, 6 of which are statistically significant/borderline significant), by state, type of birth defect, month of birth, and month of conception. While these five anomalies are relatively uncommon (about 7500 cases per year in the U.S.), sometimes making statistical significance difficult to achieve, the consistency of the results lend strength to the analysis, and suggest fetal harm from Fukushima may have occurred in western U.S. states.

Keywords

Birth Defects, Fukushima, Radiation, Meltdown, Nuclear Plant

1. Introduction

The harmful effects of radiation exposure to chromosomes have been known for nearly a century, starting with the discovery of chromosomal deformities in irradiated fruit flies [1]. Experiments with mice [2] [3] and rats [4] confirmed this knowledge, and documented elevated risk for congenital defects, at relatively low doses of ex-

*Corresponding author.

posure. Populations exposed to pre-conception X-rays have been shown to have higher congenital anomalies [5] as were those living in areas with relatively high background radiation [6][7].

One form of radiation, byproducts of uranium or plutonium fission, was first introduced into the environment from weapons and reactors seven decades ago [8]-[10]. These isotopes bind with cells, tissues, and DNA of the unborn, and thus risks of congenital defects in irradiated populations have been studied. The first documented excesses of congenital anomalies were among children of survivors of the Hiroshima and Nagasaki bombings. [8]-[10]. During the 1950s, reports of various defects among newborns in the Marshall Islands, the site of 67 large-scale U.S. nuclear weapons tests, were made public. Other studies found links with between atmospheric tests and elevated birth defects, including a high rate of Down Syndrome in northwest England in 1963-1964, the peak period of global fallout from tests [11]. Another report documented elevated birth defect incidence near the Hanford nuclear weapons plant in Washington state (USA) [12].

The 1986 meltdown at Chernobyl produced numerous reports of certain congenital anomalies among populations subject to fallout from the stricken reactor. One documented a doubling of congenital developmental anomalies among infants born to fathers who worked as liquidators to contain the meltdown [13]. Various analyses presented elevated congenital anomaly rates in various parts of the Belarus region, which received the greatest doses of radioactivity from the meltdown, in the years following Chernobyl [14]-[22]. Other research also found high birth defect rates in the Ukraine [23] [24], Bulgaria [25], Croatia [26], and Germany [27]-[30] including areas with fallout levels well below those Belarussian sites closest to the reactor.

Post-Chernobyl studies also identified elevated rates of specific anomalies, the most-analyzed of which was Down syndrome (Trisomy-21), mostly in Germany [31]-[39]. Other conditions included neural tube defects in Turkey [40]-[43], cleft lip/palate in Germany [44] [45], and anencephaly in Turkey [46]. Meta-analyses concluded that a pattern of elevated congenital anomaly rates was associated with exposure to the Chernobyl meltdown [47]-[49].

No published reports exist on the change in congenital defects rates in Japan after the March 2011 meltdown at Fukushima. However, at least one report examines morphological abnormality rates in aphids in the first sexual reproduction period after the meltdown, and found a 13.2% rate close to Fukushima vs. 3.8% in seven control areas [50].

Changes in the rate of one type of birth defect, congenital hypothyroidism, have been reported. In the five U.S. states bordering on the Pacific Ocean, with the most elevated levels of environmental radiation after the meltdown, a 16% increase in incidence of the disorder was observed in the nine months following the meltdown, compared to a 3% decrease in 36 other U.S. states [51]. The gap was particularly large (28% increase vs. a 4% decrease) in the first 14 weeks after the arrival of fallout. In addition, the rate of California newborns with a Thyroid Stimulating Hormone score of 19 micro international units per milliliter of blood during initial screening, was 27% greater in the nine months after the meltdown compared to other periods in 2011-2012 [52]. The known affinity for radioactive iodine to attack cell membranes and DNA in the thyroid gland indicates a potential link between Fukushima fallout and congenital hypothyroidism.

Historical reports linking exposure to ionizing radiation with congenital anomaly risk, plus the initial reports on congenital hypothyroidism in the western U.S. suggest further analysis be conducted on other birth defects.

The U.S. Centers for Disease Control and Prevention (CDC) publishes national data collected by state health departments on incidence of five congenital anomalies in the nation. These include Anencephaly, Cleft Lip/Palate, Down Syndrome, Omphalocele/Gastroschisis, and Spina Bifida/Meningocele [53]. Approximately 7500 cases of these five defects occur in the U.S. each year. As of mid-2014, the CDC web site contained complete birth defect data for the years 2007 to 2012.

These five specific anomalies to be addressed in this report, merit some discussion, including their suspected link with radiation exposure.

Anencephaly is a type of neural tube defect in which the baby is missing major portions of the brain and skull, resulting in stillbirths or death within the perinatal period. Neural tube defects, which begin during the first month of pregnancy, have been reduced by increased intake of folic acid during pregnancy. Conversely, risk of anencephaly has been found to increase due to exposure to X-rays and neutrons in mouse zygotes [54].

Cleft palate or cleft lip are marked by a (usually unilateral) separation of the upper lip and palate, due to faulty fusion of the medial, nasal, and maxillary processes. The condition can be surgically repaired in some cases, but requires special care of the infant to prevent choking or aspiration until the surgery can be performed. Among the risk factors identified for cleft palate/lip are environmental pollutants, including radiation exposure [55].

Down syndrome, also Trisomy-21, features growth delays, similar facial and hand features and substantial intellectual deficits. The majority of cases detected during pregnancy in the developed world result in abortion. Known causes are still emerging, but exposure to radiation and other chemical toxins have been established as one. Down syndrome is the most-studied congenital defect after the Chernobyl meltdown.

Gastroschisis occurs when the muscles of the abdomen do not close along the mid-ventral line and the intestines and liver remain outside the abdomen. Omphalocele, a related condition in which the intestines and liver remain outside the body at birth, is a defect much larger than gastroschisis. It occurs when the viscera occupy a thin sac of peritoneum located at the base of the umbilical cord. Gastroschisis risk has been found to be elevated after maternal irradiation, even at relatively low doses [56].

Spina Bifida/meningocele is a prenatal failure of the embryonic neural tube to close over the spinal cord, leaving the cord unprotected by the bony cover and open to trauma and infection. When only the membrane covering the spinal cord encloses the protruding fluid-filled sac, the condition is known as menigocele. Surgical repair is sometimes successful, but many with the disorder suffer mental, neurological, and other physical disabilities. Radiation exposure has been linked with risk of this disorder [57].

Our hypothesis is that the 2010-2011 rate change of these five anomalies increased more sharply in the five Pacific/West Coast states than the rest of the U.S., based on the presence of elevated levels of fallout from the Fukushima meltdown in the period following March 2011, and the well-documented pattern of risk to humans irradiated *in utero*.

2. Materials and Methods

One important component of the methodology identifies areas of the U.S. with the greatest exposure levels after Fukushima fallout entered the environment. Unfortunately, official measurements of isotope-specific concentrations are very limited. For example, the U.S. Environmental Protection Agency (EPA) measured just 77 samples of Iodine-131 in precipitation in the U.S. during spring 2011, of which 70 revealed a detectable amount—with no such samples in the same period of 2010—far short of a reliable sample. The number of other isotope-specific samples is well below 77 for 2011, and virtually zero in 2010 [58].

The only measure of radioactivity with large numbers of measurements in the period just after Fukushima, when environmental radiation was highest (March 15-April 30, 2011), along with the prior year, is not a specific isotope, but airborne beta emitters, or "gross beta". During this 47 day period, well over 1000 samples with detectable concentrations were collected by the EPA at over 100 U.S. stations. Because gross beta is a broad measure, it is reasonable to use it as a proxy for relative exposures in this report. The most elevated levels of environmental radioactivity in the U.S. after Fukushima occurred in the states bordering the Pacific Ocean (California, Oregon, and Washington), plus Alaska and Hawaii. **Table 1** shows the increase in airborne gross beta radioactivity for 18 sites in the five states, compared to 31 other U.S. sites with the most frequently reported data (typically 1 - 2 measurements per week). We also present the increase for 10 of the 18 sites in the five states that consistently report data (1 - 2 measurements per week), which show similar patterns.

In a previous report, we summarized EPA measurements on the 2010 and 2011 gross beta from January 1 to October 4 [51]—the most recent data at the time, and a reasonable measure of relative dose to the U.S. population in the two years in the period of highest Fukushima fallout and other periods.

For most of the period January 1 to October 4, the ratio of 2011 to 2010 beta averages was similar across the U.S. (0.983 for 18 sites in the western states, 1.018 for 31 non-western U.S. sites). But in the period March 15 to April 30, immediately after Fukushima fallout arrived, the 2011/2010 ratio for the 18 sites in the western states (7.345), was considerably higher than the 31 non-western U.S. sites (2.397). Although this is not a comprehensive assessment of dose by geographic area, it supports the belief that the greater exposures from the meltdown occurred in the five western states, using a broad measure of radiation such as gross beta. Appendix 1 shows the radiation measurement sites used.

The group that will be most susceptible to damage are those *in utero* during the period of highest environmental radioactivity levels (March 15 to April 30, 2011). March 2011 births were not included because those born early in the month were born before Fukushima. December 2011 births were not included, since 5% were not conceived by April 30, and another 5% were conceived in late April, when radiation levels were elevated, but well below those in late March.

This report will compare 2010 and 2011 rates of five birth defects for births during the eight months of April to November. The five Pacific/West Coast states will be compared with the other 45 states (plus the District of Columbia). Virtually all 2011 births in these months were *in utero* during the period of highest fallout in the spring of 2011, testing the hypothesis that elevated congenital anomaly rates occurred as fetuses were exposed to Fukushima radiation. The birth defect rates are given in cases per 100,000 births. Only those births in which a "yes" or "no" is given for presence of a birth defect in the CDC web site are included in the denominator; excluded are 0.80% of 2010 and 2011 births with the anomaly status "not stated".

Included in the analysis will be the total of all births in the eight-month period, along with subsets (by month of birth, state, type of birth defect, month of conception, and birth weight). Birth defect rates by month of conception will include live births conceived in September, October, November, and December 2010, meaning they were in their 3rd, 4th, 5th, and 6th month *in utero* when the Fukushima meltdown occurred. These will be compared with cohorts conceived at the same time for the prior year (conceived September to December 2009). To obtain month of conception, the month of birth and weeks of gestation at birth were matched (**Table 2**). Only those births of at least 29 weeks gestation, including about 97% of live births, are included, since some of those April-November 2011 births with shorter gestation periods were born before the meltdown.

Table 1. Change in average airborne gross beta concentrations, five pacific/west coast states vs. other U.S., 2010-2011.

Year	Average Airborne Gross Beta Concentrations (n)		
	5 States (18 Sites)	5 States (10 Sites)	Other U.S.
March 15-April 30			
2010	0.005112 (190)	0.005130 (132)	0.008527 (401)
2011	0.033016 (225)	0.029563 (138)	0.020204 (378)
2011/2010 Ratio**	7.345	5.253	2.397
Other Dates January 1-October 4			
2010	0.006027 (853)	0.006184 (660)	0.009573 (1810)
2011	0.005526 (858)	0.005550 (564)	0.009670 (1679)
2011/2010 Ratio**	0.983	0.0889	1.018
3/15-4/30 ratio/ Other Dates ratio	7.472	5.909	2.355

*Ten sites in West Coast/Pacific states report gross beta regularly (at least 11 measurements for each site in spring 2010 and 2011, and at least 44 measurements for other January 1-October 4 in 2010 and 2011); the column with 18 sites includes those with less regular measurements; **Ratios represent total gross beta averages for all sites divided by number of sites; Source: United States Environmental Protection Agency. Envirofacts. http://oaspub.enviro/erams.gov_query.simple_query. All averages in picocuries of gross beta per cubic meter of air.

Table 2. Computation of month of conception, by birth month and weeks gestation at birth.

Conceived		Weeks Gestation at Birth				
		29 - 32	33 - 36	37 - 40	41 - 44	45 - 47
Sept. 2010	Born	4/11	5/11	6/11	7/11	8/11
Oct. 2010	Born	5/11	6/11	7/11	8/11	9/11
Nov. 2010	Born	6/11	7/11	8/11	9/11	10/11
Dec. 2010	Born	7/11	8/11	9/11	10/11	11/11
Sept. 2009	Born	4/10	5/10	6/10	7/11	8/10
Oct. 2009	Born	5/10	6/10	7/10	8/11	9/10
Nov. 2009	Born	6/10	7/10	8/10	9/11	10/10
Dec. 2009	Born	7/10	8/10	9/10	10/11	11/10

Source: U.S. Centers for Disease Control and Prevention (http://wonder.cdc.gov/natality.html).

The statistical significance of differences in 2010-2011 changes between the two groups of states will be tested using a formula (below) that creates a 95% confidence interval of the differences [59]. If the upper and lower bounds of the confidence interval both exceed zero, the difference is statistically significant.

$$\text{VAR SIR}_1 = [(5 \text{ State } \text{SE}_1^2 * \text{Other US } \text{Rate}_1^2) + (\text{Other US } \text{SE}_1^2 * 5 \text{ State } \text{Rate}_1^2)) / \text{Other US } \text{Rate}_1^4]$$

$$\text{VAR SIR}_2 = [(5 \text{ State } \text{SE}_2^2 * \text{Other US } \text{Rate}_2^2) + (\text{Other US } \text{SE}_2^2 * 5 \text{ State } \text{Rate}_2^2)) / \text{Other US } \text{Rate}_2^4]$$

SIR stands for Standard Incidence Ratio, SE for Standard Error, and Rate for Cases of a Defect per 100,000. The subscript of $_1$ represents the year 2010, while the subscript of $_2$ represents the year 2011. To convert a confidence interval to a p-value (any value under 0.05 is considered statistically significant), an exponential function using the z-score in the following formula (inverse of a logarithm) is used:

$$p = \exp((-0.717 * (\text{absolute value z})) - (0.416 * z^2))$$

The z score is obtained by subtracting the lower limit from the upper limit of the confidence interval, and dividing the result by the Standard Error.

3. Results

The 2010-2011 change in incidence rates of all five birth defects combined, for births during the eight months of April to November, along with the two four-month periods, are given in **Table 3**.

The birth defect rate for all five defects combined increased +13.00% in the five Pacific/West Coast states for births from April to November. During this time, the number of diagnosed cases rose from 600 to 672. The corresponding rate for the rest of the U.S. decreased −3.77%, as the number of cases declined from 4378 to 4180. This difference was statistically significant (CI 0.030 - 0.205, p < 0.008). For births in the two four month periods, the rates increased for western states and declined for all other U.S. states (+10.85% vs. −3.38% for April-July births, and +15.12% vs. −1.26% for August-November births). Differences were statistically significant for the earlier four months (CI 0.004 - 0.246, p < 0.05) and of borderline significance for the latter four months (CI −0.006 - 0.230, p < 0.07).

These 2010-2011 changes in all defects combined for April-November births are presented for each of the five states (residency of mother at birth) in **Table 4**.

A 2010-2011 increase in birth defect rates was observed for each of the five states, including Alaska (+69.52%), California (+11.88%), Hawaii (+3.90%), Oregon (+8.87%), and Washington (+15.53%). Compared to the −3.77% decline for all other U.S. states, only the California increase achieved statistical significance (CI

Table 3. Change in incidence rates, five birth defects combined, April/November 2010 vs. April/November 2011 births, five pacific/west coast states vs. other U.S.

Birth Date	Rate/100,000 (n) 5 States	Rate/100,000 (n) Other U.S.	95% CI/ Significance
April-November (8 months)			
2010	133.22 (600)	196.90 (4378)	
2011	150.54 (672)	189.47 (4180)	
% Ch. Rate	13.00%	−3.77%	0.030 - 0.205 (p < 0.008)
April-July (4 months)			
2010	134.61 (297)	197.93 (2178)	
2011	149.22 (331)	190.36 (2018)	
% Ch. Rate	10.85%	−3.38%	0.004 - 0.246 (p < 0.05)
August-November (4 months)			
2010	131.90 (303)	195.89 (2200)	
2011	151.84 (341)	193.43 (2162)	
% Ch. Rate	15.12%	−1.26%	−0.006 - 0.230 (p < 0.07)

Source: U.S. Centers for Disease Control and Prevention (http://wonder.cdc.gov/natality.html).

Table 4. Change in incidence rates, five birth defects combined, April-November 2010 vs. April-November 2011 births, each of five pacific/west coast states vs. other U.S.

State	Rate/100,000 (n)	% Ch. Rate	95% CI/ Significance
Alaska			
2010	152.30 (10)		
2011	258.18 (15)	69.52%	
California			
2010	101.73 (349)		
2011	113.81 (385)	11.88%	0.001 - 0.167 (p < 0.05)
Hawaii			
2010	250.39 (32)		
2011	260.15 (33)	3.90%	
Oregon			
2010	304.15 (94)		
2011	331.13 (102)	8.87%	
Washington			
2010	201.56 (115)		
2011	232.86 (137)	15.53%	
Other U.S.			
2010	196.90 (4378)		
2011	189.47 (4180)	−3.77%	

Source: U.S. Centers for Disease Control and Prevention (http://wonder.cdc.gov/natality.html).

0.001 - 0.167, p < 0.05), as 58% of the birth defects in the five states occur to California residents. The unusually large rise in Alaska is countered by the small number of cases (10 and 15 for each year), rendering the change not statistically significant.

In addition to each state, changes for each type of birth defect are analyzed. **Table 5** compares 2010-2011 incidence changes for the five West Coast/Pacific states combined with those of all other U.S. states, for April-November births.

For each of the five defects, we observe an increase from 2010-2011 in the five West Coast/Pacific states and a decline in the remaining states. However, none of the differences were statistically significant. The largest difference in the change of the two areas occurred for Anencephaly (+41.24% vs. −3.13%); however, this defect is the rarest of the five (in the Pacific/West Coast states, the 2010 total of 30 cases rose to 42 the following year), and thus is not significant. The difference in changes was also substantial for Omphalocele/Gastroschisis (+23.86% vs. −0.55%); the difference was the closest of the five to achieve statistical significance (p < 0.17).

Changes in congenital anomaly incidence are also analyzed according to the number of weeks of gestation at birth. **Table 6** provides this information, for births at 17 - 32 weeks, 33 - 36 weeks, 37 - 40 weeks, and 41 - 47 weeks.

Again, incidence in the West Coast/Pacific states increased, and declined for all other U.S. states, for each of the four gestation groups. The difference for those births within the normal gestation of 37 - 40 weeks (+16.05% vs. −3.52%) was statistically significant (CI 0.015 - 0.257, p < 0.03), as 64% of the five birth defects occur in this group. Gaps in the differences in changes of the two groups of over 20 percentage points were observed for the lowest (17 - 32 weeks) and highest (41 - 47 weeks) gestation groups, although neither was statistically significant.

Table 5. Change in incidence rates, each of five birth defects, April-November 2010 vs. April-November 2011 births, five pacific/west coast states vs. other U.S.

Birth Defect	Rate/100,000 (n)	Rate/100,000 (n)
	5 States	Other U.S.
Anencephaly		
2010	6.66 (30)	11.56 (257)
2011	9.41 (42)	11.20 (247)
% Ch. Rate	41.24%	−3.13%
Cleft Lip/Palate		
2010	56.84 (256)	76.05 (1691)
2011	59.59 (266)	72.03 (1589)
% Ch. Rate	4.83%	−5.29%
Down Syndrome		
2010	38.63 (174)	51.09 (1136)
2011	43.91 (196)	50.00 (1103)
% Ch. Rate	13.64%	−2.14%
Omphalocele/Gastroschisis		
2010	22.43 (101)	40.75 (906)
2011	27.78 (124)	40.52 (894)
% Ch. Rate	23.86%	−0.55%
Spina Bifida/Meningocele		
2010	8.86 (39)	17.00 (378)
2011	9.86 (44)	15.82 (349)
% Ch. Rate	13.82%	−6.94%

Source: U.S. Centers for Disease Control and Prevention (http://wonder.cdc.gov/natality.html).

We also address 2010-2011 changes in birth defect rates for the pre- and post-Fukushima birth cohorts by month of conception. In the methods section, the number of birth defects and live births for those conceived September, October, November, and December 2009 and 2010, with gestation periods 29 - 47 weeks, are identified. **Table 7** compares the changes in rates for the four sets of birth cohorts.

For newborns conceived in October and December, the 2010-2011 change in the congenital anomaly rate was roughly equal for the West Coast/Pacific states and the remainder of the U.S. For those conceived in November, the rate change in the west (+33.64%) was much higher than the other U.S. states (−1.41%). Those conceived in November 2010 were four months *in utero* when the Fukushima meltdown occurred. The difference was of borderline significance (CI −0.024 - 0.478, p < 0.08). The difference for those conceived in September was substantial (+20.35% vs. −7.68%), but fell short of statistical significance.

4. Discussion

This report addresses changes in rates of certain birth defects after the Fukushima nuclear meltdown. While we await the critical data from Japan, where the greatest exposures occurred, we focus on the USA. Our hypothesis that areas in the U.S. which received elevated levels of environmental radioactivity from the Fukushima meltdown are at risk for increased birth defects is based on the documented evidence of cellular damage from radiation exposure, the particular sensitivity of the fetus to radiation, and numerous reports of elevated congenital

Table 6. Change in incidence rate, five birth defects, April-November 2010 vs. April-November 2011 births, five pacific/west coast states vs. other U.S. by weeks gestation at birth.

	Rate/100,000 (n)	Rate/100,000 (n)	95% Conf. Int./
			Significance
Weeks	5 States	Other U.S.	
17 - 32 weeks			
2010	441.66 (38)	502.32 (296)	
2011	539.21 (46)	516.84 (296)	
% Ch Rate	22.09%	2.89%	
33 - 36 weeks			
2010	358.92 (128)	441.81 (942)	
2011	376.06 (129)	440.72 (909)	
% Ch Rate	4.78%	−0.25%	
37 - 40 weeks			
2010	110.57 (377)	165.31 (2729)	
2011	128.32 (435)	159.48 (2612)	
% Ch Rate	16.05%	−3.52%	0.015 - 0.257 ($p < 0.03$)
41 - 47 weeks			
2010	87.50 (57)	136.78 (411)	
2011	96.01 (62)	119.10 (363)	
% Ch Rate	9.73%	−12.93%	

Source: U.S. Centers for Disease Control and Prevention (http://wonder.cdc.gov/natality.html).

anomaly rates after exposure to fallout from atomic bomb detonations and nuclear reactor meltdowns.

We find a consistent pattern of excess 2010-2011 increases in birth defect rates in the five West Coast/Pacific states, compared to the rest of the U.S., for the eight-month period April-November. The April-November 2011 birth cohort was exposed to Fukushima radioactivity while *in utero*. Analyses are presented by birth month, state, defect, gestation length, and conception month. There was a greater increase in the five West Coast/Pacific states in 20 of 21 comparisons. There were four categories that achieved statistical significance at $p < 0.05$ or less, including all defects combined ($p < 008$), April-July births ($p < 0.05$), California births ($p < 0.05$), and births 37 - 40 weeks gestation ($p < 0.03$). Two others were borderline significant at $p < 0.10$, including August-November births ($p < 0.07$) and births conceived the prior November ($p < 0.08$). Changes in categories with relatively small numbers of anomalies, such as individual months, are consistently elevated for the West Coast/Pacific state but vary greatly, often fail to achieve significance, and demonstrate no consistent pattern.

The relatively small number of events in many of the 21 comparisons makes it difficult to achieve statistical significance. However, the consistency of results, namely that the increase in the five West Coast/Pacific states is greater in 20 of 21 comparisons, lends strength to the analysis.

This is just the first attempt to analyze post-2010 changes in U.S. congenital anomaly rates, and proposes a hypothesis that one potential factor—radioactive fallout from a nuclear reactor meltdown—might account for temporal increases in the most-affected areas. The results need to be augmented by consideration of the many other potential factors that might contribute to such trends. Just a few examples of these many factors include access to medical care, poverty status, preventative measures prior to birth, and exposure to other environmental toxins. We strongly encourage analyses of other factors.

These trends merit further analysis. The annual rate of cases per 100,000 live births (April to November) for the five West Coast/Pacific states moved from 150.71 (2009), to 133.22 (2010), to 150.04 (2011). Thus, the rise from

Table 7. Change in incidence rates, five birth defects, April-November 2010 vs. April-November 2011 births, five pacific/west coast states vs. other U.S. by month conceived, Sept.-December 2010.

Conceived	Rate/100,000 (n)	Rate/100,000 (n)	95% CI/
	5 States	Other U.S.	Significance
December, prior to year below			
2010	143.99 (84)	186.58 (525)	
2011	149.04 (84)	194.17 (542)	
% Ch Rate	3.51%	4.07%	
November, prior to year below			
2010	119.61 (70)	187.22 (534)	
2011	159.85 (93)	184.58 (537)	
% Ch Rate	33.64%	−1.41%	−0.024 - 0.478 (p < 0.08)
October, prior to year below			
2010	142.05 (81)	198.30 (558)	
2011	129.82 (74)	176.72 (504)	
% Ch Rate	−8.61%	−10.88%	
September, prior to year below			
2010	140.38 (77)	206.69 (570)	
2011	168.89 (94)	190.82 (526)	
% Ch Rate	20.35%	−7.68%	

Source: U.S. Centers for Disease Control and Prevention (http://wonder.cdc.gov/natality.html).

2010-2011, representing those births *in utero* at the time of Fukushima, was preceded by a decline from 2009-2010. Potential long-term changes after exposure to Fukushima fallout after 2011 should be addressed in future reports.

The five birth defects included in this analysis are relatively uncommon, accounting for about 7500 annual cases among 4,000,000 U.S. births, but are unmistakable in diagnosis. We note that rates of the five birth defects are lower in the West Coast/Pacific states than that in the U.S. as a whole. Identifying reasons that may account for this pattern—such as racial and ethnic distribution, poverty, access to health care, and medical risk factors—should be made. However, it is unlikely that changes in these potential causes over a short time (2010 vs. 2011) would account for such large and consistent differences in temporal changes between areas with different levels of irradiation.

Since changes in birth defect rates after Fukushima is a yet-unaddressed topic, a number of additional analyses can be made, which we present here.

Defining pre- and post-Fukushima periods is one area of further analysis. We selected the years 2010 and 2011, as we believe that the best representation of a period prior to an event like a meltdown is that immediately before it occurs. However, future reviews might expand on these time periods. Data on birth defect rates beginning 2007 are available, so two-, three-, and four-year baselines can be used, and birth defect data after 2011 merit consideration as they become available.

We present 2010-2011 gross beta data comparisons not just after Fukushima when fallout was highest, but also in the relatively unexposed time frame of all but 47 days of the 277 days from January 1 to October 4. In future analyses, contrasting these data for shorter periods, such as individual months, might be helpful to assess any changes from year to year.

Another major issue raised by studies such as this is defining relative doses or exposures to populations. We use airborne gross beta measurements as a proxy for relative exposure to Americans soon after Fukushima. While the number of gross beta measurements in the selected U.S. sites are large (591 and 603 in the period March 15 to April 30, in 2010 and 2011), we acknowledge the lack of other frequently-conducted radiation measures. In particular, specific isotope concentrations in air, water, soil, and food are virtually non-existent (which also occurred after the 1986 Chernobyl meltdown, with even larger fallout levels than post-Fukushima). It is critical that officials need to expand future sampling programs in order to enable greater ability in assessing dose-response relationships. Until that happens, however, we recognize that any health study, using the most meaningful data possible, is crucial to better understanding of this most important topic—even if a precise dose-response is still in its early phases. The much greater rise in airborne gross beta in the west coast and Pacific states (vs. the rest of the U.S.) from spring 2010 to spring 2011 is a clear indicator of relatively greater exposures occurring in this area from fallout after the Fukushima catastrophe. The linear no-threshold model has been accepted by many to be most consistently observed in studies [60], but further studies of effects of overall doses are needed to possibly further refine the relationship.

Evidence to better understand the link between radiation exposure and birth defects has been evolving for decades. The biomedical basis for irradiated organisms causing defects in the fetus dates back to the experiments on fruit flies in the late 1920s [1] [61] [62]. Genetic changes to wild and domestic animals, birds, fish, rodents, mushrooms, insects, spiders, and bacteria after the 1986 Chernobyl meltdown corroborate these earliest discoveries [63] [64]. A lengthy number of reports cited earlier have identified unusually elevated birth defect rates among irradiated human populations.

Documentation of elevated congenital anomaly levels include those exposed to relatively high doses of radiation, including atomic bomb survivors at Hiroshima and Nagasaki, those irradiated by atmospheric nuclear weapons tests in the Marshall Islands, and those living near the Chernobyl reactor that underwent a total meltdown. The research community awaits analyses of congenital anomaly patterns among those exposed *in utero* to radiation from the Fukushima meltdown. Efforts to establish a consistent association between relatively low dose exposures and congenital anomaly risk are still evolving. The research establishing a risk of cancer death by age 10 after pelvic X-rays during pregnancy represents one form of a fetal insult resulting in subsequent manifestation of disease [65]-[67].

Birth defects result from damage to genes prior to fertilization or damage to the growing cells and tissues in the womb. Fetal insults that can result in defects in the unborn are associated with a number of chemicals, not just radiation. For example, multiple brain defects, as well as eye, facial, heart, genital and limb abnormalities resulted from exposure to the common pesticide chlorpyrifos [68]. Moreover, synergistic effects after exposure to multiple toxins occur. Biologist Rachel Carson's seminal work *Silent Spring*, which chiefly addressed effects of pesticides, also noted this synergy, specifically mentioning radiation: "In this now universal contamination of the environment, chemicals are the sinister and little recognized partners of radiation in changing the very nature of the world—the very nature of life" [69].

Continued analyses of congenital defects for those exposed to Fukushima fallout are critical. Such defects can include infant and perinatal deaths, stillbirths, low weight births, prematurity, cancer in very young children, and other anomalies. Understanding the short-term consequences to the very young can establish a basis for studies of longer-term effects on persons of all ages, which may only manifest after a latency of up to several decades.

The study of birth abnormalities should emphasize cause as much as detection and therapy, with the eventual goal of prevention. Each affected child causes not just physical and behavioral ramifications to the child, but huge economic and social burdens to the family and society, which may be responsible for the affected person's well-being for decades. A large-scale nuclear meltdown such as the Fukushima disaster presents one such opportunity to better understand cause and means of prevention. Building on the considerable epidemiological evidence of a radiation-congenital anomaly link, plus the knowledge of biochemical actions by radiation that lead to *in utero* anomalies, a much stronger effort is called for to better quantify the relative doses and the corresponding risk involved in radiation-induced birth defects.

References

[1]   Muller, H.J. (1928) The Effects of X-Radiation on Genes and Chromosomes. *Science*, **67**, 82.

[2]   Michel, C. and Fritz-Niggli, H. (1977) Radiation Damage in Mouse Embryos Exposed to 1 Rad X-Rays or Negative Pions. *Fortschr Roentgenstr*, **127**, 276-280. http://dx.doi.org/10.1055/s-0029-1230701

[3]   Rugh, R. and Grupp, E. (1959) X-Irradiation Exencephaly. *Radiation Therapy, Nuclear Medicine*, **81**, 1026-1052.

[4] United Nations Scientific Committee on the Effects of Atomic Radiation (UNSCEAR). Genetic and Somatic Effects of Ionizing Radiation. Report to the General Assembly. United Nations, New York, 1986.

[5] Goldberg M.S., Mayo, N.E., Levy, A.R., *et al.* (1998) Adverse Reproductive Outcomes among Women Exposed to Low Levels of Ionizing Radiation from Diagnostic Radiography for Adolescent Idiopathic Scoliosis. *Epidemiology*, **2**, 271-278. http://dx.doi.org/10.1097/00001648-199805000-00010

[6] Kochupillai, N., Verma, I.C., Grewal, M.S., *et al.* (1976) Down's Syndrome and Related Abnormalities in an Area of High Background Radiation in Coastal Kerala. *Nature*, **262**, 60-61. http://dx.doi.org/10.1038/262060a0

[7] Padmanabhan, V.T., Sugunan, A.P., Brahmaputhran, C.K., *et al.* (1994) Heritable Anomalies among the Inhabitants of Regions of Normal and High Background Radiation in Kerala: Results of a Cohort Study, 1988-1994. *International Journal of Health Services*, **34**, 483-515. http://dx.doi.org/10.2190/3XYE-QJPU-01BF-8YKE

[8] Yamazaki, N.J. and Schull, W.J. (1990) Perinatal Loss and Neurological Abnormalities among Children of the Atomic Bomb. *Journal of the American Medical Association*, **264**, 605-609.
http://dx.doi.org/10.1001/jama.1990.03450050063029

[9] Sawada, S. (2007) Cover-Up of the Effects of Internal Exposure by Residual Radiation from the Atomic Bombing of Hiroshima and Nagasaki. *Medicine, Conflict and Survival*, **23**, 58-74. http://dx.doi.org/10.1080/13623690601084617

[10] Schull, W.J., Otake, M. and Neel, J.V. (1981) Genetic Effects of the Atomic Bombs: A Reappraisal. *Science*, **213**, 1220-1227. http://dx.doi.org/10.1126/science.7268429

[11] Bound, J.P., Francis, B.J. and Harvey, P.W. (1995) Down's Syndrome: Prevalence and Ionizing Radiation in an Area of Northwest England, 1957-91. *Journal of Epidemiology and Community Health*, **49**, 164-170.
http://dx.doi.org/10.1136/jech.49.2.164

[12] Sever, L.E., Hessol, N.A., Gilbert, E.S. and McIntyre, J.M. (1988) The Prevalence at Birth of Congenital Malformations in Communities Near the Hanford Site. *American Journal of Epidemiology*, **127**, 243-254.

[13] Lyaginskaya, A.M., Tukov, A.R., Osypov, V.A., *et al.* (2007) Genetic Effects on the Liquidators. *Radiation Biology and Radioactivity*, **47**, 188-195. In: Yablokov, A.V., Nesternenko, V.B. and Nesterenko, A.V., Eds., *Chernobyl: Consequences of the Catastrophe for People and the Environment*, New York Academy of Sciences, New York.

[14] Lasjuk, G.I., Nykolaev, D.L. and Khmel, R.D. (1996) Absolute Number and Frequency of Congenital Malformations, Strict Accounting in Some Belarus Regions. *Biomedical Aspects of the Chernobyl Accident*, **1**, 15-17.

[15] Lazjuk, G.I., Nikolaev, D.L. and Novikova, I.V. (1997) Changes in Registered Congenital Anomalies in the Republic of Belarus after the Chernobyl Accident. *Stem Cells*, **15**, 255-260. http://dx.doi.org/10.1002/stem.5530150734

[16] Feshchenko, S.P., Schroeder, H.C., Miller, W.E.G. and Lazjuk, G.I. (2002) Congenital Malformations among Newborns and Developmental Abnormalities among Human Embryos in Belarus after Chernobyl Accident. *Cellular and Molecular Biology*, **48**, 423-426.

[17] Bogdanovich, I.P. (1997) Comparative Analysis of the Death Rate of Children, Aged 0 - 5, in 1994 in Radiocontaminated and Conventionally Clean Areas of Belarus. Medico-Biological Effects and the Ways of Overcoming the Chernobyl Accident Consequence. *Collected Book of Scientific Papers Dedicated to the 10th Anniversary of the Chernobyl accident*, Ministry of Emergency and Chernobyl Problems of Belarus and Academy of Sciences of Belarus, Minsk-Vitabsk.

[18] Savchenko, V.K. (1995) The Ecology of the Chernobyl Catastrophe. Scientific Outlines of an International Programme of Collaborative Research: Man and the Biosphere series. UNESCO, Paris.

[19] Petrova, A., Gnedko, T., Maistrova, I. and Zafranskaya, M. and Dainiak, N. (1997) Morbidity in a Large Cohort Study of Children Born to Mothers Exposed to Radiation from Chernobyl. *Stem Cells*, **15**, 141-150.

[20] Kulakov, V.I., Sokur, T.N., Volobuev, A.I., *et al.* (1993) Female Reproductive Function in Areas Affected by Radiation after the Chernobyl Power Station Accident. *Environmental Health Perspectives*, **101**, 117-123.

[21] Shidlovskii, P.R. (1992) General Morbidity of the Population in Districts of the Brest Region. *Zhravoohranenie Belorussii (Minsk)*, **1**, 8-11. (In Russian)

[22] Shevchuk, V.F. and Gurachevsky, V.L., Eds. (2006) Twenty Years after the Chernobyl Catastrophe: Consequences for Belarus Republic and Its Surrounding Area. *National Belarussian Report*, Minsk, Belarus.

[23] Godlevsky, I. and Nasvit, O. (1998) Dynamics of Health Status in Residents of Lugyny District after the Accident of the ChNPR. In: Imanaka, T., *et al.*, Eds., *Research Activities about the Radiological Consequences of the Chernobyl NPS Accident and Social Activities to Assist the Sufferers by the Accident*, Research Reactor Institute, Kyoto University, Kyoto, KURRI-KR-21.

[24] Stepanova, E.I., Vdovenko, V.Iu. and Misharina, Zh.A. (2007) Postnatal Effects in Children Irradiated during the Intra-Uterine Development, as a Result of Failure at the Chernobyl NPP. *Radiatsionnaia Biologiia, Radioecologiia*, **47**, 523-529. (In Russian)

[25] Moumjiev, N., Nedkova, V., Christova, V., *et al.* (1994) Influence of the Chernobyl Reactor Accident on the Child Health in the Region of Pleven, Bulgaria. *Paper presented at* 20*th International Congress on Pediatrics*, 6-10 September 1992. Cited by: Akar, N., Further Notes on Neural Tube Defects and Chernobyl. *Paediatric and Perinatal Epidemiology*, **8**, 456-457.

[26] Kruslin, B., Jukic, S., Kos, M., Simić, G. and Cviko, A. (1998) Congenital Anomalies of the Central Nervous System at Autopsy in Croatia in the Period before and after Chernobyl. *Acta Medica Croatica*, **52**, 103-107.

[27] Korblein, A. (2004) Fehlbildungen in Bayern nach Tschernobyl. *Strallentelex*, **416-417**, 4-6.

[28] Scherb, H. and Weigelt, E. (2003) Congenital Malformations and Stillbirth in Germany and Europe before and after the Chernobyl Nuclear Power Plant Accident. *Environmental Science and Pollution Research*, **10**, 117-125.

[29] (1987) Government of Berlin West, Section of Health and Social Affairs. Annual Health Report.

[30] Lotz, B., Haerting, J. and Schulze, E. (1996) Veranderungen im Fetalen und Kindlichen Sektionsgut im Raum Jena nach dem Reaktorrunfall von Tschernobyl. *Oral Presentation at the International Conference of the Society for Medical Documentation, Statistics, and Epidemiology*, unpublished manuscript available on request, Bonn, Germany.

[31] Lazjuk, G.I., Zastsepin, I.O., Verger, P., Gagniere, V., Robert, E., Kravchuk, Zh.P. and Khmel, R.D. (2002) Down Syndrome and Ionizing Radiation: Causal Effect or Coincidence? *Radiatsionnaia Biologiia, Radioecologiia*, **4**, 678-683. (In Russian)

[32] Zatsepin, I.O., Verger, P., Gagniere, B. and Khmel, R.D. (2004) Cluster of Down's Syndrome Cases Registered in January 1987 in Republic of Belarus as a Possible Effect of the Chernobyl Accident. *International Journal of Radiation Medicine*, **6**, 57-71.

[33] Ramsay, C.N., Ellis, P.M. and Zealley, H. (1991) Down's Syndrome in the Lothian Region of Scotland—1978 to 1989. *Biomedicine & Pharmacotherapy*, **45**, 267-272. http://dx.doi.org/10.1016/0753-3322(91)90028-R

[34] Sperling, K., Pelz, J., Wegner, R.-D., Schulzke, I. and Struck, E. (1991) Frequency of Trisomy 21 in Germany before and after the Chernobyl Accident. *Biomedicine & Pharmacotherapy*, **5**, 255-262. http://dx.doi.org/10.1016/0753-3322(91)90026-P

[35] Sperling, K., Pelz, J., Wegner, R.-D., Dorries, A., Gruters, A. and Mikkelsen, M. (1994) Significant Increase in Trisomy 21 in Berlin Nine Months after the Chernobyl Reactor Accident: Temporal Correlation or Causal Relation? *British Medical Journal*, **309**, 158-162. http://dx.doi.org/10.1136/bmj.309.6948.158

[36] Sperling, K., Neitzel, H. and Scherb, H. (2012) Evidence for an Increase in Trisomy 21 (Down Syndrome) in Europe after the Chernobyl Reactor Accident. *Genetic Epidemiology*, **36**, 48-55. http://dx.doi.org/10.1002/gepi.20662

[37] Burkart, W., Grosche, B. and Schwetzan, A. (1997) Down Syndrome Clusters in Germany after the Chernobyl Accident. *Radiation Research*, **147**, 321-328. http://dx.doi.org/10.2307/3579339

[38] Verger, P. (1997) Down Syndrome and Ionizing Radiation. *Health Physics*, **73**, 882-893. http://dx.doi.org/10.1097/00004032-199712000-00001

[39] Ericson, A. and Kallen, B. (1994) Pregnancy Outcome in Sweden after Chernobyl. *Environmental Research*, **67**, 149-159. http://dx.doi.org/10.1006/enrs.1994.1070

[40] Akar, N., Cavdar, A.O. and Areasoy, A. (1988) High Incidence of Neural Tube Defects in Bursa, Turkey. *Paediatric and Perinatal Epidemiology*, **2**, 89-92. http://dx.doi.org/10.1111/j.1365-3016.1988.tb00181.x

[41] Akar, N., Ata, Y., Aytekin, A.F. (1989) Neural Tube Defects and Chernobyl? *Paediatric and Perinatal Epidemiology*, **3**, 102-103.

[42] Caglayan, S., Kayhan, B., Mentesoglu, S., *et al.* (1990) Changing Incidence of Neural Tube Defects in Aegean Turkey. *Paediatric and Perinatal Epidemiology*, **4**, 264-268.

[43] Guvene, H., Uslu, M.A., Ozekici, U., Kocabay, K. and Bektaş, S. (1993) Changing Trend of Neural Tube Defects in Eastern Turkey. *Journal of Epidemiology & Community Health*, **47**, 40-41. http://dx.doi.org/10.1136/jech.47.1.40

[44] Zieglowski, V. and Hemprich, A. (1999) Facial Cleft Birth Rate in Former East Germany before and after the Reactor Accident in Chernobyl. *Mund-, Kiefer- und Gesichtschirurgie*, **3**, 195-199. (In German) http://dx.doi.org/10.1007/s100060050129

[45] Scherb, H. and Weigelt, E. (2004) Cleft Lip and Cleft Palate Birth Rate in Bavaria before and after the Chernobyl Nuclear Power Plant Accident. *Mund-, Kiefer- und Gesichtschirurgie*, **8**, 106-110. (In German)

[46] Mocan, H., Bozkaya, H., Mocan, Z.M. and Furtun, E.M. (1990) Changing Incidence of Anencephaly in the Eastern Black Sea Region of Turkey and Chernobyl. *Paediatric and Perinatal Epidemiology*, **4**, 264-268. http://dx.doi.org/10.1111/j.1365-3016.1990.tb00649.x

[47] Dolk, H. and Nichols, R. (1999) Evaluation of the Impact of Chernobyl on the Prevalence of Congenital Anomalies in 17 Regions of Europe. EUROCAT Working Group. *International Journal of Epidemiology*, **28**, 941-948. http://dx.doi.org/10.1093/ije/28.5.941

[48] Busby, C., Lengfelder, E., Pflugbeil, S. and Schmitz-Feuerhake, I. (2009) The Evidence of Radiation Effects in Embryos and Fetuses Exposed to Chernobyl Fallout and the Question of Dose Response. *Medicine, Conflict, and Survival*, **25**, 20-40. http://dx.doi.org/10.1080/13623690802568954

[49] Hoffmann, W. (2001) Fallout from Chernobyl Nuclear Disaster and Congenital Malformations in Europe. *Archives of Environmental Health*, **56**, 478-484. http://dx.doi.org/10.1080/00039890109602895

[50] Akimoto, S. (2014) Morphological Abnormalities in Cell Forming Aphids in a Radiation-Contaminated Area near Fukushima Daiichi: Selective Impact of Fallout? *Ecology and Evolution*, **4**, 355-369. http://dx.doi.org/10.1002/ece3.949

[51] Mangano, J. and Sherman, J. (2013) Elevated Airborne Beta Levels in Pacific/West Coast US States and Trends in Hypothyroidism among Newborns after the Fukushima Nuclear Meltdown. *Open Journal of Pediatrics*, **3**, 1-9.

[52] Mangano, J., Sherman, J. and Busby, C. (2013) Changes in Confirmed Plus Borderline Cases of Congenital Hypothyroidism in California as a Function of Environmental Fallout from the Fukushima Nuclear Meltdown. *Open Journal of Pediatrics*, **3**, 370-376. http://dx.doi.org/10.4236/ojped.2013.34067

[53] U.S. Centers for Disease Control and Prevention. CDC Wonder. http://wonder.cdc.gov/natality.html.

[54] Pampfer, S. and Streffer, C. (1988) Prenatal Death and Malformations after Irradiation of Mouse Zygotes with Neutrons or X-Rays. *Teratology*, **37**, 599-607. http://dx.doi.org/10.1002/tera.1420370609

[55] Jaikrishan, G., Sudheer, K.R., Andrews, V.J., *et al.* (2013) Study of Stillbirth and Major Congenital Anomaly among Newborns in the High-Level Natural Radiation Areas of Kerala, India. *Journal of Community Genetics*, **4**, 21-31. http://dx.doi.org/10.1007/s12687-012-0113-1

[56] Bastout, S., Jackuet, P., Michaux, A., *et al.* (2002) Developmental Abnormalities Induced by X-Irradiation in p53 Deficient Mice. *In Vivo*, **16**, 215-221.

[57] Castilla, E.E. and Orioli, I.M. (1985) Epidemiology of Neural Tube Defects in South America. *American Journal of Medical Genetics*, **22**, 695-702. http://dx.doi.org/10.1002/ajmg.1320220406

[58] U.S. Environmental Protection Agency. Office of Radiation Protection. http://oaspub.epa.gov/enviro/erams_query.v2.simple

[59] Tiwari, R.C., Clegg, L.X. and Zou, Z.H. (2006) Efficient Interval Estimation for Age-Adjusted Cancer Rates. *Statistical Methods in Medical Research*, **15**, 547-569. http://dx.doi.org/10.1177/0962280206070621

[60] Committee on the Biological Effects of Ionizing Radiation (1990) Health Effects of Exposure to Low Levels of Ionizing Radiation: BEIR V. National Research Council, National Academy Press, Washington DC.

[61] Muller, H.J. (1927) The Problem of Genetic Modification. *Zeit ind. Abst. und Vereb*, Supp. 1, 234-260.

[62] Muller, H.J. (1927) Artificial Transmutation of the Gene. *Science*, **66**, 84-87. http://dx.doi.org/10.1126/science.66.1699.84

[63] Møeller, A.P. and Mousseau, T.A. (2007) Determinants of Interspecies Variation in Population Declines of Birds after Exposure to Radiation at Chernobyl. *Journal of Applied Ecology*, **44**, 909-919. http://dx.doi.org/10.1111/j.1365-2664.2007.01353.x

[64] Møeller, A.P., Mousseau, T.A., de Lope, F. and Saino, N. (2007) Elevated Frequency of Abnormalities in Barn Swallows from Chernobyl. *Biological Letters of the Royal Society*, **3**, 414-417. http://dx.doi.org/10.1098/rsbl.2007.0136

[65] Stewart, A., Webb, J., Giles, D. and Hewitt, D. (1956) Malignant Disease in Childhood and Diagnostic Irradiation in Utero. *The Lancet*, **268**, 447. http://dx.doi.org/10.1016/S0140-6736(56)91923-7

[66] Stewart, A., Webb, J. and Hewitt, D. (1958) A Survey of Childhood Malignancies. *British Medical Journal*, **1**, 1495-1508. http://dx.doi.org/10.1136/bmj.1.5086.1495

[67] MacMahon, B. (1962) Prenatal X-Ray Exposure and Childhood Cancer. *Journal of the National Cancer Institute*, **28**, 1173-1192.

[68] Sherman, J.D. (1999) Chlorpyrifos (Dursban) Exposure and Birth Defects: Report of 15 Incidents, Evaluation of 8 Cases, Theory of Action, and Medical and Social Aspects. *European Journal of Oncology*, **4**, 653-659.

[69] Carson, R. (1962) Silent Spring. Crest Books, New York.

Appendix

Appendix 1. Sites used to calculate gross beta in air, 2010 and 2011.

PACIFIC/WEST COAST	OTHER U.S.
*Anchorage AK	Montgomery AL
Anaheim CA	Little Rock AR
*Bakersfield CA	Tucson AZ
Eureka CA	Denver CO
Fresno CA	Washington DC
Los Angeles CA	Des Moines IA
Richmond CA	Indianapolis IN
*Riverside CA	Kansas City KS
*Sacramento CA	Topeka KS
*San Bernardino CA	Lexington KY
San Diego CA	Baton Rouge LA
San Francisco CA	Worcester MA
San Jose CA	Bay City MI
*Hilo HI	Detroit MI
*Honolulu HI	Jefferson City MO
*Portland OR	Springfield MO
*Olympia WA	Jackson MS
*Spokane WA	Charlotte NC
	Edison NJ
	Trenton NJ
	Albany NY
	Cleveland OH
	Cincinnati OH
	Pierre SD
	Oak Ridge TN
	Dallas TX
	San Angelo TX
	Salt Lake City UT
	Lynchburg VA
	Richmond VA

*Sites with the most frequent (at least 24) measurements for March 15-April 30 in 2010 and 2011, and at least 100 for all other dates in the period January 1-October 4 in 2010 and 2011.

Permissions

All chapters in this book were first published in OJPED, by Scientific Research Publishing; hereby published with permission under the Creative Commons Attribution License or equivalent. Every chapter published in this book has been scrutinized by our experts. Their significance has been extensively debated. The topics covered herein carry significant findings which will fuel the growth of the discipline. They may even be implemented as practical applications or may be referred to as a beginning point for another development.

The contributors of this book come from diverse backgrounds, making this book a truly international effort. This book will bring forth new frontiers with its revolutionizing research information and detailed analysis of the nascent developments around the world.

We would like to thank all the contributing authors for lending their expertise to make the book truly unique. They have played a crucial role in the development of this book. Without their invaluable contributions this book wouldn't have been possible. They have made vital efforts to compile up to date information on the varied aspects of this subject to make this book a valuable addition to the collection of many professionals and students.

This book was conceptualized with the vision of imparting up-to-date information and advanced data in this field. To ensure the same, a matchless editorial board was set up. Every individual on the board went through rigorous rounds of assessment to prove their worth. After which they invested a large part of their time researching and compiling the most relevant data for our readers.

The editorial board has been involved in producing this book since its inception. They have spent rigorous hours researching and exploring the diverse topics which have resulted in the successful publishing of this book. They have passed on their knowledge of decades through this book. To expedite this challenging task, the publisher supported the team at every step. A small team of assistant editors was also appointed to further simplify the editing procedure and attain best results for the readers.

Apart from the editorial board, the designing team has also invested a significant amount of their time in understanding the subject and creating the most relevant covers. They scrutinized every image to scout for the most suitable representation of the subject and create an appropriate cover for the book.

The publishing team has been an ardent support to the editorial, designing and production team. Their endless efforts to recruit the best for this project, has resulted in the accomplishment of this book. They are a veteran in the field of academics and their pool of knowledge is as vast as their experience in printing. Their expertise and guidance has proved useful at every step. Their uncompromising quality standards have made this book an exceptional effort. Their encouragement from time to time has been an inspiration for everyone.

The publisher and the editorial board hope that this book will prove to be a valuable piece of knowledge for researchers, students, practitioners and scholars across the globe.

List of Contributors

J. M. Chinawa, P. C. A. E. Aronu and H. A. Obu
College of Medicine, Department of Pediatrics, University of Nigeria, Nsukka, Nigeria University of Nigeria Teaching Hospital (UNTH), Ituku, Nigeria

Manyike
College of Medicine, Ebonyi State University, Abakalki, Nigeria
Department of Pediatrics, Federal Teaching Hospital, Abakiliki (FETHA), Abakiliki, Nigeria

A. T. Chinawa
College of Medicine, Department of Community Medicine, Enugu State University of Science and Technology, Enugu, Nigeria

Fawaz Al-Refaee, Sarah Al-Enezi, Enamul Hoque and Assad Albadrawi
Department of Pediatrics, Al-Adan Hospital, Ministry of Health, Kuwait, Kuwait

Sri Endah Rahayuningsih, Rahmat Budi Kuswiyanto, Mira Haryanti and Evelyn Phangkawira
Department of Child Health, Faculty of Medicine, Padjadjaran University/Hasan Sadikin General Hospital, Bandung, Indonesia

George M. Gilly, Donald E. Harmon, Eric H. Busch, Bobby D. Nossaman and David M. Broussard
Department of Anesthesiology, Ochsner Clinic Foundation, New Orleans, LA, USA

Walter J. Hoyt
Division of Pediatric Cardiology, University of Virginia, Charlottesville, VA, USA

Christopher S. Snyder
Department of Pediatrics, Division of Pediatric Cardiology, Rainbow Babies and Children's Hospital, Case Western Reserve School of Medicine, Cleveland, OH, USA

Fatemeh Nayeri and Mamak Shariat
Maternal, Fetal and Neonatal Research Center, Tehran University of Medical Sciences, Tehran, Iran

Hosein Dalili, Farima Raji and Akram Karimi
Breast Feeding Research Center, Tehran University of Medical Sciences, Tehran, Iran

Bijay Upadhyay, Xuedong Wu, Jun Li, Ning Wang, Shanshan Zhang and Na Li
Department of Pediatric Surgery, Affiliated Hospital of Dali University, Dali, China

Kisito Nagalo
Service of Pediatrics, Clinique El Fateh-Suka, Ouagadougou, Burkina Faso

Isso Ouédraogo and Kisito Nagalo
Training and Research Unit of Health Sciences, University of Ouagadougou, Ouagadougou, Burkina Faso

Isso Ouédraogo
Department of Pediatric Surgery, Charles De Gaulle Pediatric University Teaching Hospital, Ouagadougou, Burkina Faso

Jean Turgeon, Louise Caouette-Laberge and Jean-Martin Laberge
Mission Sourires d'Afrique, Montreal, Canada

Jean-Martin Laberge
Department of Pediatric Surgery, McGill University, Montreal, Canada

Louise Caouette-Laberge
Department of Surgery, University of Montreal, Montreal, Canada

Jean Turgeon
Department of Pediatrics, University of Montreal, Montreal, Canada

Uruwan Yamborisut
Human Nutrition Unit, Institute of Nutrition, Mahidol University, Salaya, Thailand

Wanphen Wimonpeerapattana, Nipa Rojroongwasinkul and Sayamon Senaprom
Biostatistics Unit, Institute of Nutrition, Mahidol University, Salaya, Thailand

Atitada Boonpraderm
Community Nutrition Unit, Institute of Nutrition, Mahidol University, Salaya, Thailand

Wiyada Thasanasuwan
Nutrition Physiology Unit, Institute of Nutrition, Mahidol University, Salaya, Thailand

Ilse Khouw
Friesland Campina, Amersfoort, The Netherlands

Paul Deurenberg
Nutrition Consultant, Langkawi, Malaysia

Fla Koueta, Kisito Nagalo, François Housseini Tall and Diarra Ye
The Burkinabe Pediatrics Society, Ouagadougou, Burkina Faso

Kisito Nagalo, Fla Koueta, Leatitia Ouedraogo and Diarra Ye
Training and Research Unit of Health Sciences, University of Ouagadougou, Ouagadougou, Burkina Faso

Fla Koueta and Diarra Ye
Service of Medical Pediatrics, Charles De Gaulle Pediatric University Teaching Hospital, Ouagadougou, Burkina Faso

Kisito Nagalo
Service of Pediatrics, Clinique El Fateh-Suka, Ouagadougou, Burkina Faso

Maen Mahfouz
Department of Orthodontics and Pediatric Dentistry, Dental School, Arab American University, Jenin, Palestine

Ismail Masri
Department of Basic Biomedical Sciences, Dental School, Arab American University, Jenin, Palestine

Haneen Mahfouz
Biomedical Department, Central Public Health Lab, Palestinian Ministry of Health, Ramallah, Palestine

Yara Mahfouz
Dental Department, Al Zafer Hospital, Najran, Saudi Arabia

Thi Hoa Chu and Thi Hoa Duong
National Hospital of Pediatrics, Hanoi, Vietnam

Thi Hoa Duong
Centre for Person-Centred Care (GPCC), Institute of Health and Care Sciences, Sahlgrenska Academy, University of Gothenburg, Gothenburg, Sweden

Daniela Simoncini, Anna Peirolo, Stefania Porcu, Daniela Graziani and Luigi Nespoli
Department of Clinical and Experimental Medicine, University of Insubria c/o Ospedale Filippo del Ponte, Varese, Italy

Alberto Macchi
Otorhinolaryngology Clinic University of Insubria Varese, AICNA, c/o Ospedale di Circolo, Varese, Italy

Hassan Aguenaou
Joint Research Unit in Nutrition and Food URAC 39, (Ibn Tofaïl University – CNESTEN), Regional Designated Center of Nutrition Associated with AFRA/IAEA, Kénitra, Morocco

Mohammed Amine Radouani, Naima Chahid, Loubna Benmiloud, Aicha Kharbach and Amina Barkat
Department of Medicine and Neonatal Resuscitation, National Center for Neonatology and Nutrition, Rabat, Morocco
Faculté de Medicine et de Pharmacie de Rabat, Université Mohammed V de Rabat, Rabat, Morocco

Khalid Lahlou, Leila El Ammari, Larbi Rjimati and Laila Acharrai
Population Department, Ministry of Health, Rabat, Morocco

Xiangyu Hu and Lina Hu
Pingdingshang City Hospital of Traditional Chinese Medicine, Pingdingshan, China

Mohamed Amine Radouani, Salem Ananou, Aicha Kharbach and Amina Barkat
Research Team on Health and Nutrition of Mother and Child, Faculty of Medicine and Pharmacy of Rabat, Mohammed V University of Rabat, Rabat, Morocco

Mustapha Mrabet
Teaching and Research Unit of Public Health, Research Team on Health and Nutrition of Mother and Child, Faculty of Medicine and Pharmacy of Rabat, Mohammed V University of Rabat, Rabat, Morocco

Hassan Aguenaou
Joint Research Unit in Nutrition and Food URAC 39 (Ibn Tofaïl University – CNESTEN), Designated Regional Center of Nutrition Partner of AFRA/IAEA, Kenitra, Morocco

Amina Barkat
Department of Medicine and Neonatal Resuscitation, National Center for Neonatology and Nutrition, Rabat, Morocco

Jia-Feng Chang and Wei-Ning Lin
Graduate Institute of Basic Medicine, Fu Jen Catholic University, Taipei, Taiwan

Jia-Feng Chang
Division of Nephrology, Department of Internal Medicine, Far Eastern Memorial Hospital, New Taipei City, Taiwan

Chien-Chen Tsai
Department of Anatomic Pathology, Far Eastern Memorial Hospital, New Taipei City, Taiwan

Dedi Rachmadi
Department of Child Health, Faculty of Medicine, Universitas Padjadjaran Bandung, Bandung, Indonesia

Ani Melani
Medical Faculty, Health Research Unit, Universitas Padjadjaran Bandung, Bandung, Indonesia

Leo Monnens
Department of Pediatrics, Radboud University Medical Centre Nijmegen, Nijmegen, The Netherlands

A. Sánchez Andrés and J. I. Carrasco Moreno
Pediatric Cardiology Unit, Hospital Universitario y Politécnico La Fe, Valencia, Spain

C. González Miño
Pediatric Intensive Care Unit, Hospital General de Castellón, Castellon, Spain

E. Valdés Diéguez and L. Boni
Pediatric Surgery Unit, Hospital Universitario y Politécnico La Fe, Valencia, Spain

Shakeel Ahmed, Syed Rehan Ali and Farhana Tabassum
Department of Paediatrics and Child Health, Aga Khan University Hospital, Karachi, Pakistan

Shakeel Ahmed
Department of Paediatrics, Bahria University Medical and Dental College, Karachi, Pakistan

Alexander K. C. Leung
University of Calgary, Calgary, Canada
Alberta Children's Hospital, Calgary, Canada

Benjamin Barankin
Toronto Dermatology Centre, Toronto, Canada

Nur Dian Firmani, Tetty Yuniati and Dedi Rachmadi
Department of Child Health, Faculty of Medicine, Universitas Padjadjaran, Bandung, Indonesia

Jeff Maotela Kabinda and Ahuka Serge Miyanga
Provincial Blood Transfusion Centre of Bukavu, Bukavu, Congo

Tony Shindano Akilimali and Jeff Maotela Kabinda
Catholic University of Bukavu, Bukavu, Congo

Dramaix-Wilmet Michèle and Jeff Maotela Kabinda
Research Centre in Biostatistics and Epidemiology, Brussels, Belgium

Philippe Donnen and Dramaix-Wilmet Michèle
Free University of Brussels, Brussels, Belgium

Philippe Donnen and Dramaix-Wilmet Michèle
School of Public Health, Brussels, Belgium

Philippe Donnen
Centre for Policy and Health Systems/International Health, Brussels, Belgium

Gülsen Meral, Ayşegül Uslu and Faruk Akçay
Department of Children Health and Disease, Kagithane State Hospital, Istanbul, Turkey

Ali Ünsal Yozgatli
Department of Obstetrics & Gynecology, Kagithane State Hospital, Istanbul, Turkey

Edy Novery, Susi Susanah and Dedi Rachmadi
Department of Child Health, Faculty of Medicine, Universitas Padjadjaran, Bandung, Indonesia

Conceição Costa and Teresa Torres
Departments of Pediatrics—Centro Hospitalar Vila Nova de Gaia/Espinho, Vila Nova de Gaia, Portugal

Andreia Teles
Departments of Pediatrics, Neonatology Unit—Centro Hospitalar Vila Nova de Gaia/Espinho, Vila Nova de Gaia, Portugal

Osama Almadhoun
University of Kansas Medical Center, Kansas City, USA

Teresa Rivera-Penera
Division of Pediatric Gastroenterology, St. Joseph's Children Hospital, Paterson, USA

Lauren Lipeski
Division of Pediatric Endocrinology, Upstate Medical Center, Golisano Children Hospital, Syracuse, USA

Irina Livshitz
University Hospitals Case Medical Center, Cleveland, USA

Peyman Hashemian
Psychiatry and Behavioral Sciences Research Center, Ibn-e-Sina Hospital, Faculty of Medicine, Mashhad University of Medical Sciences, Mashhad, Iran

Mansoureh Mohammadi
Islamic Azad University, Ghochan, Iran

Dorothy Mbaya
Chuka District Hospital, Chuka, Kenya

Lucy Kivuti Bitok, Anna K. Karani and Dorothy Mbaya
School of Nursing Sciences, College of Health Sciences, University of Nairobi, Nairobi, Kenya

Boniface Osano
Department of Pediatrics and Child Health, School of Medicine, College of Health Sciences, University of Nairobi, Nairobi, Kenya

Michael Habtu
Institute of Tropical Medicine and Infectious Diseases, Jomo Kenyatta University of Agriculture and Technology, Nairobi, Kenya

Zsuzsa I. Bartik, Sofia Sjöström, Rune Sixt and Ulla Sillén
The Pediatric Uro-Nephrologic Centre, The Queen Silvia Children's Hospital, Sahlgrenska Academy, University of Gothenburg, Gothenburg, Sweden

Agneta Nordenskjöld
Department of Women and Children Health, Karolinska Institutet and Center of Molecular Medicine, Karolinska University Hospital, Stockholm, Sweden

Patricia Bernal, Johanna Montaña, Rocio Acosta and Yonathan Rojas
Universidad de San Buenaventura, Bogotá, Colombia

Ayala Yahav, Yaakov Shachter, Aryeh Simmonds, Yakov Shiff and Nechama Sharon
Department of Pediatrics, Laniado Hospital, Netanya, Israel

Chaim Kaplinsky
Department of Pediatric Hemato-Oncology, Sheba Hospital, Tel Hashomer, Israel

Miguel M. Glatstein
Divisions of Pediatric Emergency Medicine and Clinical Pharmacology and Toxicology, Dana-Dwek Children Hospital, Tel Aviv Sourasky Medical Center, Affiliated to the Sackler Faculty of Medicine, Tel Aviv, Israel

Dennis Scolnik
Divisions of Pediatric Emergency Medicine and Clinical Pharmacology and Toxicology, Department of Pediatrics, The Hospital for Sick Children, University of Toronto, Toronto, Canada

Nechama Sharon
Pediatric Hemato-Oncology, Laniado Hospital, Netanya, Israel

A. Sánchez Andrés and J. I. Carrasco Moreno
Pediatric Cardiology Unit, Hospital Universitario y Politécnico La Fe, Valencia, Spain

C. González Miño
Pediatric Intensive Care Unit, Hospital General de Castellón, Castellon, Spain

E. Valdés Diéguez and L. Boni
Pediatric Surgery Unit, Hospital Universitario y Politécnico La Fe, Valencia, Spain

Joseph Mangano and Janette D. Sherman
Radiation and Public Health Project, New York, USA